Women's Empowerment
and Global Health

Women's Empowerment and Global Health

A Twenty-First-Century Agenda

EDITED BY

Shari L. Dworkin, Monica Gandhi, and Paige Passano

UNIVERSITY OF CALIFORNIA PRESS

University of California Press, one of the most
distinguished university presses in the United States,
enriches lives around the world by advancing scholarship
in the humanities, social sciences, and natural sciences. Its
activities are supported by the UC Press Foundation and
by philanthropic contributions from individuals and
institutions. For more information, visit www.ucpress.edu.

University of California Press
Oakland, California

Library of Congress Cataloging-in-Publication Data

Names: Dworkin, Shari L., editor. | Gandhi, Monica,
    editor. | Passano, Paige, editor.
Title: Women's empowerment and global health : a
    twenty-first-century agenda / edited by Shari L.
    Dworkin, Monica Gandhi, and Paige Passano.
Description: Oakland, California : University of
    California Press, [2017] | Includes bibliographical
    references and index.
Identifiers: LCCN 2016030545 (print) | LCCN 2016032540
    (ebook) | ISBN 9780520272873 (cloth : alk. paper) |
    ISBN 9780520272880 (pbk. : alk. paper) | ISBN
    9780520962729 (Epub)
Subjects: LCSH: Women's rights—Case studies. |
    Women—Health and hygiene—Case studies. |
    Women—Political activity—Cross-cultural studies. |
    Medical policy—Case studies. | Women—Social
    conditions—Case studies.
Classification: LCC HQ1236 .W598 2017 (print) | LCC
    HQ1236 (ebook) | DDC 305.42—dc23
LC record available at https://lccn.loc.gov/2016030545

Manufactured in the United States of America

25 24 23 22 21 20 19 18 17
10 9 8 7 6 5 4 3 2 1

Contents

Illustrations

TABLES

Introduction

Empowering Women for Health

GITA SEN

In the lexicon of gender equality, there are probably no two words as common as *women's empowerment*. Ever since its early usage (Sen and Grown 1987, p 89) in the mid-1980s, few terms have so captured the imagination of activists, scholars, advocates, scientists, intervention experts, and policy makers alike as the term *empowerment*. Early authors on empowerment (Batliwala 1994; Kabeer 1994, 1999; Oxaal and Baden 1997; Sen and Batliwala 2000; Stromquist 2002) and more recent ones (Cornwall and Edwards 2014) have pointed to the risks inherent in the rapid spread of this term. As Presser and Sen (2000) have argued, "while the rhetoric about women's empowerment is pervasive, the concept has remained ill-defined" (p 3).

Is the term acceptable because it is vague enough to allow people to interpret it as they please, filling it with content that can be radical, objective, or simply business-as-usual? Is its wide usage due to its appearance of promoting strong action without any intrinsic policy accountability for actually doing so? Despite ongoing worries about the term and its use, empowerment continues to be a powerful concept to understand and use to advocate for social and political transformation. For example, after an extensive global debate over development priorities, the 2030 Agenda for Sustainable Development selected "Achieve gender equality and empower all women and girls" as the fifth of seventeen Sustainable Development Goals (Sustainable Development Knowledge Platform, https://sustainabledevelopment.un.org/post2015/transformingourworld).

Although discrepancies remain over the definition of the term *empowerment*, programs aiming to enhance women's empowerment continue to spring up across the globe—and researchers are increasingly deploying the term and designing studies to better measure it. Given this growing interest, the editors of the current volume requested contributing authors to define what they mean by *empowerment*, describe interventions that have been designed to change the factors that lead to empowerment, and think carefully about how empowerment affects health outcomes. In some chapters, authors also discuss the reverse: how health impacts empowerment. But how does one measure empowerment? And why does it matter for health?

MEASURING EMPOWERMENT

The central meaning of *empowerment* in early writing is "the process by which the powerless gain greater control over the circumstances of their lives" (Sen and Batliwala 2000, p 18). Power is central both to the word itself and to the concept. Feminist activist-scholars, searching for an appropriate word to express what was being discussed within the rapidly growing discourse and practice of gender equality and development, gravitated towards the term primarily because it contained the word *power*. They recognized the pervasiveness of the power relations that govern women's lives in *families* (through unfair division of resources, labor, access to health and education, constraints on mobility and decision making, and control over women's sexuality), *communities* (through discrimination on the basis of gender as well as on factors such as caste, ethnicity, race, sexual orientation, gender identity, disability, age, indigeneity, and cultural norms, beliefs, and practices), *markets* (inequitable access to markets for labor, land, credit, technology, and other resources), and *the state* (discriminatory laws, institutions, policies and practices; poorly funded or poor quality government programs) (ibid., p 21).

Importantly, empowerment implies more than just formal equality between women and men as a matter of law. Empowerment is a way for previously powerless women to gain control over material resources—physical, human, financial, and intellectual—and over ideology (beliefs, values, and attitudes) (Batliwala 1994). It therefore includes both extrinsic control and growing internal confidence and capabilities—a transformation of women's beliefs and consciousness. For many feminists, empowerment is largely something women must do for themselves (Rowlands 1997). It is not simply something to be done for them from outside by governments, corporate actors, development agencies, or even non-governmental organizations, whose role is to create enabling environments and, if needed, to act as catalysts of change (Sholkamy 2010). It is women's own actions and awareness that hold the key to their empowerment. This kind of thinking is certainly reflective of several works in this book. For example, Victor Robinson, Theresa Hwang, and Elisa Martínez (chapter 5) meticulously detail how sex worker collectivization in India shaped empowerment and health-related processes recursively, producing outcomes well beyond what individual-level action could ever achieve. Kate Grünke-Horton and Shari Dworkin (chapter 12) detail how women at the grassroots level in Nyanza, Kenya, worked to secure women's access to land using community mobilization, mediation to resolve land disputes, and collaboration with government officials and traditional leaders. These efforts not only improved women's voice and agency but shifted their status in the community—and reduced their risk of HIV and gender-based violence.

These examples also highlight the importance of groups and group processes. Groups have been stressed as providing strength and support for individual women who feel subordinated and oppressed by power relations (Bisnath and Elson 1999). Indeed, it was personal involvement in group processes that catalyzed much of the original work by feminist scholars (Sen and Grown 1987; Batliwala 1994). But group processes are not enough. As Kabeer (2001) emphasizes, women must be able to exercise agency (the ability to use their new resources to create new opportunities), leading to achievements (new social outcomes). In the context of this volume, achievements include health and social and economic outcomes. Most authors in this volume indeed draw upon and deploy Kabeer's definition of empowerment, which is significant because it highlights the limitations not only of individual-level analysis (knowledge, information, skills) but also reveals the ways in which newly gained resources amplify women's voices and spark social change. In short, resources coupled with collective action and voice lead to a catalytic and internally transformative process within women, creating in them the ability not only to "speak truth to power" but to be able to change the practice of the power relations that constrain their lives (Klugman 2000). Megan Dunbar's research (chapter 8) reveals that adolescents in Zimbabwe who are at high risk of acquiring HIV can be supported in their process of empowerment through a combination of group-based vocational training, life skills education, and economic and livelihood opportunities to reduce their HIV risks. Abigail Hatcher and her colleagues (chapter 9) highlight the importance of merging resources (microfinance) with gender equity training and community-level action. The chapter reveals the specific mechanisms that shaped empowerment-related processes—and these include both control over resources and collective action (among others).

Such a transformation can be rejected by families, communities, and male partners, but this need not be a zero-sum game (such as the assumption that when women gain, men lose), as others have argued (Dworkin et al. 2012, Dworkin 2015; Sen and Batliwala 2000, p 20). While it is generally accepted that gender inequities constrain women's opportunities and yield poor health outcome among women, the impact of this gendered power imbalance on men is less understood. The literature on masculinities bears evidence that unequal gender power relations, while giving men greater control over and access to a variety of resources, can also be damaging to men's own health and well-being, resulting in narrowed emotional and cognitive experiences, violence, substance abuse, and premature death (Baker et al. 2014; Courtenay 2000; Dworkin et al. 2012; Hatcher et al. 2014). The central importance of masculinities based gender-transformative health programs, such as the one described in chapter 7, shows us that we can simultaneously work towards a social environment that sets the stage for women's health and empowerment alongside men's social transformation—because this shift in inequitable social norms improves not just women's health but also men's health.

The discussion above also highlights how much of the foundational writing on empowerment conceptualizes it as both process and outcome. But if women's empowerment, while not a zero-sum game, is a complex and perhaps open-ended process, where does that leave researchers who need to rigorously trace cause and effect or to clearly specify variables? Can outcomes be attributed to particular causes if complex, layered processes are at play? A number of authors (Kabeer 1999; Dixon-Mueller and Germain 2000; Jejeebhoy 2000; Kishor 2000; Kritz, Makinwa-Adebusoye, and Gurak 2000) have grappled with this question, and some of the authors in this volume continue to press this debate forward. To engage the complexity of these processes, the editors asked each of the authors in this volume to discuss the promises and limitations of their research and its implementation. In addition, each chapter contains boxes that summarize the successes or challenges that arose during program implementation or an explanation of how the program diverge from previous assumptions about health and empowerment in favor of a more contemporary approach. The work in this volume shows that, with a skillful mix of quantitative and qualitative methods, it is indeed possible to measure inputs, processes, and outcomes in innovative ways that lead to new insights. One of these critical insights is how empowerment is linked to health.

GENDER, POWER, AND HEALTH

Recent decades have seen an explosion of academic and policy writing on women and health in both high, middle, and low-income countries (Doyal 1995; Sen, George, and Östlin 2002). These multiple strands of literature are often built on a core hypothesis that gender inequality has adverse effects on the health of women and girls, of infants and small children, and even of men. These two concepts—women's empowerment and gender equality—are deeply intertwined with a third concept: universal human rights.

Gendered power relations are a central basis of gender inequality. Sen, Östlin, and George (2007) posit that gendered power is embedded in structural determinants, impacting health through four pathways: (1) discriminatory values, norms, practices, and behaviors; (2) differential exposures and vulnerabilities to disease, disability, and injuries; (3) biases in health systems; and (4) biases in health research. These various biases and forms of discrimination are themselves interlinked, a product of structural determinants of health, including multiple and intersecting power relationships, demographic factors, economic realities, and legal frameworks and institutions, which result in different health outcomes by gender.

The impact of gendered power on health is complex and multifaceted. Power imbalances are exacerbated by discriminatory belief systems and values, such as the belief that a girl should be married off at the onset of puberty (often coupled with the belief that she therefore doesn't need education) or that women who do not obey their husband deserve violence. Changing regressive gender norms is empowering for both young men and young women and can lead to improved health for both. In this volume, the case study by Shelly Grabe, Anjali Dutt, and Carlos Arenas (chapter 13) on Xochilt Acalt demonstrates how discriminatory beliefs and practices keep women from owning land. The authors show how breaking restrictive gender ideologies can embolden women to assume greater power and economic autonomy in the household while simultaneously safeguarding their health. Leslie Brody, Sannisha Dale, Gwendolyn Kelso, Ruth Cruise, Kathleen Weber, Lynissa

Stokes, and Mardge Cohen (chapter 6) demonstrate how HIV-positive women who question traditional gender norms and connect with a supportive community of peers fare better in terms of adherence to antiretroviral medications and broader health outcomes.

Exposures and vulnerabilities also differ by gender. For example, women are more exposed to kitchen smoke and thus more vulnerable to acquiring respiratory disease than men in many parts of the world. These vulnerabilities are further exacerbated by gendered biases in health care. In chapters 1 and 11, Pallavi Gupta, Kirti Iyengar, Sharad Iyengar, and Gustavo Ortiz Millán vividly illustrate the harsh repercussions of poor access to abortion services on poor and rural women—and the children who depend on them. Both chapters call upon governments to take action to protect women's health, showing that as higher quality, safe abortion services become available, women no longer need to risk their lives to control their fertility.

Biases in research funding and research methodologies can also play a significant role in health outcomes of marginalized groups. Indeed, in practice, health systems rarely recognize the multiple challenges to accessing health care that girls and women often face (e.g., lack of income, restrictions on mobility, or the disproportionate burden of caring for others). In the second chapter of this volume, Lindsey Pollaczek, Paula Tavrow, and Habiba Mohamed reveal how weaknesses in the health-care infrastructure, paired with stigma linked to obstetric fistula within rural communities, required empathetic community insiders to find and assist the women whose basic reproductive rights had been denied. In chapter 10, Carroll Estes reveals how political and economic processes, alongside broader societal norms, shape assumptions about whether politicians even view women as deserving of health care, Medicare, and social security—and discusses the challenges associated with multisectoral collaborative social movements for social change.

Govender and Penn-Kekana (2010) argue that gender has a profound impact on interactions between patients and health-care providers. However, empowerment of both patients and providers (who are themselves marginalized) can alter and improve the health consequences related to these interactions. Khan's (2014) study of Pakistan's "lady health worker" (LHW) program also shows that empowerment may be bidirectional and long-term. Her case studies show that "within the private sphere and her own family, the LHW is redressing gender balances without directly confronting this most patriarchal of institutions. . . . [H]er work has earned her increased agency[:] . . . decision-making over her own reproductive health, the schooling and marriage decisions of her children, and the management of her own and family finances" (p 120). Pallavi Gupta, Kirti Iyengar, and Sharad Iyengar in chapter 1 of this volume provide further evidence of bidirectional empowerment. By training health workers from castes and communities similar to those of the rural women they intended to reach, trust and acceptability was enhanced while the new knowledge empowered both health workers and rural women who needed information and services.

The authors in this volume show how this kind of bidirectionality matters outside the health system as well. In chapter 3, Daniel Perlman, Fatima Adamu, Mairo Mandara, Olorukooba Abiola, David Cao, and Malcolm Potts reveal the potential for multigenerational health impacts in communities where the gender imbalance in rural secondary education is slowly shifting towards improving girls' access to and retention in secondary school. Through extensive engagement with adolescent girls and their communities, patriarchal norms are being influenced subtly, but profoundly. As girls exert greater influence over critical life decisions, they will become different types of role models for their children. As a result, their children's health and educational trajectories are likely to be impacted. In chapter 4, Karen Austrian, Judith Bruce, and M. Catherine Maternowska discuss a unique intervention that targets organizations that aspire to serve vulnerable populations of adolescent girls. The intervention helps organizations rethink the content of their programs, strengthening the organizations' ability to support girls in building assets that will protect them as they transition through adolescence and into adulthood. By training program designers and implementers to be more strategic and accountable when designing interventions and outreach strategies, program planners can reverse common mistakes that tend to deepen the marginalization of the poorest girls, thereby improving their chances to participate fully in society and realize their human rights.

EMPOWERMENT AND THE HUMAN RIGHT TO HEALTH

The international human rights framework addresses gender equality and health, as well as the interconnectedness between them. From the early 1990s on, first through the vehicle of major United Nations conferences (the International Conference on Human Rights in Vienna in 1993; the International Conference on Population and Development [ICPD] in Cairo in 1994; and the Fourth World Conference on Women in Beijing in 1995), a human rights-based approach to women's health came into its own (Chavkin and Chesler 2005; Sen 2014). Although the right to health was enshrined in the Constitution of the World Health Organization; the Universal Declaration on Human Rights; the International Covenant on Economic, Social and Cultural Rights (ICESCR); and the Alma-Ata declaration, it was not until the flurry of international activity in the 1990s, spurred largely by women's rights organizations from around the globe, that international instruments recognized the links between women's health and gender equality. For example, these instruments began to recognize sexual and reproductive health and rights and the right to be free from gender-based violence as key components to full realization of women's human rights. The approach of the 1990s represented a more inclusive approach, emphasizing the right to health services as well as the right to access key material and social determinants such as clean water and adequate housing, sanitation, and nutrition.

This human rights–based approach to health used sexuality and reproduction as central themes in shaping gender inequality, while also addressing violations of women's human rights by directing attention to the issue of bodily integrity. It emphasized laws, policies, and programs that would both advance gender equality and advance sexual and reproductive health and rights. The Programme of Action of the ICPD included a central chapter titled "Gender Equality, Equity and Empowerment of Women" (United Nations Population Fund 2004, chapter 4). More recently, advocacy for sexual rights has included claims beyond those for reproductive rights and gender equality. Examples include the right to sexual autonomy outside of one's reproductive capacity (i.e., nonprocreative sex) and equality rights based on sexual orientation and gender identity (the *Yogyakarta Principles* in 2007, the UNHCHR Sexual Orientation and Gender Identity [SOGI] declaration in 2011, and additional developments that emerged from the 2014 Human Rights Council Resolution). The 2000 ICESCR's General Comment on the Right to Health also articulated a broader conceptualization of rights, asserting states' obligations to respect, protect, and fulfill the right to health for all people. The UN Political Declarations on HIV/AIDS from 2001, 2006, and 2011 asserted that gender inequality can place women and girls at risk for HIV. While too long to list, there have been numerous other general comments and international recommendations related to women's health and empowerment, including ones that are focused on female genital mutilation, child marriage, and violence, several of which emerged out of the UN Convention on the Elimination of All Forms of Discrimination Against Women (CEDAW).

Have the approaches that link gender equality, women's empowerment, and human rights been assessed rigorously enough to conclude that empowerment interventions affect the realization of the right to health? Some of the literature cited earlier (Kishor 2000; Jejeebhoy 2000; Kritz, Makinwa-Adebusoye, and Gurak 2000; as well as other chapters in Presser and Sen 2000) has begun such an assessment, and more recent work is beginning to grapple more thoroughly with measuring rights and examining the causal links between rights-based interventions and health outcomes (Gruskin and Ferguson 2013; Polet et al. 2015; Unnithan 2015). And although there were multiple assessments of the achievements of the ICPD agenda occasioned by its twentieth-year review processes in 2014, they tended to be broad, partially due to the broad nature of the ICPD agenda itself.

In this context, the UN Population Fund's global review (UNPF 2014) demonstrates that, while much has been achieved, major challenges remain. These include considerable inequalities both within and between countries in relation to sexual and reproductive health outcomes and significant shortfalls in the fulfillment of women's human right to health overall. But these results also come with caveats about the inadequacy of data and the paucity of strong empirical research, even as theory has advanced and political commitments continue to be made. Importantly, this volume helps fill the gaps in the empirical research base by providing detailed descriptions and lessons learned from both science-based interventions and advocacy programs that strive towards the achievement of fundamental human rights.

Part of the challenge of linking health, human rights, and gender equality is the sometimes stark difference in perspectives, approaches, methodologies, and language used by those in the health sciences and the social sciences and those working in the realms of law, policy, and human rights advocacy. This is why the University of California Global Health Institute's (UCGHI) Center of Expertise (COE) on Women's Health and Empowerment (WHE) was established. The editors of this book are situated in different disciplines (medicine, public health, medical sociology) and seek to address the major gap in cross-disciplinary communication and action related to women's empowerment and health. The COE works to achieve this through integrated research, educational initiatives, and knowledge dissemination—pushing scholars and practitioners across the ten University of California campuses and beyond to engage in discussions, expand their perspectives, and work collaboratively to produce knowledge and educational programs that benefit from a multidisciplinary perspective. This book represents one concrete step towards translating the goals of the Center of Expertise in Women's Health and Empowerment into a reality. It is written for a general audience, with particular relevance for upper-level undergraduates and graduate students across disciplines and for practitioners implementing health and empowerment programs. In addition, instead of being focused only on academic research studies or only on work carried out by community-based organizations, many of the chapters in this book represent an intersection between theory and practice: a collaboration between academic researchers or policy experts and community-based organizations or non-governmental organizations.

A basic reason for the slowness in developing a multidisciplinary perspective may lie in the politics of research on women and health. To date, research politics have downplayed research on gender in favor of research on biologic sex (Kreiger 2003; Springer 2012). Far too little funding has been earmarked for the combination of biomedical and social science research that can uncover their complex connections (Sharman and Johnson 2012; Springer, Stellman, and Jordan-Young 2012). These internal biases in research do not incentivize innovative cross-disciplinary research or recognize the value of social science research in relation to biomedical research. To explore newer hypotheses about the links between health, human rights, and gender in this context is not easy.

Thus, the editors and authors of this volume offer a timely and valuable contribution to bridging three existing divides: between empowerment and health, between theory and practice, and between science and advocacy. *Empowering Women for Global Health: A Twenty-First-Century Agenda* provides a much needed, in-depth examination of specific women's health and empowerment interventions and programs implemented across the world. The case studies provide readers with a window into these programs—enabling them to see, in different contexts, what works, what doesn't, and how. Several of the chapters are complemented by short videos that take readers right into the setting, bringing them closer to the work, eliciting the feel of the context, and highlighting some of the promises and challenges of carrying out actual programs on the ground.

The first section of the book explores sociocultural, educational, and health systems' interventions as tools for empowerment, with each chapter describing an attempt to alter the factors that lead to disempowerment and poor health. The cases in section 1 reveal the importance of reaching out directly to "community insiders" who have the most at stake and perhaps the greatest incentive to lift binding constraints to transform their communities. The second section of the book presses beyond individual, group, educational, and organizational processes to explore broader economic, policy, and structural interventions as tools for empowerment. The authors in this section delve into factors that structurally shape health, such as access to and control over resources and rights-based and policy-level approaches. This section delves into analyses of microfinance, property rights, and land tenure to demonstrate the powerful influence that factors outside of health have on health and empowerment. This section illustrates the importance of law and policy to secure human rights and emphasizes the need for strong advocates working across multiple sectors to ensure that these laws and policy changes translate into a reality for people on the ground. This volume shows that the time is ripe to provide some answers and raise new questions about how women's empowerment improves health—and to light the path leading us there.

Box 0.1. Videos

Seven of the chapters in this edited volume have short films that have been produced by local filmmakers in the context in which the chapter is focused. The films offer students, researchers, practitioners, and policy makers insight into the specificities of the context, the nuts and bolts of interventions examined in the text of the chapter, and highlight the promises and limitations of program implementation. Each short film helps readers to "see" empowerment and health programs in action so as to extend their understanding of not just what works in such interventions but how these work.

Chapter 1: Action Research and Training for Health (ARTH), Rajasthan, India—https://youtu.be/mObfWwc6Gmk

Chapter 2: Let's End Fistula Project: A Holistic Approach from Kenya—https://youtu.be/YCsD-Tcywoo

Chapter 6: Women Organized to Respond to Life-Threatening Disease (WORLD), United States—https://youtu.be/FgYzjR3VfUY

Chapter 7: Sonke Gender Justice and One Man Can, South Africa—https://youtu.be/HWTGTUc3Yho

Chapter 8: The SHAZ! HUB: Serving the Needs of Adolescent Women and Girls in Zimbabwe—https://youtu.be/WTeLwR1HZqg

Chapter 11: Legal Interruption of Pregnancy (ILE), Mexico City—https://youtu.be/36fcRyGNQjk

Chapter 13: Xochilt Acalt Women's Center, Nicaragua—https://youtu.be/Gzxz7jdNhzI

REFERENCES

Alsop, R., and Heinsohn, N. 2005. *Measuring Empowerment in Practice: Structuring Analysis and Framing Indicators.* Washington, DC: World Bank. Policy Research Working Paper 3510. (accessed 14 April 2014). http://siteresources.worldbank.org/INTEMPOWERMENT/Resources/41307_wps3510.pdf.

Baker, P., Dworkin, S. L., Tong, S., Banks, I., and Yamey, G. 2014. Global action on men's health could benefit men, women, and children. *WHO Bulletin.* 92:618–620.

Barker, G., Ricardo, C., Nascimento, M., Olukoya, A., and Santos C. 2010. Questioning gender norms with men to improve health outcomes: Evidence of impact. *Global Public Health.* 5: 539–553.

Batliwala, S. 1994. The meaning of women's empowerment: new concepts from action. In *Population Policies Reconsidered: Health, Empowerment and Rights,* ed. G. Sen, A. Germain, and L. C. Chen, 127–138. Cambridge, MA: Harvard Center for Population and Development Studies.

Bisnath, S., and Elson, D. 1999. *Women's Empowerment Revisited.* Background paper, Progress of the World's Women. New York (NY): UNIFEM. www.unifem.undp.org/progressww/empower.html.

Chavkin, W., and Chesler E. 2005. *Where Human Rights Begin: Health, Sexuality and Women in the New Millennium.* New Brunswick, NJ: Rutgers University Press.

Cornwall, A. and Edwards, J. 2014. Introduction. In *Feminisms, Empowerment and Development: Changing Women's Lives,* ed. A. Cornwall and J. Edwards, 1–31. London: Zed Press.

Courtenay, WH. 2000. Constructions of masculinity and their influence on men's well-being: A theory of gender and health. *Social Science and Medicine.* May 50(10): 1385–1401.

Dixon-Mueller, R., and Germain, A. 2000. Reproductive health and the demographic imagination. In *Women's Empowerment and Demographic Processes: Moving beyond Cairo,* ed. H. B. Presser and G. Sen, 69–94. Oxford (UK): Oxford University Press.

Doyal, L. 1995. *What Makes Women Sick: Gender and the Political Economy of Health.* New Brunswick, NJ: Rutgers University Press.

Dworkin, S. L. 2015. *Men at Risk: Masculinity, Heterosexuality, and HIV/AIDS Prevention.* New York, NY: New York University Press.

Dworkin, S. L., Colvin, C., Hatcher, A., and Peacock, D. 2012. Men's perceptions of women's rights and changing gender relations in South Africa: Lessons for working with men and boys in HIV and anti-violence programs. *Gender and Society.* 26: 97–120.

Dworkin, S. L., Hatcher, A., Colvin, C., and Peacock, D. 2013. Impact of an anti-violence and HIV program on masculinities and gender ideologies in Limpopo and the Eastern Cape. *Men and Masculinities.* 16: 181–202.

Dworkin, S. L,. Kagan, S., and Lippman, S. 2014. Are gender-transformative interventions to reduce violence and HIV risks with heterosexually active men successful? What do we know? What else needs to be done? *AIDS and Behavior.* 17: 2845–2863.

Ferguson, A. 2004. Can development create empowerment and women's liberation? Paper presented at 2004 Center for Global Justice Workshop Alternatives to Globalization. (accessed 6 April 2014). www.globaljusticecenter.org/wp-content/dev1.pdf.

Govender, V., and Penn-Kekana, L. 2010. Challenging gender in patient-provider interactions. In *Gender Equity in Health: the Shifting Frontiers of Evidence and Action,* ed. G. Sen and P. Östlin, 184–209. New York, NY: Routledge.

Gruskin, S., and Ferguson, L. 2013. Using indicators to determine the contribution of human rights to public health efforts. In *Health and Human Rights in a Changing World,* ed. M. Grodin, D. Tarantola, G. Annas, and S. Gruskin, 202–211. New York, NY: Routledge.

Hatcher, A., Colvin, C., Ndlovo, N., and Dworkin, S. L. 2014. Intimate partner violence among rural South African men: Alcohol use, sexual decision making and partner communication. *Culture, Health, and Sexuality.* 18: 1–17.

Israel, B., Checkoway, B., Schulz, A., and Zimmerman, M. 1994. Health education and community empowerment: Conceptualizing and measuring perceptions of individual, organizational and community control. *Health Education Quarterly.* 21(2):149–170.

Jejeebhoy, S. 2000. Women's autonomy in rural India: Its dimensions, determinants, and the influence of context. In *Women's Empowerment and Demographic Processes: Moving Beyond Cairo,* ed. H.B. Presser and G. Sen, 204–238. Oxford, UK: Oxford University Press.

Kabeer, N. 1994. *Reversed Realities: Gender Hierarchies in Development Thought.* London: Verso.

———. 1999. Resources, agency, achievements: Reflection on the measurement of women's empowerment. *Development and Change.* 30 (3): 435–464.

———. 2001. Resources, Agency, Achievements: Reflections on the Measurement of Women's Empowerment. In *Discussing Women's Empowerment—Theory and Practice,* ed. A. Sisask, Sida Studies No. 3, 17–59. Stockholm, Sweden: Swedish International Development Agency.

Keleher, H. 2010. Gender norms and empowerment: "What works" to increase equity for women and girls. In *Gender Equity in Health: The Shifting Frontiers of Evidence and Action,* ed. G. Sen and P. Östlin, 161–183. New York: Routledge.

Khan, A. 2014. Paid work as a pathway of empowerment: Pakistan's Lady Health Worker programme. In *Feminisms, Empowerment and Development: Changing Women's Lives,* ed. A. Cornwall and J. Edwards, 104–122. London: Zed Press.

Kishor, S. 2000. Empowerment of women in Egypt and links to the survival and health of their infants. In *Women's Empowerment and Demographic Processes: Moving Beyond Cairo,* ed. H.B. Presser and G. Sen, 119–158. Oxford, UK: Oxford University Press.

Klugman, B. 2000. Empowering women through the policy process: The making of health policy in South Africa. In *Women's Empowerment and Demographic Processes: Moving Beyond Cairo,* ed. H.B. Presser and G. Sen, 95–118. Oxford, UK: Oxford University Press.

Kreiger, N. 2003. Gender, sexes, and health: What are the connections—and why does it matter? *International Journal of Epidemiology*. 32: 652–657.

Kritz, M., Makinwa-Adebusoye, P., and Gurak, D T. 2000. The role of gender context in shaping reproductive behaviour in Nigeria. In *Women's Empowerment and Demographic Processes: Moving Beyond Cairo*, ed. H. B. Presser and G. Sen, 239–260. Oxford, UK: Oxford University Press.

Malhotra, A., Schuler, S. R., and Boender, C. 2002. *Measuring Women's Empowerment as a Variable in International Development*. Washington, DC: World Bank, Gender and Development Group. www.icrw.org/docs /MeasuringEmpowerment_workingpaper_802.doc.

Moghadam, V. M., and Senftova, L. 2005. Measuring women's empowerment: Participation and rights in civil, political, social, economic, and cultural domains. *International Social Science Journal*. 57 (2): 389–412.

Oxaal, Z., and Baden, S. 1997. *Gender and Empowerment: Definitions, Approaches and Implications for Policy*. Brighton (UK): University of Sussex, Institute of Development Studies, Gender and Sexuality Cluster, BRIDGE. Report No. 40. (accessed 12 January 2014). www.bridge.ids .ac.uk/Reports/R40%20Gen%20Emp%20Policy%202c.doc.

Pathways of Women's Empowerment. n.d. Brighton (UK): University of Sussex, Institute of Development Studies, Pathways of Women's Empowerment. www.pathwaysofempowerment.org

Polet, F., Malaise, G., Mahieu, A., Utrera, E., Montes, J., Tablang, R., Aytin, A., Kambale, E., Luzala, S., al-Ghoul, D., et al. 2015. Empowerment for the right to health: The use of "most significant change" methodology in monitoring. *Health and Human Rights Journal*. 17: 71–82.

Pollack, W. 1998. *Real Boys: Rescuing our Sons from the Myths of Boyhood*. New York: Random House.

Pradhan, B. 2003. Measuring empowerment: A methodological approach. *Development*. 46 (2): 51–57.

Presser, H. B., and Sen, G. 2000. Women's empowerment and demographic processes: Laying the groundwork. In *Women's Empowerment and Demographic Processes: Moving Beyond Cairo*. ed. H. B. Presser and G. Sen, 3–11. Oxford, UK: Oxford University Press.

Rowlands, J. 1997. *Questioning Empowerment: Working with Women in Honduras*. Oxford, UK: Oxfam Publishing.

Sardenberg, C. 2009. *Liberal vs. Liberating Empowerment: Conceptualising Women's Empowerment from a Latin American Feminist Perspective*. Pathways Working Paper No. 7. Brighton (UK): University of Sussex, Institute of Development Studies, Pathways of Women's Empowerment.

Sen, G. 2014. Sexual and reproductive health and rights in the post-2015 development agenda. *Global Public Health*. 9: 599–606.

Sen, G., and Batliwala, S. 2000. Empowering women for reproductive rights. In *Women's Empowerment and Demographic Processes: Moving beyond Cairo*, ed. H. B. Presser and G. Sen, 15–36. Oxford, UK: Oxford University Press.

Sen, G., and Grown C. 1987. *Development, Crises and Alternative Visions: Third World Women's Perspectives*. New York: Monthly Review Press.

Sen, G., George, A., and Östlin, P. 2002. *Engendering International Health: The Challenge of Equity.* Cambridge, MA: MIT Press.

Sen, G., Östlin, P., and George, A. 2007. *Unequal, Unfair, Ineffective and Inefficient—Gender Inequity in Health: Why It Exists and How We Can Change It.* Final report of the Women and Gender Equity Knowledge Network to the WHO Commission on Social Determinants of Health. Bangalore and Stockholm: Indian Institute of Management Bangalore and Karolinska Institute.

Sharman, Z., and Johnson, J. 2012. Towards the inclusion of gender and sex in health research and funding: An institutional perspective. *Social Science and Medicine.* 74: 1812–1816.

Sholkamy, H. 2010. Power, politics and development in the Arab context: Or how can rearing chicks change patriarchy? *Development.* 53: 254–258.

Snow R. 2010. The social body: Gender and the burden of disease. In *Gender Equity in Health: The Shifting Frontiers of Evidence and Action,* ed. G. Sen and P. Östlin, 47–69. New York: Routledge.

Springer, K. 2012. Gender and health: Relational, intersectional, and biosocial approaches. *Social Science and Medicine.* 74: 1661–1666.

Springer, K. Stellman, J. M., and Jordan-Young, R. 2012. Beyond a catalogue of differences: A theoretical frame and good practice guidelines for researching sex/gender in human health. *Social Science and Medicine.* 74: 1817–1824.

Stromquist, N. 2002. Education as a means for empowering women. In *Rethinking Empowerment: Gender and Development in a Global/Local World,* ed. J. Parpart, S. Raj, and K. Staudt, 22–38. London: Routledge.

United Nations Population Fund (UNPF). 2004. Programme of Action. Adopted at the International Conference on Population and Development, Cairo, 5–13 September 1994.

———. 2014. *Framework of Actions for the Follow-Up to the Programme of Action of the ICDP beyond 2014.* (accessed 20 April 2014). http://icpdbeyond2014.org/upload/browser/files/icpd_global_review_report.pdf.

Unnithan, U. 2015. What constitutes evidence in human rights-based approaches to health: Learning from lives experiences of maternal and sexual reproductive health. *Health and Human Rights Journal.* 17: 45–56.

UN Women. 2013. *A Transformative Stand-Alone Goal on Achieving Gender Equality, Women's Rights and Women's Empowerment: Imperatives and Key Components.* (accessed 14 January 2014). www.unwomen.org/en/digital-library/publications/2013/7/post-2015-long-paper#view

Wallerstein, N. 2006. *What is the evidence on effectiveness of empowerment to improve health?* Health Evidence Network Report. Copenhagen: WHO Regional Office for Europe.

Yogyakarta Principles. 2007. www.yogyakartaprinciples.org/principles_en.pdf.

Sociocultural, Educational, and Health Service Interventions as Tools of Empowerment

Introduction

DALLAS SWENDEMAN AND PAULA TAVROW

Moving from Gita Sen's excellent overview of complex definitions and measures of empowerment and their links to health to thinking about what an empowered woman is or does is more challenging than it seems. While it might appear to be easy at first glance to describe a powerful woman, the process of achieving greater power—or empowerment—is much more complex and profoundly contextual. For instance, what may be a key determinant of empowerment for women in one context, such as greater mobility, may not be a defining factor for women elsewhere. Empowerment as a concept is operationalized and understood in diverse ways, and as is noted elsewhere in this volume, it can be viewed as a *process* for achieving power or goals and as the *outcome* of such processes (Israel et al., 1994; Zimmerman, 2000). Unfortunately, it is all too common for educational or behavioral interventions—and global health interventions overall—to be labelled as "empowering" if they simply focus on increasing women's knowledge or self-efficacy. Interventions that lead to greater knowledge and self-efficacy can be considered empowering at the individual or personal level by enhancing agency (Israel et al., 1994; Zimmerman, 2000), but unless they are combined with enhanced access to resources at a broader level (e.g., familial, organizational, community, societal), they are unlikely to lead to sustainably better outcomes for women (Kabeer, 1999).

In the chapters in this section, the empowerment approaches to achieving improvements in women's health have strong emphases on sociocultural factors and educational strategies, including bundling such strategies with innovations in the delivery of health services. These programs and the multiple intervention strategies embedded within them represent resource inputs or structural changes at local levels of program implementation, but the primary aims of the programs are to enhance the agency and status of women through education, training, community mobilization, and enhanced access to critical health or education services. By contrast, the case studies in section 2 of this book focus primarily on structural interventions, such as legal or policy changes, rights-based approaches, and economic security as tools of empowerment and health. Each case study in this section focuses on a different women's health and empowerment issue across the life course—educational access, fertility decisions, child marriage and early childbearing, community support (or lack thereof), prevention of HIV/STI transmission, coping positively with HIV, and gender-based violence—all exemplify how empowerment-oriented interventions can impact women's agency at various levels (individual, interpersonal, family, community, society) and domains (health, education, marketplace, etc.).

Importantly, education or training in the traditional sense is not sufficient for empowerment. Rather, as Gita Sen highlighted in the introduction to the book, and as theorist Paolo Freire (1973) has noted, what is needed for empowerment is for people to develop a "critical consciousness"—in other words, to have an education that nurtures a critical understanding of power relations and sources of inequality. Information alone will not empower women to be able to make strategic life choices. The truism that "knowledge is power" is unsatisfactory because it fails to take into account the broader socioeconomic factors that either facilitate or close down opportunities to apply knowledge or skills to achieve goals.

The most empowering interventions, then, simultaneously shift structural conditions (i.e., institutional, social, and political contexts within which actors make choices; Samman and Santos, 2009) while enhancing the agency (i.e., the capacity to exercise purposeful choice; Alsop and Heinsohn, 2005) of individuals, organizations, or communities to act upon new opportunities presented by these structural changes. Section 2 of this volume picks up on this idea and focuses solely on structural interventions as tools of empowerment, while the case studies in this section tend to focus on educational, sociocultural, or health services interventions that enhance women's agency. In these case studies, accompanying structural changes are limited to the local context of intervention implementation. Several phases of girls' and women's lives are included in the case studies in this section of our volume: young women, adolescents, and middle-aged women are featured.

In chapter 1, "Taking Services to the Doorstep: Providing Rural Indian Women Greater Control over Their Fertility," Pallavi Gupta, Kirti Iyengar, and Sharad Iyengar describe how the seemingly simple strategy of providing urine screen pregnancy tests to community health workers (CHWs) doing home visits in rural Rajasthan, India, requires a bundle of multilevel intervention components to address individual and local structural barriers that hinder women from making informed decisions about fertility. This intervention focuses on the major gaps in training, healthcare infrastructure, and service linkages to enable women to achieve desired reproductive health goals. The authors also acknowledge larger structural barriers to reproductive health at the legal, policy, and marketplace levels, most specifically on the skewed emphasis on sterilization as the preferred family planning method. Men were also engaged in education or mobilization activities to mitigate barriers to the program.

This chapter also illustrates the recursive dynamism inherent in empowerment practice and research: Gupta and her coauthors note that while the influence of women's empowerment on fertility is relatively well established, the potential impact of empowering women with greater control over their fertility on subsequent empowerment outcomes over the life course is a topic worthy of greater attention. Few women in rural Rajasthan have control over their reproductive decisions, which the authors assert both reflects and compounds their social disempowerment. Increasing access to pregnancy tests through CHWs served as an entry point to empower pregnant women to understand their options, make critical decisions at an early stage in their pregnancy, and be linked to appropriate services. The chapter makes a compelling case for enabling rural women to have greater control over their reproductive decisions and, by extension, the trajectory of their lives.

Also focused on health services, Lindsey Pollaczek, Paula Tavrow, and Habiba Mohamed in chapter 2, "Obstetric Fistula in Kenya: A Holistic Model of Outreach, Treatment, and Reintegration," describe a program built on empowerment principles to achieve secondary and tertiary prevention of obstetric fistula in Western Kenya. The structural factors most proximal to risk for fistula are lack of access to emergency obstetric care for women with obstructed labor, lack of knowledge about fistula risks, and social norms that may impede use of services. More distal structural factors include early childbirth that increases risk of fistulas, and low status and power of women that might constrain any action (choice) to prevent fistula. Once women have fistula, they become further disempowered by social stigma and marginalization and their subsequent psychological and economic consequences, which are major barriers to treatment. The intervention described uses a number of empowering processes. First, local women who have had their fistulas repaired are trained to take on leadership roles by actively working to identify fistula sufferers in the community. By engaging in community mobilization and home visits to encourage other women to undergo surgical repair, these survivors become empowered in the same localities where they had once been pariahs. The program further recognizes that repair itself is not sufficiently empowering, so it also has an important reintegration component to build women's self-reliance upon returning to their communities after reparative surgery. The reintegration component aims to improve women's psychological well-being, help them to control their fertility (reducing the risk of fistula recurrence), increase their income, develop a critical consciousness about their situation, and participate once again in community life. Although the chapter demonstrates that a program can support women suffering from a serious health condition to obtain treatment and reintegrate into society, it is worth noting that the program did not make many inroads in primary prevention of fistulas. Intervening to address the more distal factors that could prevent obstetric fistulas, such as societal norms about early childbearing or financial constraints around service availability, is often beyond the reach of programs focused mainly on education and treatment.

By contrast, chapter 3, "Pathways to Choice: Delaying Age of Marriage through Girls' Education in Northern Nigeria," by Daniel Perlman, Fatima Adamu, Mairo Mandara, Olorukooba Abiola, David Cao, and Malcolm Potts, takes its starting point not from a specific health issue but from the structural factor of early marriage, which is linked to multiple health problems, including maternal mortality and morbidities such as fistulas. The chapter serves to remind us that health funding streams often require interventions to be framed around a specific disease (such as HIV/AIDS), even though an empowerment-focused intervention should ultimately reduce morbidity and mortality from many sources. Although the intervention described in this chapter is focused on girls' education in northern Nigeria, the ultimate aim of the program is to prevent early marriage and early childbearing while also supporting young women to achieve higher levels of education and greater economic opportunities. Specific empowerment intervention strategies highlighted in this chapter include community engagement and advocacy with power brokers such as religious leaders, traditional leaders, and parents; financial incentives (reduced school fees) to offset the costs to families for supporting daughters' education; and after-school mentored support groups for girls, which include critical reflection and consciousness-building activities in addition to remedial literacy and numeracy support. Overall, this work highlights the interplay of structure and agency at multiple levels by acknowledging the root causes of disempowerment (low status of women, gender bias in education, child marriage) and by its use of empowerment strategies that address structural factors (e.g., advocacy within communities to gain support for girls' education, providing scholarships to address parents' financial barriers). At the same time, the program emphasizes the process of empowerment by supporting girls' to achieve critical consciousness about the value of education, their long-term vision and dreams for their own future, and their potential role to spark change within their communities.

Chapter 4, "Early Empowerment: The Evolution and Practice of Girls' 'Boot Camps' in Kenya and Haiti," by Karen Austrian, Judith Bruce, and M. Catherine Maternowska, provides a somewhat unique approach among the case studies in this book by targeting programs that support vulnerable and marginalized adolescent girls, rather than the girls themselves. The chapter describes adolescent girls' programming boot camps, a participatory, data-driven process of designing and/ or tailoring programs to serve marginalized adolescent girls. At the boot camps, program staff are matched with "girl experts" to develop or strengthen programs that emphasize multisectoral asset building, to share knowledge of best practices across organizations and programs, and to develop or revise program plans and funding applications. The chapter focuses on two formative experiences in Kenya and Haiti, which despite the geographic divide, uncover similar disadvantages associated with being both young and female, which can be severely exacerbated in contexts of political and environmental crises. One critical point about this chapter that readers should note is that because the boot camp model focuses on the process of program development rather than specific intervention strategies, it is highly generalizable across a broad range of contexts and programs. The chapter's results highlight three core elements of successful programs identified over years of cross-context comparisons and evaluations: safe and supportive girls-only spaces, female mentors as role models, and a focus on building social networks. Austrian and her coauthors emphasize the importance of safe and supportive spaces for adolescent girls, arguing that such spaces are rare in many contexts, including the home, the school, and the community. Safe spaces can be mapped and fostered in a variety of locations (i.e., not just in a typical NGO or youth center), and these spaces can create the platform from which girls can engage with mentors and build supportive social networks. Safe spaces, mentors or role models, and social-network building are evident in many of the other chapters in this section: for example, in the after-school clubs for girls in northern Nigeria (chapter 3) and in the support groups for women with obstetric fistula in Kenya (chapter 2) as well as drop-in centers for sex workers in Bangladesh described in chapter 5. In each case, the safe spaces served as starting points for engaging vulnerable women and girls and as settings for mentoring, dialogue, social-network building and other programmatic activities to build critical consciousness and empowerment.

The chapter on CARE International's work (chapter 5), "Empowerment and HIV Risk Reduction among Sex Workers in Bangladesh," by Victor Robinson, Theresa Hwang, and Elisa Martínez, highlights the need to listen to marginalized populations define the problems that affect them and for them to participate actively in the solutions that shape their empowerment and health. The chapter focuses on the multiple structural factors that marginalize female sex workers. The case study focuses on brothel-based and street-based sex workers at risk of contracting HIV and other sexually transmitted infections (STIs). Throughout South Asia, sex workers struggle with poverty, low literacy, lack of economic opportunities, and a low status of women in general, compounded by the stigma and marginalization of sex work. Addressing such deeply rooted and distal (upstream) structural factors is often beyond the scope or ability of health interventions focused on more immediate health threats. Yet, intervention strategies that focus simply on increasing knowledge, risk perception, condom use, and negotiation skills are typically insufficient to result in sustained and consistent behavioral changes among sex workers and their clients. Without shifts in norms and power relations among peers, power brokers (madams, brothel owners), clients, and sex workers, the use of condoms, HIV testing, and HIV treatment and support services will be sporadic. The chapter highlights how multiple levels and domains affect sex workers' empowerment, such as the legal and social context for sex work in Bangladesh, the role of brothels, and the development of collective identity and leadership among sex workers. Recognizing these multiple influences, the CARE empowerment initiative used innovative strategies to establish an environment for sex workers' empowerment in conjunction with HIV/STI testing, treatment and condom availability. Most notable were the introduction of drop-in center safe spaces, support for community-based "self-help" organizations, and activities to build critical reflection among sex workers. By simultaneously valuing the voices of sex workers and targeting behaviors and structural conditions in a multi-component program, synergistic impacts occurred and sex workers reported feeling empowered to take meaningful action to reduce their vulnerability to HIV and STIs.

In chapter 6, "Gender Roles in U.S. Women with HIV: Intersection with Psychological and Physical Health Outcomes," Leslie R. Brody, Sannisha Dale, Gwendolyn Kelso, Ruth Cruise, Kathleen Weber, Lynissa Stokes, and Mardge Cohen illustrate that challenges related to women's empowerment and health are not limited to developing or lower-income countries. In this chapter, the context of empowerment among HIV-positive or at-risk women is illustrated in an analysis of a survey conducted among a cohort of middle-aged women (average age 43 years) in the National Institutes of Health (NIH)–funded Women's Interagency HIV Study (WIHS) in the United States. This research indicated that empowerment-related constructs such as gender roles and agency-oriented, or "agentic," coping strategies are linked to health outcomes that vary by women's age. For example, agentic coping strategies, such as persistence and making meaning by finding the positive value in traumatic experiences, are related to more egalitarian gender role behaviors, which in turn are related to higher resilience in women with and at risk for HIV. Middle-aged women in this survey displayed less egalitarian gender role behaviors than younger women, which were associated with higher levels of depression and lower levels of resilience in the older cohort. These results suggest that generational factors, or perhaps factors associated with aging, may intersect with empowerment and health for women. The results of the survey are followed in this chapter by the description of an organization in Oakland, California, called Women Organized to Respond to Life Threatening Diseases (WORLD), which aims through its interventions to improve access to psychosocial support to improve coping strategies, resilience, and empowerment among its clients, women living with HIV infection in the San Francisco Bay Area. WORLD's programming includes a mix of peer advocacy, support groups, and educational programs that focus on strategies identified in the WIHS-based survey that can increase empowerment, including helping clients gain insight into their lives and take active steps, such as leaving abusive situations, living with more mindfulness and optimism, seeking education, practicing self-reliance, and setting realistic goals. These outcomes, framed under the umbrella of empowerment, are notably psychological in emphasis, in contrast to most other chapters in this section. This may reflect the dominant sociobehavioral sciences paradigm in U.S. health research while also suggesting that women's empowerment in high-resource settings may entail more emphasis on psychological barriers to realize the potentially greater levels of resources and opportunities available than in low- and middle-income countries.

Finally, whereas the previous chapters all seek to achieve improved women's health through empowering activities targeting girls and women, chapter 7, by Shari Dworkin, Abigail Hatcher, Christopher Colvin, and Dean Peacock, "Examining the Impact of a Masculinities-Based HIV Prevention and Antiviolence Program in Limpopo and Eastern Cape, South Africa," describes a collaboration between the University of California at San Francisco (UCSF), the University of Cape Town (UCT), and a South African non-governmental organization (NGO) known as Sonke Gender Justice. Sonke aims to shift men in the direction of more gender equality in order to improve women's empowerment and health outcomes, while also assisting men through critical reflection on narrow and constraining aspects of masculinity that shape both women's and men's health outcomes. In South Africa, due to extremely high rates of domestic and sexual violence, and one of the world's highest HIV prevalence rates, this linkage is of particular concern. Moreover, young women in South Africa have a disproportionately higher rate of HIV than young men. The program works with communities of men to change men's social norms about masculinities (what it means to be a man) and to present alternatives to a variety of health behaviors, including violence against women. The organization also used empowering processes such as community mobilization, advocacy strategies, and media campaigns. The chapter examines the effects of the program as perceived by participants of Sonke's small-group workshops, which were intended to build critical reflection among men on links between HIV and gender, power, and other health risks. These reflections occurred through a social justice framework, paired with personal and community-level action. By focusing on men and boys, the program aims to promote women's equality and health, while at the same time demonstrating to men that they stand to gain, personally and collectively, as well. Notably, the activities never directly target women, although it is possible that they might be strengthened if they included a complementary program on women's views on masculinities, including women's expectations about men.

Overall, the chapters in this section demonstrate a diverse range of social and educational programs to achieve improvements in women's health and empowerment. Rather than relying on a single health, educational, or social change strategy, all of the programs include activities aimed to enhance women's agency, with multiple components targeting proximal structural barriers, as well as the root causes of disempowerment and ill health that are embedded in societies. All interventions seek to build not only skills and self-efficacy but also critical consciousness to frame and motivate change. This bundling of strategies enhances these programs' potential to have a more lasting impact on women's empowerment and health.

REFERENCES

Alsop, R., and Heinsohn, N. 2005. *Measuring Empowerment in Practice: Structuring Analysis and Framing Indicators.* Washington, DC: World Bank. Policy Research Working Paper 3510. http://siteresources.worldbank.org/INTEMPOWERMENT/Resources/41307_wps3510.pdf.
Freire, P. 1973. *Education for Critical Consciousness.* Continuum, vol. 1. New York: Seabury Press.
Israel, B., Checkoway, B., Schulz, A., and Zimmerman, M. 1994. Health education and community empowerment: Conceptualizing and measuring perceptions of individual, organizational and community control. *Health Education Quarterly.* 21 (2): 149–170.
Kabeer, N., 1999. Resources, agency, achievements: Reflections on the measurement of women's empowerment. *Development and change,* 30(3), pp.435–464.
Samman, E., and Santos, M.E. 2009. *Agency and Empowerment: A Review of Concepts, Indicators and Empirical Evidence.* Oxford, UK: Oxford Poverty

and Human Development Initiative. Prepared for the 2009 Human Development Report in Latin America and the Caribbean. www.ophi.org.uk /wp-content/uploads/OPHI-RP-10a.pdf.

Zimmerman, M. A. 2000. Empowerment theory: Psychological, organizational, and community levels of analysis. In *Handbook of Community Psychology*, ed. J. Rappaport and E. Seidman, 43–63. New York: Springer Science.

Taking Services to the Doorstep

Providing Rural Indian Women Greater
Control over Their Fertility

PALLAVI GUPTA, KIRTI IYENGAR, AND SHARAD IYENGAR

Empowerment has been defined by Kabeer as the expansion of the ability to make strategic life choices. Such choices include those related to education, marriage, childbearing, and livelihood.[1] While augmenting women's empowerment has been shown to result in a decline in fertility because their choices expand,[2] the inverse effect of fertility control on empowerment has not been adequately explored.[3] Various pathways have been theorized to explain the relationship between fertility control and subsequent empowerment. Some hypothesize that women who enjoy greater control over their fertility may experience greater gender equality because they are better able to balance and time their sexual, reproductive, and nonreproductive aspirations, thus facilitating access to emerging opportunities in the workplace and beyond.

A woman's ability to control her own fertility is likely to be crucial to her empowerment. If a woman can have control over the timing and spacing of her pregnancies, she can plan how many and which years of her life will be free from childbearing, and she may have the freedom to participate more fully and equally in economic and nonreproductive activities. Our intervention aimed to enable young women and adolescents in India to gain greater control over their fertility by improving access to pregnancy tests at the village level and linking women to quality reproductive health services. Pregnancy tests were made available to women residing in the organization's field program, which covers a rural population of about 60,800, in forty-nine villages of Udaipur and

Rajsamand districts in the state of Rajasthan, India. Women in this area have very low levels of literacy, a very early median age of marriage, and limited decision-making ability and financial autonomy.[4] Further, while family planning programs have been recognized to play a key role in improving women's reproductive health, it is difficult to make family planning (and abortion) accessible to young women living in socially conservative societies where young women are often disempowered. Through this program, we found that using pregnancy tests as an entry point to improve reproductive health made it easier to make both contraceptive and safe abortion services more accessible for women.

CONTEXT

Rajasthan, located in the northwest of India (figures 1.1 and 1.2), is the country's largest state in terms of area (342,239 square kilometers, 10.41% of the country's total area) and is home to about 68 million people according to the 2011 national census.

Like other north Indian states, Rajasthan is marked by patrilineal, patrilocal, and patriarchal social systems. The union government counts it among India's "empowered action group" (EAG) states, which entails high governmental priority for development initiatives.[5] Development indicators of the state are among the most adverse in the country, especially for women. Barely 46% of rural women were literate in 2011,[6] and 62% were married before the age of 18 years.[7] Women also have low autonomy in terms of mobility and decision making: an International Institute for Population Sciences survey revealed that only 32% of women were allowed to go to three specified places alone—the market, the health facility, and places outside the village/community; the rest could not go anywhere alone.[8] Young women are at the bottom of social hierarchy, and the use of modern methods of family planning is still rare: only 4.6% couples in 2005–2006 used a modern method of contraception before the first child, and only 16.5% did so between their first and second child.[9] The total fertility rate in the state is 3.1,[10] while the maternal mortality ratio, at 318 per 100,000 live births, is much higher than the overall national figure (212 per 100,000 live births).[11] Women shoulder a heavy work burden—their days are spent fetching fuel, fodder, and water and in activities of farming, housework, and wage labor.

Action Research & Training for Health (ARTH), a private, nonprofit public health organization based in Udaipur, Rajasthan, has been work-

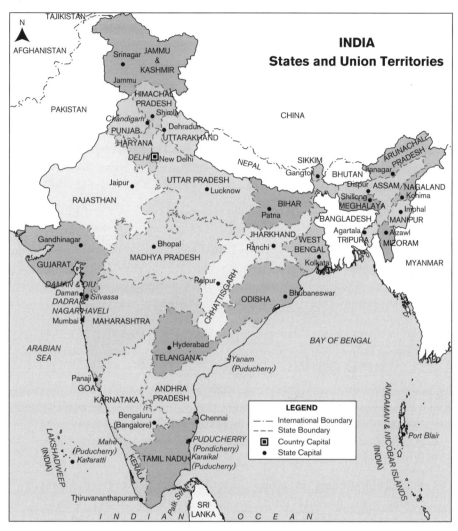

FIGURE 1.1. Map of India. Source: Indira Gandhi Conservation Monitoring Centre, WWF India.

ing in interior rural areas of two southern districts of the state since 1997. ARTH's field service program covers a population of 60,800 people within forty-nine villages, nearly half of which belong to an underprivileged tribal community. The hilly terrain of this area, coupled with the low autonomy of women in the region, makes it difficult for women to access health care services. ARTH operates two reproductive and child health centers in this area that provide a range of reproductive and

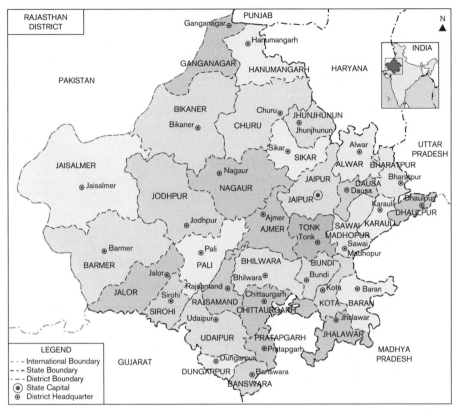

FIGURE I.2. Map of Rajasthan. Source: Indira Gandhi Conservation Monitoring Centre, WWF India.

child health services, including twenty-four-hour delivery and maternal care services, antenatal care, first-trimester abortions, and reversible methods of contraception (including intrauterine devices [IUDs], inject-able contraceptives, oral pills, condoms, and emergency contraceptive pills). ARTH also provides community-based education and services through its outreach workers.

The public health system in rural India comprises health subcenters, each staffed by an auxiliary nurse-midwife (ANM), who serves a group of villages with approximately 3,000–5,000 individuals; primary health centers staffed by one or two doctors and two nurse-midwives, serving 15–30 villages (a population of about 25,000); and community health centers (CHCs), serving 120–200 villages (a population of about 175,000). Although pregnancy test kits have been available in developed countries since 1977 and in urban areas of developing countries since the late 1980s, they have not been available to rural women until very recently.[12] Therefore, there are few reliable mechanisms for rural women to confirm their pregnancy status. From interactions with women in our field area, we learned that ANMs procure the tests from the market and perform each test for INR 50 (approximately USD 1). Apart from the high cost to women, the ANMs irregular presence in the villages means that women are often unable to access this service when it is most needed.

AVAILABILITY OF CONTRACEPTION AND ABORTION SERVICES

India has been promoting family planning through its Family Welfare Programme (FWP) since 1951. Despite policy commitment to a target-free approach, the FWPs of many states (including Rajasthan) continue to impose targets and set local goals, now called "expected levels of achievement" (ELAs), which essentially means that health workers are expected to find a certain number of contraceptive acceptors.[13] Thus, the program in practice continues to be heavily biased in favor of incentives and targets, with a skewed emphasis on female sterilization.[14] Since frontline workers are penalized for not attaining their ELA for sterilization, they tend to avoid providing information about reversible methods (in favor of permanent methods), especially to women who have two or more children. Studies by ARTH have shown that even women who wish to limit their pregnancies may not want to use an irreversible contraceptive method because they might be afraid of the side effects of sterilization, or they might wish to maintain their fertility potential since they fear the possibility of widowhood, remarriage, or the death of a child. These women, who have achieved their desired family size but are not willing to be sterilized, have restricted access to reversible contraceptives under current family planning programs. They remain at risk for unwanted pregnancies.

A review of the National Rural Health Mission (NRHM)[15] commissioned by the government of India in 2009, observed that female sterilization continued to be the most prevalent method of contraception in Rajasthan, and that the use of spacing methods needed to increase. The authors of the review observed that some Information, Education, and Communication (IEC) materials produced by the Rajasthan government promoted the two-child norm, a practice that could be considered a violation of reproductive rights. They recommended that the IEC materials be modified to encourage the use of family planning methods in general, rather than focusing on how many children families should have.[16] Another evaluation of NRHM in 2009 found that awareness of reversible methods of family planning remains low in Rajasthan—only 19% of 15- to 49-year-old currently married women were aware of IUDs, and only 12% knew about emergency contraceptive pills.[17] Hence, it is not surprising that the majority of contraceptive users in India continue to choose female sterilization.[18] Out of the 44.4% currently married women using modern contraceptives in Rajasthan, 34.2% adopted female sterilization.[19]

In 1971, the Medical Termination of Pregnancy (MTP) Act legalized abortions performed up to twenty weeks of gestation, under specific circumstances including risk to the woman's life or grave injury to her physical or mental health. The latter clause includes pregnancy resulting from rape, risk of physical or mental abnormalities in the child, and failure of contraceptive method used by a married woman or her husband. Even though the MTP Act is an enabling piece of legislation, the availability of safe abortion services, especially in rural areas of the country, remains extremely limited. In 1999, there were no health facilities that were certified to provide safe abortions in the block where ARTH worked (comprising a population of 150,000). A study of licensed facilities in Rajasthan between 2007 and 2010 revealed only 0.85 certified abortion facilities per 100,000 rural people, as compared to 3.65 facilities per 100,000 urban people. The same study revealed that the government facility in the block in which ARTH worked had reported performing no abortions over a three-year period.[20] Going to the city for abortion is not an option for most rural women, because of lack of familiarity with the city and the cultural expectation that a male should accompany a woman on such a journey. Male accompaniment is often not feasible, both because of the high costs of travel and the high rates of male migration. These conditions limit women's mobility, resulting in a higher incidence of women undergoing unsafe abortions or continuing with unwanted pregnancies.

Poor access to pregnancy tests has meant that rural women either wait weeks before they seek an abortion or have to travel to a block health facility located several kilometers away just to confirm a pregnancy. If they are late in approaching an abortion provider in terms of week of pregnancy, they are likely to be denied the service because most rural health facilities provide only first-trimester abortion services. On the other hand, women's lack of knowledge of pregnancy status can be exploited by abortion providers. In the course of providing services, the ARTH team came across two women with secondary amenorrhea, due to lactation and injectable contraceptives respectively, who had been informed by private doctors that they were pregnant and hence needed an abortion. When they came to our health center to confirm their pregnancies, ARTH learned that neither woman was pregnant.

METHODS

In 2007, ARTH began an intervention in its field service program to offer urine pregnancy tests to village women, counsel them about their options (depending on the result of the pregnancy test) and subsequently help them access the reproductive health services of their choice. We trained two kinds of community health workers—government-appointed Accredited Social Health Activists (ASHAs)[21]—one ASHA per 1,000 population—and ARTH-appointed village health workers (VHWs)—one VHW per 4,000–5,000 population. Both categories of health workers were mainly locally residing women who were educated at least up to class 8.

ASHAs and VHWs underwent two days of training that covered the following topics:

· Counselling skills
· Process of conception
· Methods of contraception including emergency contraception (EC)
· How to use a urine pregnancy test kit
· Importance of early antenatal check-ups
· Dangers of unsafe abortion
· Where to go for a safe abortion

At the end of training, community health workers were expected to conduct pregnancy tests, and based on the results of the test and the woman's fertility intentions, provide each woman with the desired services or referrals (figure 1.3). If the result of the pregnancy test was positive and the woman wanted to continue the pregnancy, the health worker referred her to antenatal care services. If the test was positive but she did not want to continue the pregnancy, the health worker referred her to ARTH's health centers for safe abortion services. If the

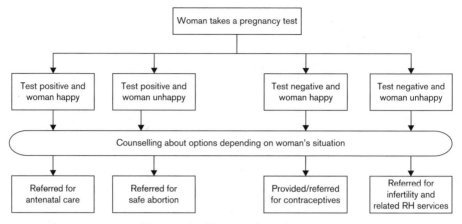

FIGURE 1.3. Conceptual framework of the intervention by ARTH.

pregnancy test was negative and the woman did not wish to become pregnant, then the health worker counseled her about contraceptives. The health worker was authorized to offer oral contraceptive pills, condoms, and emergency contraceptives; women interested in injectable contraception, IUDs, or sterilization were referred to appropriate facilities. If the pregnancy test was negative and the woman wanted to become pregnant, the health worker would subsequently refer her to services for preconception counseling, infertility, or childlessness.

Due to attrition, we trained seventy ASHAs and nineteen VHWs over the four-year period. Of the ASHAs, eighteen proved to be inactive and stopped coming to review meetings; eleven VHWs stopped working after having been trained. Overall, there was attrition of eighteen out of seventy ASHAs from this intervention and eleven out of nineteen VHWs.

Each pregnancy test strip cost around INR 5 (approximately USD 0.1). The tests were priced at INR 10 (approximately USD 0.2) for the user. Health workers reported that some women did not have money to pay for the tests. Because our organization did not want to restrict access, we advised the health workers to continue to provide the service irrespective of whether women paid or not. In the last year of the intervention, the service was provided free of cost to women after we started using the kits made available via the public health system.

Initial training was followed by a monthly refresher training-review meeting, during which we discussed and addressed problems faced by

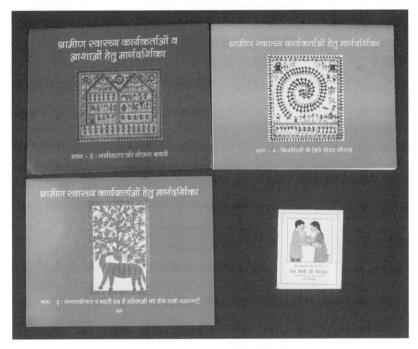

FIGURE 1.4. Educational materials used by health workers.

health workers, refreshed their knowledge and skills, and resupplied them with pregnancy test kits and contraceptives. We provided the health workers with health education material for use during individual or group interactions in the villages. These included three illustrated educational books and small take-home booklets that could easily fit in the front shirt pocket of men interested in contributing to the planning of their families (figure 1.4).

In order to create an enabling environment for health workers to be able to provide these services, project staff initially conducted 184 orientation meetings with men and village leaders in each village to explain the intervention to them and answer any questions that might arise. We also commissioned 50 color wall paintings (figure 1.5) and conducted 132 video shows and small-group meetings with young women and men in each village. For the majority of women, one-to-one contact and word of mouth were the primary ways in which they learned about the service.

To ensure that women received the services and to confirm the tests' accuracy, we carried out regular field supervision. In the first year, a

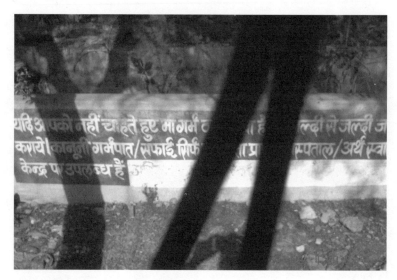

FIGURE 1.5. Wall painting by ARTH.

supervisor verified almost half (49%) of all the tests by visiting the women's homes while maintaining confidentiality. On finding that about 97% test results were accurate and recognizing the potentially intrusive nature of such verification visits, we reduced the extent of supervision in subsequent years.

RESULTS

From 2007 onward, the popularity of pregnancy tests in the region grew steadily (figure 1.6). In the last year of the program, the numbers were reduced as ARTH started sourcing the pregnancy test kits from the NRHM to dovetail our intervention with the government program, both to achieve sustainability and to avoid duplication of resources. This reliance on the government program sometimes led to disruption of the regular supply of kits, as delays in getting them from the government did occur. Between July 2007 and June 2011, health workers conducted 4,161 pregnancy tests at the village level (figure 1.6). On average, they conducted 26 tests per 1,000 population in the third year, when the intervention was running optimally. Though ASHAs outnumbered VHWs and conducted a greater proportion of the pregnancy tests (figure 1.7), the performance of VHWs surpassed that of ASHAs. On average in year 3, each VHW conducted 87 tests while each ASHA conducted only 14 tests.

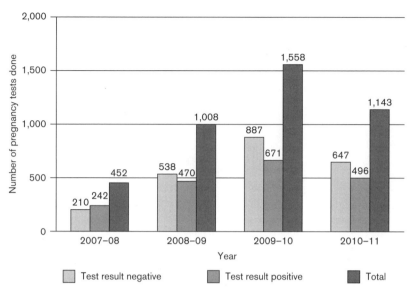

FIGURE 1.6. Number of pregnancy tests done by ARTH health workers, 2007–2011.

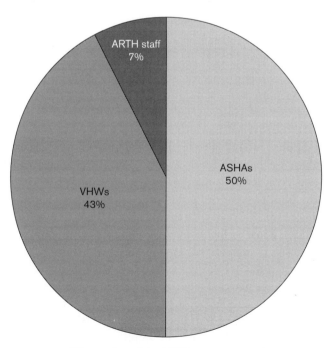

FIGURE 1.7. Who conducted the ARTH pregnancy tests?

TABLE 1.1   PROFILE OF WOMEN WHO USED THE PREGNANCY TEST SERVICE IN
THE VILLAGES

Age (N = 4,161)	<20	300 (7.2%)
	20–24	1,489 (35.8%)
	25–29	1,469 (35.3%)
	30 and above	903 (21.7%)
	Mean age	25.4 years
	Range	15–48 years
Caste (N = 4,161)	Scheduled caste[22]	420 (10.1%)
	Scheduled tribe[22]	2,091 (50.2%)
	Other	1,650 (39.7%)
No. of living children (N = 4,161)	0	985 (23.7%)
	1 to 2	1,943 (46.7%)
	3 to 4	978 (23.5%)
	5 and more	253 (6.1%)
	Not recorded	2
Education (N = 3,279)	Illiterate	2,362 (72.0%)
(February 2009 onwards)	1st to 5th	428 (13.0%)
	6th to 8th	309 (9.4%)
	9th and above	180 (5.5%)
Marital status (N = 4,161)	Married	4,098 (98.5%)
	Unmarried	56 (1.3%)
	Separated/widowed	7 (0.2%)

Nearly 43% women who took the test were under 25 years of age (table 1.1). As many as 24% did not have any living children, and 47% had either one or two children, indicating that the service was accessible to women in the early phase of their reproductive cycle.

A disproportionately high number of pregnancy test users belonged to the otherwise hard-to-reach groups—60.3% women belonged to socially and economically marginalized communities, who constitute 45% of the total population in the intervention area, according to the 2001 India census.[22] Nearly three-fourths of these women had never been to school. Most of the women were married, although a minority (1.5%) were single (unmarried, separated, or widowed). Married adolescents who had not yet started cohabiting with their husbands were included among the married women. As per local tradition, in the event of marriage during childhood, a girl may wait for two to five years before joining her husband's home. During this transition period, she may visit her husband's home on family occasions, where sexual

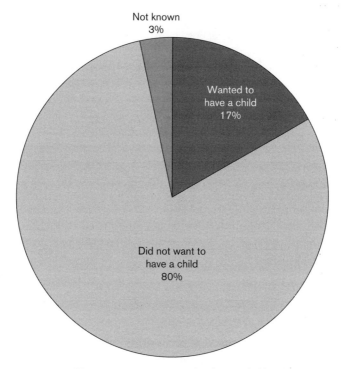

FIGURE 1.8. How many women wanted to have a child at the time of their pregnancy test?

contacts might result in pregnancy. She also might also become pregnant through intercourse with another person. However, pregnancy during this phase is considered stigmatizing; these young girls are expected to be sexually inactive, which makes it difficult for them to access reproductive health services.

Women Who Tested Negative (n = 2,282)

A high proportion of the total tests conducted resulted in a negative pregnancy outcome (54.8%). Of those women, 79.8% (1,821) did not want to have a child at the time (figure 1.8), and 64.7% (1,178) of them either had no children or one or two children. Of the women who did not want to have a child, 50.8% (925) initiated a reversible contraceptive soon after the test was performed, with oral contraceptives pills being the most popular among the users (46.8%), followed by condoms (30.9%), emergency contraceptive (EC) pills (8.1%), and injectable contraceptives (7.1%). The health worker who conducted the test gave the women the choice of all contraceptive options and informed the women where to access each option. The health worker was also able to provide oral pills, condoms, and ECs immediately following the test in the village; for clinic-based methods of contraception, the woman was referred to an appropriate health facility.

In the event that a woman who desired pregnancy was not pregnant (16.8%, 383), the health workers referred her to an obstetrician/gynecologist at ARTH's health center (see example 1.1). The gynecologist would examine the patient and advise on a first round of tests before making a referral to an infertility center when needed. We do not have information about how many of these women sought further medical advice for infertility.

Women Who Tested Positive (n = 1,879)

A total of 45.1% of women tested positive for pregnancy. Of these, 61% wanted to continue the pregnancy, and 39% did not (figure 1.9).

Example 1.1. Pemli Gameti's Story

Pemli Gameti, an illiterate 35-year-old woman belonging to the tribal community, missed her period. She lived in a village about 35 kilometers from the nearest town where she could access reproductive health services. When the village health worker (VHW) was on one of her regular visits to Pemli's village, Pemli saw her and called her. Pemli informed the VHW that she had not had her period for the last two months and was concerned that she might be pregnant. The VHW conducted a urine pregnancy test for Pemli, which revealed that she was not pregnant. Pemli was relieved as she already had five children and did not want any more. The VHW counselled her and told her that her amenorrhea could be due to lactation. The VHW advised her to come to the clinic and also told her about the various contraceptive options. After a visit to the clinic and meeting with the physician, Pemli decided to start oral contraceptive pills. Subsequently, she took her supply of pills from the VHW whenever she visited the village.

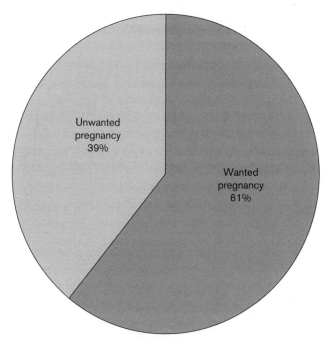

FIGURE 1.9. How many women wanted to continue their pregnancy?

The women who reported that they wanted to continue the pregnancy were referred for early antenatal checkups to either the ARTH health centers or to the government ANM.

A follow-up of the 735 women who did not wish to continue the pregnancy revealed that the majority (72%) reported having an induced abortion, and 9% reported spontaneous abortions. However, 18% women who expressed that the pregnancy was unwanted subsequently continued their pregnancies (figure 1.10). We did not record the reasons for carrying unwanted pregnancies to term. However, discussions with women in the villages revealed that financial constraints or inability to go out of the home to seek abortion services were among the reasons for continuing unwanted pregnancies. The team was unable to follow 1% of women who migrated out of their village, usually to be with their husband who worked in a city.

Among the women who reported induced abortions, 70.4% (371) underwent safe abortions at certified facilities (figure 1.11). Such a high proportion of safe abortions is not a reality for many Rajasthani women.

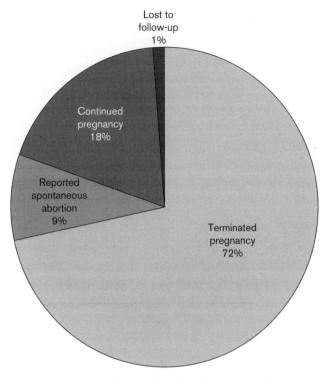

FIGURE 1.10. What did women do in case of an unwanted pregnancy?

While some women went to government or private health facilities in the city (20–65 kilometers away), most of them (64.4%, 239 women) obtained safe abortion services from one of ARTH's two health centers in their immediate vicinity. (See examples 1.2 and 1.3.) Thus, the availability of good-quality, subsidized services at ARTH's health centers, close to women's villages, provided an important follow-up service to the field level service being provided by the health workers. Over a quarter of the women (27%, 145) underwent unsafe abortion—either by consuming tablets for medical abortion (bought over the counter from pharmacy shops) or by seeking services from unauthorized providers or by consuming a traditional herbal concoction on their own. Two percent of the women (11) did not reveal the provider of their abortion. Nearly half of the women (49.6%, 365) who did not want to continue the pregnancy (735) had either none, one or two children already.

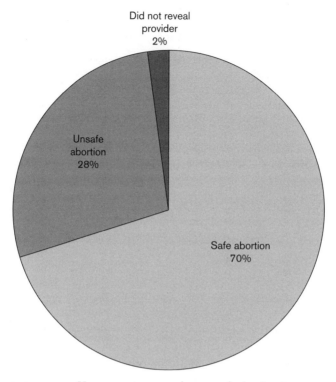

FIGURE 1.11. How many women underwent safe abortions?

Example 1.2. Pushpa Singh's Story

Pushpa Singh, an illiterate 35-year-old mother of four children, belonging to one of the higher castes, had missed her period. She saw the VHW in her village when the VHW had come to make a postpartum visit to another woman. Pushpa called the VHW to her house and asked her what materials she could share. Along with other demonstrations, the VHW showed her the urine pregnancy test kit. Pushpa then told the VHW that she had not had her period for the last two months and asked her to do the test. The test was positive. Pushpa did not want to continue the pregnancy and asked the VHW for some tablets to abort. The VHW referred her to ARTH's health center for abortion services, which was located 8 kilometers from her village. Pushpa obtained a safe abortion from ARTH and subsequently chose to use an IUD to prevent further unwanted pregnancies.

Example 1.3. Mohini Gameti's Story

Mohini Gameti was an illiterate woman belonging to a tribal community and lived in a village 25 kilometers from the city. Mohini became a mother at the age of 16. At the age of 18, when her daughter was one-and-a-half years old, she missed her period again. When a village health worker (VHW) visited her village, Mohini obtained a pregnancy test and learned that she was pregnant. She did not want to have another baby so soon. However, she could not tell her husband or in-laws, who would pressure her to carry the pregnancy to term. Mohini managed to take money from her husband on the pretext that she had to return it to someone from whom she had borrowed. Mohini went with the VHW and had a safe abortion. Thereafter, she continued to take oral contraceptive pills from the village health worker.

DISCUSSION

The decision to reproduce, paired with the freedom to regulate one's own fertility, has been identified as one of the mainstays of reproductive health. Reproductive health is affected by a variety of sociocultural and biological factors on one hand and by the quality and responsiveness of the health-care delivery system on the other.[23] Women's ability to control their fertility is also fundamental to their empowerment: if a woman can plan her family, it will be easier for her to plan her nonreproductive choices as well. Prevention of unwanted fertility protects a woman's health, and when a woman is healthy, she becomes more productive and better able to care for her existing children. When her reproductive rights are protected, she has the freedom to participate more fully and equally in society. Our experience shows that training community health workers to provide pregnancy tests at the village level is an important step to empowering rural women in India to take charge of their reproductive health.

In our intervention, the pregnancy test served as an entry point to talk to women about broader aspects of their reproductive and sexual health. The service made it possible for women to know their pregnancy status at an early stage without having to leave their village. Seventy percent of the users of the pregnancy test service were women with no children or with one or two children. Given that younger women in rural Rajasthan have very limited autonomy and mobility, this doorstep service was crucial for them. The majority of these women did not want to have a child (or more children) at that point in their lives, and thus knowing their pregnancy status and subsequently having access to contraceptives or abortion was a direct pathway to make an informed choice.

In southern Rajasthan, where this intervention was carried out, there is a considerable social distance between health care providers (mostly urban, well-educated, and of higher socioeconomic status) and women (mostly rural, illiterate, and socioeconomically disadvantaged). This social distance makes women hesitate to approach or talk frankly with trained health providers. Unscrupulous providers who come to know about a woman's pregnancy status before she herself knows that she is pregnant have at times exploited this asymmetry of power and information. Providing the pregnancy test service through a woman-to-woman outreach program has changed this dynamic, enabling women to *gain important information about their own health and bodies in time to make informed decisions.* Women were excited to be able to see the strip and to learn how it could tell them if they are pregnant or not. Furthermore, the convenience of being able to get this information without leaving the village saved them a lot of time and effort.

There have been efforts in other parts of India to provide pregnancy tests at the village level, primarily through non-governmental organizations. One program provided urine pregnancy tests in the villages, followed by registering new pregnancies and providing family planning services at the field level.[24] Another program offered a urine pregnancy test kit as one of the items in the reproductive health tool kit of its village health workers.[25] However, we did not find any published information about a program that linked the urine pregnancy test with other reproductive health services. A small study conducted in the central Indian state of Madhya Pradesh among two hundred newly married women who used the pregnancy test kit followed their pregnancy outcomes until their delivery.[26] The study found an increase in early registration of pregnancies and an increase in deliveries performed at healthcare facilities among women who used the pregnancy test kit. However, our data shows that a higher proportion of women who underwent the pregnancy test did not want to be pregnant at that time. Thus, while early pregnancy registration and increased institutional delivery are potential advantages of the home-based pregnancy test, our experience suggests that the service also holds a high potential to address the needs of those women who do not want to be pregnant. This is further validated by the findings of a retrospective cross-sectional study conducted in Cape Town, South Africa, that found that women who had obtained a urine pregnancy test of their own accord presented 3.6 weeks and 1.4

weeks earlier for antenatal care and abortion services respectively, independent of all other factors.[27] Thus, easy access to pregnancy confirmation seems to be associated with earlier care seeking for antenatal care and abortion.

Access to a service may be promoted or hindered by the provider's attitude, as was found in the South Africa study.[28] Half of the seventy-eight public health-care providers interviewed thought that they should not perform tests on young teenagers because "they should not be sexually active or using contraception anyway." Reasons given for not promoting the pregnancy test service were "irresponsible client behavior," "decreased contraceptive use," and the "possibility of clients abusing the service."[29] Thus, access to technology, especially among more vulnerable groups, may be restricted by providers' own values. Our findings reveal that some women as young as 15 years old were sexually active. These young women utilized the pregnancy test service when it was provided in a nonjudgmental and adolescent-friendly manner. Other studies in India have shown that compared to married women, single women face a more complex process when deciding to undergo an abortion, with others often deciding on their behalf. As a result, single women are more likely to approach informal providers who are perceived to be better at maintaining confidentiality.[30] Hence, if the service is to be scaled up in a large program, it would be crucial that service providers are trained and guided to respect the reproductive health needs of adolescents, young people, and single women, irrespective of their own values and perceptions.

One feature of our intervention was that the performance of health workers was not consistent. The performance of ASHAs, appointed by the government, varied widely. Some ASHAs conducted only two pregnancy tests over a one-year period, while others conducted up to twenty tests in the same time frame. On average, the village health workers conducted more pregnancy tests than did the ASHAs. While ARTH staff provided similar supervisory support to both ASHAs and VHWs, encouraging both groups to offer the service in the villages, pregnancy testing was not the government's priority at the time.[31] We suspect that since pregnancy testing was not a priority for the government, ASHAs did not focus much attention on this activity. In 2009 (two years after we started this intervention), the government of India started providing urine pregnancy tests (*nishchay* kits) at the village level through ASHAs, in a phased manner.[32] Although the government intended the pregnancy test kit to act as an entry point to reproductive health and family planning services, there were problems with the supply chain and with the supervision of ASHAs. As a result, the test kits have not become easily accessible to a majority of the women who are its intended beneficiaries. The third review of NRHM observed that the nishchay pregnancy kits were not being used to rule out pregnancy and provide contraceptives to women.[33] Additionally, an evaluation of the ASHA program in Rajasthan revealed low levels of counseling being offered by ASHAs, and in terms of referral for services, female sterilization has remained the central focus.

A qualitative study done with ASHAs provides more evidence of the government's promotion of sterilization over reversible contraceptive methods. ASHAs report facing pressure to meet sterilization targets and being penalized by their supervisors for not meeting the targets. It may be the case that our intervention has the potential to enable women to fulfill their reproductive rights by gaining access to a full range of health services. However, this will be possible only when the performance monitoring of frontline workers in the public health system changes from "ELAs" to meeting the actual reproductive needs of women.

LESSONS LEARNED

We found that this intervention was an important step to help women make decisions about their sexual and reproductive health at critical junctures in their lives. It also contributed to their health by preventing unwanted pregnancies and unsafe abortions. Those with a negative pregnancy test who did not want children at that point in their lives were able to start a contraceptive in time, whereas those whose test was positive but who did not want to continue the pregnancy were counselled and helped to access safe abortion services. Women who wanted to continue their pregnancies were able to start antenatal checkups in time. This intervention also allowed us to reach hard-to-reach groups such as adolescents and young women.

Developing a suitable workforce of community health workers was a challenge. While ASHAs had limited and highly variable effectiveness, village health workers had a high turnover rate, largely because they were young (unmarried or newly married) women who did not have the autonomy to decide about their jobs. Some of them moved from paternal homes to husband's homes and were asked to quit their jobs, while others had to leave within a few months of training either because their families were not happy that they had to "roam around in villages" or because their families needed them to attend to household chores.

Our experience suggests that systematic, effective referral links to clinic-based services such as long-term family planning methods or safe abortion are essential for the effectiveness of community-based services. We linked the compensation for village health workers to the services they provided, which we believe contributed to higher performance. In order to take the intervention to scale, it would be crucial to develop a robust resupply system for getting test strips, oral pills, condoms, and emergency contraceptive pills to health workers. In a large government system, it will be equally important to orient village volunteers (e.g., ASHAs) to provide nonjudgmental services to unmarried and newly married adolescents and women and to women who might be seen as "candidates for sterilization." Further, a system of monitoring and supervision will be important to avoid misreporting and to ensure that even women living in remote villages receive services.

CONCLUSION

In rural Rajasthan, very few women have genuine control over their fertility decisions, which reflects and compounds their social disempowerment. Our organization views the relationship between fertility and empowerment to be synergistic: by bringing fertility management under women's control, this can be one small step towards empowering women in other aspects of their health and well-being. Our project's door-to-door pregnancy testing service marked the first step of this process.

Given that the use of reversible methods of contraception in the country is low and there is a high unmet need for contraceptives for spacing,[34] conducting a pregnancy test provides an opportunity to meet the reproductive health needs of women and couples, as has been shown by this pilot intervention. The intervention has potential to be scaled up because it involves a safe, low-cost, low-technology service that can be provided by low-literate health workers who lack formal medical training. The components of the intervention are easy to use at the community level and can therefore be integrated with other community-based distribution (CBD) programs.[35] In communities where women have difficulty accessing contraceptives, safe abortion, and timely antenatal care, a community-based pregnancy testing service could provide the much needed "pull" for uptake of other reproductive health services (as against the current "push" by the public health system for women to choose sterilization).

Although we have not systematically evaluated the impact of this intervention on reproductive outcomes and women's ability to control their fertility, we believe it offers promise for scale-up and integration into the government's current family planning programs. The results may also be relevant for program planning in other countries where women have limited reproductive autonomy. Because this intervention has excellent potential to reach adolescents and younger women in need of birth spacing, it could be a viable strategy to promote reproductive rights and health among hard-to-reach populations.[36]

Box 1.1. Summary

Geographic area: Rural population of about 60,800 people living in forty-nine villages across Udaipur and Rajsamand districts in the northwestern state of Rajasthan, India.

Global importance of the health condition: Limited mobility and autonomy of rural women in low-income countries makes it difficult for them to access reproductive health care services, often leading to adverse health consequences.

Intervention or program: Action Research & Training for Health (ARTH) trained community health workers to provide a doorstep urine pregnancy test service at a minimal cost followed by counseling and referrals to help women make their own reproductive health decisions and obtain the required products and services (condoms, oral pills, emergency contraceptive pills, or a safe abortion) at the village level or at a health facility.

Impact: Large numbers of illiterate young women belonging to socioeconomically disadvantaged communities learned their pregnancy status at a minimal cost within their village and sought follow-up services of their choice—particularly contraception and safe abortion.

Lessons learned: This low-cost, door-to-door pregnancy test service provided an entry point to address the broader reproductive health needs of women. It was greatly appreciated by rural women, especially the younger ones. Nonjudgmental delivery of such services, coupled with a robust system of supervision, resupply, and effective referrals were important factors in the success of this community-based intervention.

Link between empowerment and health: The decision to reproduce, when paired with the freedom to regulate one's own fertility, has been identified as one of the mainstays of reproductive health. Empowerment has been defined as the expansion of the ability to make strategic life choices—choices that are critical for people to live the lives they want. These choices include those related to education, marriage, childbearing, and livelihood. Prevention of unwanted pregnancy is directly linked to women's health and also enables them to balance and time their reproductive and nonreproductive aspirations, thus facilitating their access to emerging opportunities. When women's reproductive rights are promoted and protected, they have the freedom to participate more fully and equally in society.

For a video about Action Research and Training for Health (ARTH), see https://youtu.be/mObfWwc6Gmk.

Box 1.2. Factors behind the Success of Village-Based Reproductive Health Services in India

- The intervention demonstrated that a safe, low cost, low technology intervention designed to support women's fertility preferences can be provided by *community-based health workers* with low levels of literacy and no formal medical training.

- *Young community health volunteers, trained to provide services* in a nonjudgmental and confidential manner, were able to reach large numbers of adolescents and young women.

- *Orientation meetings* with village leaders, video shows, wall paintings, and small group meetings with young women and men helped health workers establish an enabling environment and enabled them to provide effective services.

- *A robust system of supervision, resupply, and referrals,* backed by an accessible clinic-based service, contributed greatly to the intervention's success.

- The intervention can be *easily integrated with other community-based distribution programs* as an entry point to begin a conversation with women (especially adolescents and young women) about reproductive health issues.

NOTES

1. Kabeer 2001, 19.
2. Larsen and Hollos 2003, 1111–1112.
3. Malhotra 2012, 3; Ansara et al. 2011.
4. IIPS 2010a, 2010b.
5. Planning Commission 2006, 8.
6. Registrar General and Census Commissioner 2011.
7. IIPS 2010a, 6.
8. IIPS and Macro International 2007, 1:473.
9. IIPS and Macro International 2008, 48.
10. Registrar General of India 2012, 48.
11. Registrar General of India 2011, 3.
12. Leavitt 2003.
13. Demography and Evaluation Cell 2012.
14. Jejeebhoy 1997, 5; Santhya 2003, 2–5.
15. NRHM is a flagship program of the government of India, launched in 2005, to improve the health status in rural parts of the country.
16. NRHM 2009, 29.
17. IIPS 2010c, 174.
18. Pachauri 2004, 16–17; Mookim 2006, 4–7.
19. IIPS and Macro International 2008, 48.
20. ARTH n.d.
21. Asha is a commonly used name for girls, it means "hope" in Hindi and several other Indian languages.
22. Taking note of the fact that certain communities in the country suffer from extreme social, educational, and economic deprivation, the first schedule of the Constitution of India has identified them as Scheduled Castes and Scheduled Tribes as per provisions contained in Clause 1 of Articles 341 and 342 of the Constitution (http://lawmin.nic.in/ld/subord/rule3a.htm, http://ncst.nic.in/index.asp?langid=1).
23. Jejeebhoy 1997, 2.
24. "Tribhuvandas Foundation" 2016.
25. Jan Swasthya Sahyog 2006, 9.
26. Saroshe, Mehta, and Dixit 2012, 46.
27. Morroni and Moodley 2006.
28. Ibid.
29. Ibid.
30. Visaria et al. 2004.
31. NHSRC, 2011, 103.
32. HLFPPT n.d.
33. NRHM 2009, 29–30.
34. IIPS and Macro International 2007, 1: 121, 159–160.
35. Price n.d., 2–3.
36. Youth Health and Rights Coalition 2011, 3.

REFERENCES

Action Research & Training for Health (ARTH). n.d. Access to Safe Abortion Services in Rajasthan, the Three Year Trend Report, 2007–2010. Unpublished.

Ansara, Donna L., Jessica D. Gipson, Socorro A. Gultiano, and Michelle J. Hindin. 2011. "Intergenerational Relationships between Fertility and Empowerment: The Cebu Longitudinal Health and Nutrition Surveys (CLHNS)." Paper presented at the Annual Meeting of the Population Association of America, Washington DC, 31 March–2 April 2011. http://paa2011.princeton.edu/papers/110711.

Directorate of Health and Family Welfare Services, Demography and Evaluation Cell. 2012. *Training Programme on Expected Level of Achievement (Target Fixation) for Family Welfare Programmes.* Bangalore, Karnataka: Government of Karnataka, 1–7. http://stg2.kar.nic.in/healthnew/demo/REV%20ELA.pdf.

Hindustan Latex Family Planning Promotion Trust (HLFPPT). n.d. "Nishchay." HLFPPT. www.hlfppt.org/images/atul_nishchay.pdf.

International Institute for Population Sciences (IIPS). 2010a. "District Fact Sheet: District Rajsamand, Rajasthan." *District Level Household and Facility Survey (DLHS 3) 2007–08.* Mumbai: IIPS. http://nrhmrajasthan.nic.in/DLHS-III/Rajsamand.xls.

———. 2010b. "District Fact Sheet: District Udaipur, Rajasthan." *District Level Household and Facility Survey (DLHS 3) 2007–08.* Mumbai: IIPS. http://nrhmrajasthan.nic.in/DLHS-III/Udaipur.xls.

———. 2010c. "Fact Sheet: States and Union Territories, 2009." *Concurrent Evaluation of National Rural Health* Mission *(NRHM).* Mumbai: IIPS.

International Institute for Population Sciences (IIPS) and Macro International. 2007. *National Family Health Survey (NFHS-3), 2005–06, India.* 2 vols. Mumbai: IIPS.

———. 2008.*National Family Health Survey (NFHS-3), India, 2005–06: Rajasthan.* Mumbai: IIPS.

Jan Swasthya Sahyog. 2006. *Appropriate Technology for Health Care.* Bilaspur, Chattisgarh: Jan Swasthya Sahyog. www.jssbilaspur.org/wordpress/wp-content/uploads/2015/07/AppropriateTechnologyCatalog.pdf.

Jejeebhoy, Shireen J. 1997. "Addressing Women's Reproductive Health Needs: Priorities for the Family Welfare Program." *Economic and Political Weekly* 32, nos. 9–10, March: 475–484.

Kabeer, Naila. 2001. "Resources, Agency, Achievements: Reflections on the Measurement of Women's Empowerment." In *Discussing Women's Empowerment—Theory and Practice, Sida studies 3,* edited by Anne Sisask, 17–57. Stockholm: Swedish International Development Agency.

Larsen, Ulla, and Marida Hollos. 2003. "Women's Empowerment and Fertility Decline among the Pare of Kilimanjaro Region, Northern Tanzania." *Social Science Medicine* 57, no.6 (September): 1099–115. doi:10.1016/S0277-9536(02)00488-4.

Leavitt, Sarah A. 2003. "A Timeline of Pregnancy Testing." *A Thin Blue Line: The History of the Pregnancy Test Kit.* Office of NIH History, December. http://history.nih.gov/exhibits/thinblueline/timeline.html.

Malhotra, Anju. 2012. *Remobilizing the Gender and Fertility Connection: The Case for Examining the Impact of Fertility Control and Fertility Declines on Gender Equality*. Fertility and Empowerment Network Working Paper Series 001–2012-ICRW-FE. Washington, DC: International Center for Research on Women. www.icrw.org/pdf_download/1587/ed2acb5 bdd778ea5a4a6655b310c9787.

Mookim, Pooja G. 2006, November 10. "Gender Preference, Fertility Choices and Government Policy in India." Unpublished manuscript. Department of Economics, Boston University. http://people.bu.edu/pgupta1/mookim_ india_nov15.pdf.

Morroni, Chelsea, and Jennifer Moodley. 2006. "The Role of Urine Pregnancy Testing in Facilitating Access to Antenatal Care and Abortion Services in South Africa: A Cross Sectional Study." *BMC Pregnancy and Childbirth* 6, no. 26. www.biomedcentral.com/1471-2393/6/26.

National Health Systems Resource Centre (NHSRC). *ASHA Which Way Forward . . . ? Evaluation of ASHA Programme*. New Delhi: NHSRC, National Rural Health Mission, 2011.

National Rural Health Mission (NRHM). 2009. *Third Common Review Mission, State Report, Rajasthan, November 2009*. New Delhi: NRHM Division, Ministry of Health and Family Welfare, Government of India.

Pachauri, Saroj. 2004. "Expanding Contraceptive Choice in India: Issues and Evidence." *Journal of Family Welfare* 50: 13–25. http://medind.nic.in/jah /t04/s1/jaht04s1p13g.pdf.

Planning Commission, Government of India. 2006. *Report of the Working Group on Population Stabilization for the Eleventh Five Year Plan (2007–2012)*. New Delhi: Government of India.

Price, Neil. n.d. "Community-Based Distribution." Paper 4. Edited by Rupert Walder. In *Service Sustainability Strategies in Sexual and Reproductive Health Programming*. London: Resource Centre for Sexual and Reproductive Health (JSI UK), Department for International Development.

Registrar General and Census Commissioner, India. 2011. "Census of India 2011, Provisional Population Totals, Rajasthan Profile." *Census of India*. New Delhi: Ministry of Home Affairs, Government of India. http:// censusindia.gov.in/2011census/censusinfodashboard/stock/profiles/en /IND008_Rajasthan.pdf.

Registrar General of India. 2011. *Sample Registration System, Special Bulletin on Maternal Mortality in India 2007–09*. New Delhi: Office of the Registrar General, Ministry of Home Affairs, Government of India, June.

———. 2012. *Sample Registration System Statistical Report 2010*. Report no. 1 of 2012. New Delhi: Office of the Registrar General, Ministry of Home Affairs, Government of India.

Santhya, K.G. 2003. *Changing Family Planning Scenario in India: An Overview of Recent Evidence*. Regional Working Papers, South and East Asia, 2003, no.17. New Delhi, India: Population Council.

Saroshe, Satish, S.C. Mehta, and Sanjay Dixit. 2012. "Assessment of Knowledge and Awareness regarding Rapid Home Pregnancy Test Kits among

Newly Married Women and Their Utilization of RCH Services." *National Journal of Community Medicine* 3, no. 1 (Jan.–March): 44–47.

"Tribhuvandas Foundation." 2016. *Wikipedia*. Page last modified 1 April 2016. http://en.wikipedia.org/wiki/Tribhuvandas_Foundation.

Visaria, Leela, Vimala Ramachandran, Bela Ganatra, and Shveta Kalyanwala. "Abortion in India: Emerging Issues from the Qualitative Studies." 2004. In *Abortion Assessment Project-India: Research Summaries and Abstracts*, 75–89. Mumbai: CEHAT, December.

Youth Health and Rights Coalition. 2011. *Promoting the Sexual and Reproductive Rights and Health of Adolescents and Youth*. Watertown, MA: Pathfinder International, August. www.pathfinder.org/publications-tools/pdfs /Promoting-the-sexual-and-reproductive-rights-and-health-of-Adolescents-and-Youth.pdf.

2

Obstetric Fistula in Kenya

A Holistic Model of Outreach, Treatment, and Reintegration

LINDSEY POLLACZEK, PAULA TAVROW,
AND HABIBA MOHAMED

Obstetric fistula is one of the most devastating injuries that a woman can suffer in childbirth. It is primarily caused by prolonged and obstructed labor, when a woman goes for days without receiving essential obstetrical care such as a cesarean section. During prolonged labor, the constant pressure of the fetal head compresses the soft tissues between the bladder and the vagina and/or rectum, causing a hole, or fistula, as the tissue dies. If untreated, a woman will experience constant and uncontrollable leakage of urine and/or feces through her vagina. In most cases of obstructed labor in which a fistula develops, the baby is stillborn.[1]

While obstetric fistula has been nearly eradicated in the industrialized world, the condition continues to afflict an estimated two million girls and women in developing countries, with approximately 50,000–100,000 new cases every year.[2] Poor, young, first-time mothers living in rural areas with limited or no access to emergency obstetric services are at highest risk. Root causes of obstetric fistula include low status of women, early marriage, poverty, and lack of knowledge about pregnancy complications—all of which impede women and their families from making timely reproductive health choices and accessing essential obstetric services.[3]

Women with fistula suffer both physically and socially. The physical afflictions can include chronic abrasion of the skin due to persistent leakage of urine; kidney disease; infertility; infection; and neurological injury, such as foot drop, due to nerve damage sustained during the prolonged labor.[4] But the social injuries—the humiliation, isolation, and stigma—can be even more damaging. Women with fistula are often abandoned by their husbands, taunted by community members, and ostracized from society.[5] Many people view fistula as witchcraft or a punishment by God, for which there is no cure.[6] Women with fistula suffer from high rates of depression, low self-esteem, and sometimes suicide ideation.[7,8]

Obstetric fistula can also be economically disempowering because it frequently impairs a woman's ability to work, often driving her into abject poverty. The physical consequences of fistula—weakness, discomfort, and constant leakage of urine—make it difficult for a woman to farm or do other manual work. The social stigma affects her ability to conduct business because many people avoid buying goods from women with fistula out of fear that everything these women touch will smell and be contaminated with urine. Women with fistula report having to buy additional soap and personal hygiene products to manage their condition.[9] With reduced or no income and limited support from their spouse or family members, some women with fistula must beg for food and money to survive.[10]

During our fieldwork in western Kenya, we met a woman who was fifty years old and had lived with fistula for thirteen years. She described vividly the hardships she had endured:

> Life has been a challenge. I tell you that it has been difficult right from the place where I was doing my selling. People would run away from me owing to the stench. Even my friends avoided me. Back in the house, my husband's attitude towards me also changed. I would soil wherever I slept and whatever I slept on. It was a lot of work to clean my bedding every day. I was unable to make many movements, for when I moved, I experienced pain and urine would pass uncontrollably . . . Whenever I went to church, it was an embarrassment. I would soil my clothes and people kept on staring at me and at times they even laughed at me. I developed fear and I cried a lot wondering what had happened to me. It got to a point where I preferred death to living with such a condition. I started praying that God would kill me. . . . I had lost hope in life and the value of continuing to live.[11]

WHAT CAN BE DONE?

Obstetric fistula can be repaired with reconstructive surgery, but most developing countries have very limited capacity to perform the surgery. Additionally, the lack of community knowledge about fistula contributes to significant delays in women getting the care they need.[12] Women often live with the condition for years, or even decades. Although fistula repair surgery can have success rates as high as 80–95%, women who suffer from fistula generally also require emotional, social, and economic support to recover from their ordeal and return to leading healthy and productive lives.[13]

Like most countries in sub-Saharan Africa, Kenya suffers from high rates of maternal mortality and morbidity. According to a 2004 needs assessment, an estimated 3,000 women develop fistula each year in Kenya, and there is a large backlog of women who need fistula repair.[14] Only 7.5 percent of women with fistula receive surgical treatment each year.[15] A 2010 Human Rights Watch report noted that there are insufficient numbers of trained surgeons in Kenya to treat women with fistula. Furthermore, low community awareness about fistula and economic constraints to accessing treatment—as well as lack of follow-up support after surgery—have hindered Kenya from dealing effectively with the problem.[16]

A NEW MODEL IN WESTERN KENYA

The Let's End Fistula Program (LEFP), a comprehensive outreach, treatment, and reintegration program in western Kenya, was launched in early 2011 to address many of these challenges. The program focuses on restoring women's health in a holistic sense. In addition to treating fistula, it helps women regain psychological well-being, control their fertility, have better access to skilled delivery care, and increase their incomes. Fistula survivors' ability to recover and remain healthy is closely tied to their empowerment. After a successful surgery, it is essential that they develop a critical consciousness about their situation and take control over their lives. Women living with fistula become extremely powerless and stigmatized; a program built on empowerment principles can help fistula survivors resume participation in community life and also have greater agency and access to resources.

In this chapter, we are using Batliwala's conceptualization of empowerment as a process of transforming power between individuals and groups in three ways: (1) by challenging the ideologies that justify social inequality; (2) by changing prevailing patterns of access to and control over economic, natural and intellectual resources; and (3) by transforming the institutions and structures that reinforce and sustain existing power structures.[17] Although the LEFP has not yet sought to challenge the inequities that lead to obstetric fistula, it has been empowering fistula survivors by changing their access to resources and their status in the community and within their own families.

The LEFP consisted of a three-pronged approach to empowering fistula survivors: (1) *outreach* and identification of women suffering from fistula and referral to care; (2) *treatment* with surgical repair and psychosocial counseling; and (3) *reintegration* assistance to help women regain their sense of self-worth, take control of their health, and improve their economic well-being. The program was a collaboration between three organizations:

> One By One, a Seattle-based organization that supports identification of and care for women with fistula;
>
> Gynocare Fistula Center in Eldoret, Kenya, that provides surgical treatment and counseling; and
>
> Women and Development against Distress in Africa (WADADIA), a grassroots organization based in Mumias, Kenya, that reintegrates fistula survivors into their communities.

This model is unique because it addresses the multiple barriers that limit women's access to treatment and also provides ongoing psychosocial and economic support following surgical repair to help women successfully reintegrate.

1. Outreach

Many women with fistula live in remote villages, far from urban treatment facilities. Because of low community knowledge and the highly stigmatizing and isolating nature of the condition, many sufferers do not think that fistula can be treated and have given up hope of being healed. This makes it difficult to track down long-time sufferers and refer them to treatment. Even when women are aware that treatment is available, fear or anxiety about the procedure or difficulty in obtaining funds for transportation and treatment can be formidable barriers.

Traditionally, outreach efforts to identify women with fistula relied on radio or TV broadcasts in the weeks prior to a fistula-repair surgical camp.[18] These broadcasts fail to reach the more isolated or disempowered women and are too short-lived to overcome women's fears and other barriers. In contrast, LEFP's strategy is to engage in continuous community mobilization and education through on-the-ground Regional Representatives, many of whom are fistula survivors (a few are spouses or relatives of survivors). The representatives were selected based on good communication skills, leadership potential, and commitment to helping other women with fistula. All received an intensive three-day training in obstetric fistula issues, data collection, public speaking, and leadership. Their main tasks are to (1) educate their communities about fistula treatment and prevention; (2) identify fistula patients and arrange their transport to Gynocare; and (3) provide follow-up of women once they return home. One By One trained the first group of thirty representatives in September 2011 and provides refresher trainings to clarify issues and troubleshoot problems. Representatives also receive a stipend for their work, plus a mobile phone and airtime.

Upon returning to their communities, the representatives conduct outreach educational events in schools, churches, and health facilities. After these meetings, community members frequently come forward with knowledge about someone potentially suffering with fistula. The representative then visits this woman and convinces her to undergo phone screening to determine if she indeed has fistula. If the woman screens positive for fistula and agrees to travel for treatment at Gynocare Fistula Center, the representative obtains funds via her phone to pay for the fistula sufferer's transportation.

In the first twelve months of the outreach program, representatives conducted nearly 3,500 community education activities and identified over 500 women to be screened for fistula. The phone screening method allows many women to be screened at relatively little cost. However, without visual inspection, this method has resulted in some women being incorrectly diagnosed, which leads to some unnecessary expenses and disappointment.

Early in the program, a few fistula sufferers declined treatment because of fear, anxiety, and lack of family permission. To overcome these barriers, the representatives now make home visits to provide detailed information about the treatment and recovery process directly to women and their families. As fistula survivors themselves, representatives serve as proof that successful treatment is possible. Incorporating family members into the educational sessions and decision-making process increases the likelihood that a woman will consent to treatment and will be reintegrated. Other researchers have found that women with fistula who have a support network are more likely to reintegrate successfully and have improved quality of life following repair than those who do not.[19]

For representatives who are themselves fistula survivors, their new role can be personally empowering. With increased knowledge of the condition, as well as resources to assist others, these formerly ostracized women become leaders and community advocates. One representative stated proudly that community members have such high regard for her that they greet her with "Welcome, Doctor." Another representative described how her new position changed the dynamics in her relationship with her husband, and helped her achieve greater confidence and agency:

> Now my husband has come back to me, and wants to be with me wherever I attend the meetings. It's unlike earlier on when I was leaking urine, if I made ugali [maize porridge], my husband refused to eat it because he says I'm stinky, even my food is stinky. But now I am very clean and I am happy for this opportunity. My husband is even ready to join up in the fight against fistula and be a Regional Representative.[20]

2. Treatment

Fistula repair is a life-transforming surgery, allowing women to regain their dignity and productivity after years of suffering. Starting as an outpatient clinic in 2009, the Gynocare Fistula Center in Eldoret, Kenya, has been providing routine fistula-repair surgery since June 2011. Previously, most rural women were able to obtain surgery only when hospitals held treatment camps, which entailed long waits and no follow-up services. In 2010, only three hospitals in Kenya provided routine fistula repair services for an estimated 1,000 women, far fewer than the need.[21,22]

In its first sixteen months, the twenty-three-bed Gynocare facility (which has only one surgeon and one small operating theater) treated more than 240 women with fistula. In comparison, Kenyatta National Hospital, the largest referral and teaching hospital in the country, treated 200 patients in 2010.[23] Donor funding has allowed Gynocare to provide fistula treatment to women at no cost, thereby removing a key barrier, while the representatives have helped maintain a steady referral of patients.

Women who reach Gynocare often feel disempowered, vulnerable, and alone in their condition. At Gynocare, they meet a group of women with the same condition. This sense of community helps the women grow emotionally stronger while they heal from the surgery. LEFP promotes friendship and joint healing by creating support groups among these women. Besides offering surgery, Gynocare provides counseling to women who have experienced severe psychological trauma caused by having fistula. Trained psychologists and social workers provide two to three sessions of counseling in individual and group formats. The counseling allows women to share their experiences and learn how to cope with trauma. It also prepares the women for what to expect during surgery, recovery, and after they return home. Gynocare counselors help women work through common anxieties such as reuniting with their spouses, regaining the community's acceptance, and starting income-generating activities.

The Gynocare staff and the representatives work together to ensure continuity of care throughout the referral, treatment, and reintegration processes. When a woman is ready for discharge—fourteen days post-surgery on average—the Gynocare staff connect with the LEFP manager to arrange her transportation home. The representative closest to the woman's home area is notified, greets her at the bus station, and escorts her home in most cases.[24]

3. Reintegration

For many women who receive fistula repair, discharge from the hospital after surgery marks the beginning of the healing process. The LEFP is the first fistula program in Kenya to provide ongoing support to women after they return to their communities. The program's reintegration component focuses on women's social and economic empowerment, increased control over their reproductive health, and improved access to health services to reduce the risk of a recurrent fistula.

WADADIA, a community-based organization with a decade of experience in empowering commercial sex workers, links fistula survivors through peer support groups, provides psychosocial support, promotes economic empowerment by teaching survivors income-generating skills, increases survivors' access to bank accounts and microloans from financial institutions, and generally helps survivors achieve better control over their health.

As of September 2012, there were over 480 fistula survivors actively participating in peer support groups in ten districts. (This includes women who received treatment at Gynocare and at other regional hospitals.) The support group is a centerpiece of the reintegration effort and provides a springboard for psychosocial and economic empowerment activities. Simply meeting with others who have similar experiences seems to enhance survivors' emotional well-being. The support groups offer women a safe environment in which to discuss ways to cope with challenges at home. For previously ostracized women, spending time with new friends, singing, dancing, laughing, and sharing stories is very meaningful.

The months immediately following surgery are a critical time for physical healing and emotional recovery. Women are encouraged to engage in specific self-care activities, such as practicing good personal hygiene and drinking fluids. They are also to abstain for six months from heavy manual labor and sexual intercourse, which could compromise their recovery. The support groups help to reinforce these recommendations, although some women still are not able to avoid sex. The women also learn about the signs of possible complications and how to get care if needed.

A key objective of the support group is to assist women to avoid a fistula recurrence. Although many women experience infertility after living with fistula, some are able to conceive after repair and desire children. The women are advised on the importance of attending antenatal care clinics and preparing a birth plan that includes delivering at a hospital where cesarean section is available, which often requires financial support from family members.

The program has sought to remove financial barriers to elective cesarean sections by enrolling fistula survivors in the Kenyan National Hospital Insurance Fund (NHIF). NHIF membership covers health services for the woman as well as for her family. As of September 2012, of the 160 who were originally registered, 92 women were active enrollees. Sustainability of the NHIF participation is an ongoing challenge, as many women who enroll are unable to maintain the monthly dues, which keep rising. The Regional Representatives, who are all members of the NHIF, promote the importance of insurance. The support groups have launched a number of income-generating activities, including poultry raising, fish farming, beekeeping, agricultural and horticultural programs, and small businesses. They have also created loan programs to give women start-up capital. In the less formal loan programs, group members contribute money monthly to a fund (typically $0.25 to $2.00), which is given to a different member each month. The larger loan programs involve microloans of $150 to $500 from well-known financial institutions, for which WADADIA acts as the guarantor.

Many of the income-generating projects are group efforts, which nurture solidarity between the women as they learn new skills and problem-solve together. One Regional Representative explained the process:

> We sat down and realized that we have no income. And so we thought we should start with chickens. We decided to each contribute a chick and we put them together at a home. But while there, they died, and then we realized we don't know how to take good care of them. So we asked the Ministry of Livestock to come in and teach us how to take care of the chickens. Then with WADADIA we submitted a proposal to start a poultry unit and the Ministry also gave us 25 more chickens. Now we have decided that every person should have a chicken in her home, and eventually everyone will have a full unit not just a chicken. We are yet to get it, but that is our dream. We are going to do it.[25]

By having a vision, working together as a team and learning from their initial failures, the women in the support groups are taking more control over income-generating activities and slowly improving their financial status.

EVALUATION

In March 2012, we carried out a brief survey among support-group members in four areas of western Kenya (Mumias, Khwisero, Bukhalarire, and Cheptais) to gain insight into how the reintegration assistance programs were affecting women's recovery and socioeconomic empowerment following fistula repair. We administered the survey face to face to forty members and also conducted a focus group discussion with four others. The average age of the respondents was 42 years old (range: 21–69 years old), and the average duration of living with fistula prior to repair was 9 years (range: 1–30 years). The average number of years since fistula repair surgery was 2 years (range: 5 months to 9 years). Unfortunately, we were not able to administer the survey to survivors not attending support group sessions, so the results are biased towards those who were regular attendees (presumably because they found the sessions useful).

The survey results suggested that the groups improved survivors' well-being. More than 90% of respondents reported that the support groups "helped [them] a lot" to make new friends, communicate with their family members, and feel happy with their lives. As one woman explained in the focus group discussion:

> This support group transformed my life greatly because before treatment, I had a lot of things in my mind that were not good, I had stress. I was

confused and I did not know what to do at times. But after treatment, we formed this group in which we regularly shared our experiences and supported each other. We received many teachings to increase our self-esteem and shed off the bad thoughts. . . . I used to be confused with self-stigma; I was not free with people. But I have learnt a lot after joining the group. The group has helped me. I now feel normal and succeeding in everything I do.[26]

The support groups also improved women's understanding about fistula: 85% of women surveyed indicated that the support groups helped them "a lot" to understand how fistula occurs and how to prevent it from recurring. Women in the focus group discussion were able to articulate the causes of fistula, could counter beliefs that it was due to witchcraft, and knew how to prevent recurrence after repair. While the participation in support groups was beneficial for most women, some reported difficulties in affording the cost of transportation to meetings.

Although support group participation appeared to significantly enhance survivors' social empowerment and emotional well-being, it had a less pronounced effect on their economic situation. Regarding the support group's income-generating activities, only 9% reported that they had been helped "a lot" with their basic needs. About 64% said that the groups helped "somewhat," and 23% said "not very much." Because income-generating projects take time to yield sufficient profits to meet the participants' daily needs, these results are not surprising.

In the focus group discussion, women who had been able to get microloans reported problems related to spoilage of perishable items, theft of supplies, requirements to pay bribes to authorities, and animal illnesses that necessitated vaccinations and medicines. However, women seemed to be overcoming some of these problems with the support and encouragement of group members, who sometimes helped each other them to meet loan payments. One woman who had experienced abject poverty while suffering from fistula, explained how her life had become transformed:

I started out small but now I am able to take large loan amounts [for my poultry business]. As soon as I clear a loan, I get a message from the banks congratulating me and encouraging me to take another loan. I do lots of stuff I couldn't do before, like I sensitize the community on fistula and I refer them to WADADIA for free treatment. I am now called big names and earn much respect, something I never thought could happen before. I am even called "Doctor" because whenever there is a fistula case, I am called to examine the case; I make referral to the office where screening is done.[27]

Our discussions with survivors in support groups revealed how health and empowerment are closely linked. For example, "Christine" was a thirty-eight-year-old survivor, who had suffered with fistula for eight years before an outreach team found her and took her in for treatment. Upon returning home, she joined a support group and was able to share experiences and develop friendships with fellow fistula survivors. She yearned to have a child, and so she enrolled in the NHIF. She delivered a healthy baby boy by elective cesarean section. With the help of the support group, she set up a poultry unit, a pond for a tilapia fish farm, and is growing bananas and traditional vegetables to sell at market. She recently convinced another fistula sufferer in her village to go for treatment and helped to refer her for care. This woman had been suffering with fistula for twenty years. When asked what she liked most about the support groups, a big smile crossed Christine's face: "I like it all. I like the farming, the business, the education, the friends. There are so many things, and it is very good for me."

CONCLUSION

Women with fistula have been referred to as "the most dispossessed, outcast, powerless group of women in the world."[28] However, an integrated model of outreach, treatment, and reintegration appeared to make a major difference in these women's lives—both physically and emotionally. In time, it may also help them financially. The holistic LEFP in western Kenya, offered through the efforts of three collaborating organizations, provided the core components necessary to help women with fistula regain their dignity and achieve greater control over their lives.

Since the evaluation of LEFP in 2012, new fistula programs have been launched in Kenya that take elements of this model and adapt them to reach women with fistula across the country. In the LEFP target communities, the number of women seeking fistula treatment has declined, suggesting that the initiative raised awareness of fistula and effectively reduced the large backlog of cases that once existed there. The survivor support groups continue to meet regularly to help members experience enhanced psychosocial and economic empowerment. The LEFP model seems most effective where there is a concentrated backlog of cases. The challenge now is to maintain LEFP's success in western Kenya and prevent new cases, while at the same time reaching women across the country who may be longtime sufferers.

Box 2.1. Summary

Geographic area: Rural women living with obstetric fistula in Rift, Nyanza, and Western Provinces in western Kenya.

Global importance of the health condition: Approximately two million girls and women in developing countries suffer from obstetric fistula, a devastating childbirth injury that can have profound physical, psychosocial, and economic consequences if left untreated.

Intervention: A multipronged approach to empower women living with fistula: (1) *outreach* and identification of women suffering from fistula and referral to care; (2) *treatment* with surgical repair and psychosocial counseling; and (3) *reintegration* assistance to help women regain their sense of value and self-worth, take control over their health, and improve their economic well-being.

Impact: An integrated fistula-care model ensures women living with fistula receive comprehensive treatment and reintegration support, which can lead to significant improvements in fistula survivors' physical, social, and emotional well-being and increased opportunities for economic empowerment.

Lessons learned: Fistula survivors who are trained to serve as community-based Regional Representatives can work effectively to improve community awareness of the condition, increase the number of women suffering with fistula who are successfully identified and referred to surgical and psychological treatment, and provide meaningful reintegration assistance that can uplift and empower women once they return home to their communities.

Link between empowerment and health: Women living with fistula are extremely powerless and stigmatized. A holistic treatment model that is built on empowerment principles can help fistula survivors develop a critical consciousness about their situation and take better control over their lives. It is important for fistula survivor's health and long-term well-being that they are able to resume participation in family and community life and also have greater agency and access to resources.

Box 2.2. Factors behind the Success of the Let's End Fistula Program in Kenya

- *A multiorganization collaboration* providing community outreach, surgical care, and reintegration support for fistula survivors draws on the respective strengths of three organizations to restore women's dignity and productivity.

- *Empowering fistula survivors to conduct community outreach* is a powerful strategy to reach the most isolated and disempowered women living with fistula. This also helps to build legitimacy, hope, and trust among fistula sufferers and their communities that treatment and rehabilitation are achievable.

- *Including family members in discussions* about what to expect during the treatment and healing process is important to maximize the number of women who consent to treatment. Such discussions can facilitate the reintegration and healing process once a woman returns home to her family and community.

- *Peer support groups* can provide fistula survivors with an opportunity to socialize with women who have faced similar challenges, enabling them to gain self-confidence and build social networks. The groups also serve as a good platform for training and education on reproductive health and income-generating opportunities.

NOTES

1. Wall, Karshima, et al. 2004, 1013.
2. UN General Assembly 2010, 4.
3. Roush et al. 2012, 789.
4. Arrowsmith, Hamlin, and Wall, 1996, 568.
5. Ahmed and Holtz 2007, S12.
6. Ibid., S12.
7. Weston et al. 2011, 31.
8. Goh et al. 2005, 1328.
9. Women's Dignity Project and EngenderHealth 2006, 29.
10. Kelly 1995, 15.
11. Interview with Western Kenya woman, March 27, 2012.
12. Bangser et al. 2011.
13. Wall, Arrowsmith, et al. 2005, 1415.
14. Ministry of Health and UNFPA Kenya 2004, 14.
15. Ibid., 14.

16. Human Rights Watch 2010, 3–5.
17. Batliwala 1993.
18. Wegner et al. 2007, S109.
19. Pope, Bangser, and Harris Requejo 2011, 869.
20. Interview with female regional representative in Western Kenya, April 7, 2012
21. Human Rights Watch 2010, 52.
22. Direct Relief, UNFPA, and Fistula Foundation 2015.
23. Ibid.
24. In 2014, the program began assessing survivors prior to discharge to determine those who might need help in reintegration. Those at higher risk include women who do not believe that their husbands will abstain from sexual intercourse for the recommended period of time, women who fear they will need to return to manual labor right away, and women who have mental health issues. Host families agree to look after the women for six to nine months during their recovery, until women are ready to return home.
25. WADADIA focus group discussion, August 27, 2015.
26. Ibid.
27. Ibid.
28. Wall 1995, 293.

REFERENCES

Ahmed, S., S. A. Holtz. 2007. "Social and Economic Consequences of Obstetric Fistula: Life Changed Forever?" *International Journal of Gynecology and Obstetrics* 99: S10–S15.
Arrowsmith, Stephen, Catherine Hamlin, and Lewis Wall. 1996. "Obstructed Labor Injury Complex: Obstetric Fistula Formation and the Multifaceted Morbidity of Maternal Birth Trauma in the Developing World." *Obstetrical & Gynecological Survey* 51, 9: 568–574.
Bangser, Maggie, Manisha Mehta, Janet Singer, Chris Daly, Catherine Kamugumya, and Atuswege Mwangomale. 2011. "Childbirth Experiences of Women with Obstetric Fistula in Tanzania and Uganda and Their Implications for Fistula Program Development." *International Urogynecolgical Journal* 22: 91–98. doi10.1007/s00192-010-1236-8.
Batliwala, Srilatha. 1993. "Women's Empowerment in South Asia—Concepts and Practices." http://opendemocracy.net/article/putting_power_back_into_empowerment_o.
Direct Relief, United Nations Population Fund (UNPFA) Campaign to End Fistula, and Fistula Foundation.2015. Global Fistula Map. www.globalfistulamap.org.
Goh, J. T. W., K. M. Sloane, H. G. Krause, A. Browning, and S. Akhter. 2005. "Mental Health Screening in Women with Genital Tract Fistulae." *BJOG* 112: 1328–1330.
Human Rights Watch. 2010. "I Am Not Dead but I Am Not Living: Barriers to Fistula Prevention and Treatment in Kenya." www.hrw.org.

Kelly, John. 1995. "Ethiopia: An Epidemiological Study of Vesico-vaginal Fistula in Addis Ababa." *World Health Statistics Quarterly* 48, no. 1: 15–17.

Ministry of Health (MOH), Division of Reproductive Health, Kenya, and UNFPA Kenya. 2004. *Needs Assessment of Obstetric Fistula in Kenya: Final Report.* Nairobi, Kenya: MOH and UNFPA Kenya, February.

Pope, Rachel, Maggie Bangser, and Jennifer Harris Requejo. 2011. "Restoring Dignity: Social Reintegration after Obstetric Fistula Repair in Ukerewe, Tanzania." *Global Public Health: An International Journal for Research, Policy and Practice* 6, no. 8: 859–873.

Roush, Karen, Ann Kurth, M. Katherine Hutchinson, and Nancy Van Devanter. 2012. "Obstetric Fistula: What about Gender Power?" *Health Care for Women International* 33, no. 9: 787–798.

United Nations General Assembly. 2010. *Supporting Efforts to End Obstetric Fistula: Report of the Secretary-General.* A/65/268. https://documents-dds-ny .un.org/doc/UNDOC/GEN/N10/479/52/PDF/N1047952.pdf?OpenElement.

Wall, Lewis. 1995. "Obstetric Fistulas: Hope for a New Beginning." *International Urogynecology Journal* 6: 292–295.

———. 2006. "Obstetric Vesicovaginal Fistula as an International Public-Health Problem." *Lancet* 368: 1201–1209.

Wall, Lewis, S. D. Arrowsmith, N. D. Briggs, A. Browning, and A. Lassey. 2005. "The Obstetric Vesicovaginal Fistula in the Developing World." *Obstetrical and Gynecological Survey* 60, no. 7: 1403–1453.

Wall, Lewis, Jonathan A. Karshima, Carolyn Kirschner, and Steven D. Arrowsmith. 2004. "The Obstetric Vesicovaginal Fistula: Characteristics of 899 Patients from Jos, Nigeria." *American Journal of Obstetrics and Gynecology* 190: 1011–1019.

Wegner, M. N., J. Ruminjo, E. Sinclair, L. Pesso, and M. Mehta. 2007. "Improving Community Knowledge of Obstetric Fistula Prevention and Treatment." *International Journal of Gynecology and Obstetrics* 99: S108-S111.

Weston, Khisa, Stephen Mutiso, Judy M. Mwangi, Zahida Qureshi, Jessica Beard, and Pavithra Venkat. 2011. "Depression among Women with Obstetric Fistula in Kenya." *International Journal of Gynecology and Obstetrics* 115: 31–33.

Women's Dignity Project and EngenderHealth. In partnership with Health Action Promotion Association, Kivulini Women's Rights Organization, and Permiho Mission Hospital. 2006. *Risk and Resilience: Obstetric Fistula in Tanzania.* New York: EngenderHealth, November. www.engenderhealth .org/files/pubs/maternal-health/risk-and-resilience-obstetric-fistula-in-tanzania.pdf.

3

Pathways to Choice

Delaying Age of Marriage through Girls' Education in Northern Nigeria

DANIEL PERLMAN, FATIMA ADAMU, MAIRO MANDARA,
OLORUKOOBA ABIOLA, DAVID CAO, AND MALCOLM POTTS

One way of thinking about power is in terms of the ability to
make choices.

—Naila Kabeer

Early marriage for girls remains a common practice in West Africa. The
consequences can be dire, including increased rates of maternal and
infant morbidity and mortality.[1,2,3] Since 2008, the Centre for Girls
Education (CGE)—a girls' education training, practice, and research
center—has worked to delay the age of marriage in rural communities
in northwestern Nigeria by reducing social and economic barriers to
female schooling and providing group-based mentoring and support.

Expanding female education and delaying age of marriage are valuable
pathways to improved well-being and health, but can they be considered
empowering? Naila Kabeer defines empowerment as an increase in the
ability to make strategic life choices in a context where this ability was
previously denied.[4] Decisions relating to education, marriage, childbearing, and livelihood are critical to the lives of rural Hausa girls in northern
Nigeria. Yet, societal norms in this region constrain a girl's input into these
decisions. Strategic decision making in this setting is usually a communal
process involving extended family members and is shaped by conservative
gender norms that constrain the life paths available to young women.

Kabeer sees the exercise of choice as incorporating three interrelated
dimensions: *resources,* the enabling factors, competencies, knowledge,

and skills that enhance the capacity to exercise choice; *agency,* the ability to define one's life goals and act upon them; and *achievements,* the outcomes of choices. Resources ("the power to") and agency ("the power within") together enhance people's potential to live the lives they desire, and achievements reflect the extent to which this potential is actually realized.[5]

Girls' education is one of the most effective means to expand choices and enhance agency. Reducing social and economic barriers to girls' education increases adolescent girls' ability to delay marriage and realize other achievements. This expands the critical years in which girls can acquire the human and social resources to self-define and act upon life goals.

CONTEXT

> I felt a sharp pain in my lower abdomen and noticed that my skirt was stained with blood. I was 13 at the time. I rushed to my mother. She smiled and held my hand and explained menstruation. When my father came home that night, he called me and asked if I had a suitor. I told him no. After some days my mother told me that I was to be married. I knew that there would be merriment and that I would be bought clothes, shoes, a bed, and a chest of drawers. I was happy about this but sad that I would be leaving my family to live at my future husband's home. I wanted to stay in school. But I could not disobey my father. (An 18-year-old rural adolescent girl, five years married)

The Centre for Girls Education (CGE) is a joint program of Ahmadu Bello University's Population and Reproductive Health Initiative (PRHI) and the University of California, Berkeley's Bixby Center for Population, Health, and Sustainability. In 2006, the Bixby Center and PRHI received funding from the National Institutes of Health (NIH) to train postdoctoral fellows from northern Nigeria to conduct community-based research on the underlying causes of maternal mortality and morbidity in the region. Notably, northern Nigeria has one of the highest maternal mortality rates in the world, especially among rural Hausa communities, an ethnic group estimated to number 40 million in West Africa.

Early Marriage in Northern Nigeria

The PRHI-Bixby postdoctoral fellows began the project with ethnographic fieldwork (participant-observation and in-depth interviewing) and a baseline household demographic and reproductive health survey.[6,7] They found the mean age of marriage to be 14.9 years and that 45% of adolescents aged 15–19 had begun childbearing in collaborating communities.[8] Married adolescent girls are a particularly vulnerable population for a number of poor outcomes due to early sexual initiation, lack of educational attainment, little knowledge of reproductive health, and strong social pressure to reproduce.[9] These social patterns, combined with poor nutritional status, lack of physical maturity of girls at first pregnancy, and poor access to family planning and emergency obstetric care, greatly increase the risks of complications during pregnancy and delivery, and the subsequent likelihood of poor health outcomes among infants. Worldwide, mothers aged 15–19 are twice as likely to die in childbirth as mothers over 19.[10]

This baseline survey also found a total fertility rate (TFR) of 8.2 and a modern contraceptive prevalence rate (CPR) of 0.05% among married women.[11,12] Using the Sisterhood Method to estimate the maternal mortality ratio (MMR), the research fellows found the MMR in participating communities to be over 1,400/100,000 live births.[13] Knowledge about maternal health was low among both men and women.[14]

Whereas an unmarried adolescent girl has a fair amount of freedom of mobility in the community, this freedom is typically constrained dramatically after marriage. Although Hausa culture pre-dated Islam, the culture has been heavily influenced by Islamic practices especially since the sixteenth century. Virtually all rural Hausa families practice a system of seclusion, in which married women are expected to conduct most activities within their compound and other private spaces.[15,16] A married woman needs the permission of the head of household to go outside the home to visit a relative or a health facility, even in the case of an obstetric emergency.[17,18] With multiple limitations on work outside the home, women engage in a variety of income-generating activities in their courtyards such as embroidering, sewing, and preparing products for sale.[19] Girls assist their mothers in a myriad of ways— going to the market, selling foodstuffs, bringing water, and minding younger siblings—so keeping a daughter in school entails significant opportunity costs for women.

The world of most rural Hausa adolescent girls is built around marriage. Being a successful wife and mother is a career to which almost all aspire. "If all of my children do well, I will have succeeded. People will refer to them as my children, and I will be proud," said one young mother. The unmarried girls reported that when they are with their closest friends, they often talk about boyfriends, suitors, and which one of them will marry first.

Despite the emphasis on marriage, virtually all of the female primary school graduates interviewed by the postdoctoral fellows said they would like to complete their secondary education before marrying. Unfortunately, there is differential access to educational opportunities by gender in the region. The baseline survey found that only 8% of women ages 18 to 24 had completed primary school and just 5% had completed secondary school. Because primary school dropout rates are high among girls, literacy and numeracy skills are low. Only 21% of women ages 15 to 49 in northwest Nigeria can read a single sentence in their mother tongue.[20] In contrast, more than twice as many boys complete primary school (17%) and secondary school (14%).[21] As a consequence, three times more men than women ages 15 to 49 in northwest Nigeria can read a sentence (60%).

The majority of parents interviewed by the postdoctoral fellows saw menarche as a sign of readiness for marriage. They view marriage as a way to keep their daughters safe and regard the social roles of wife and mother as the most viable and acceptable for a girl through puberty. The Hausa people have resisted outside interference into their religious and cultural practices in both colonial and postcolonial periods. Many rural Hausa resent external criticism of early marriage. Nonetheless, during our baseline research most parents expressed willingness to keep their daughters in school and delay their marriages if offered modest help with school fees and books. Thus, based on the findings of this baseline survey and exploratory ethnography, prolonging girls' education appeared as if it would be an effective strategy to help delay marriage and the onset of childbearing in rural northern Nigeria.

Public Education in the Region

Western education was not widely available in northern Nigeria until after the nation had obtained its independence from the United Kingdom in 1960. The indigenous leaders in the north, through whom the British ruled, associated Western education with missionary schools and saw it as a threat to Qur'anic education and an Islamic way of life. Some parents told the postdoctoral fellows they were concerned that Western education would weaken their girls' sense of propriety and undermine other Hausa and Islamic values.

Basic education in the region currently suffers from a lack of teachers, decaying infrastructure, and limited funding—all of which contribute to poor learning outcomes.[22] A learning assessment conducted in the Bauchi and Sokoto states of northern Nigeria in 2011 found that, at the end of third grade, only 6% of students were able to read a simple sentence.[23] Given the low quality of public education, many parents are reluctant to make the sacrifices—loss of labor and cost of school fees, books, uniforms, and transportation—required to send their children to school. "My first daughter graduated from primary school and can't read a word. I won't send my second daughter," said one mother. This is a sentiment that came up often in the exploratory ethnographic research and underlies CGE's emphasis on basic literary and numeracy.

FROM RESEARCH TO PRACTICE

Following the baseline survey and ethnographic research phase of the project, the postdoctoral fellows and their faculty advisors organized a series of meetings with people from the research communities to discuss how best to address barriers to girls' education. Teachers suggested that they start with girls graduating from primary school, a time when many left school to marry. The Nigerian Universal Basic Education Act of 2004 guarantees free education to every Nigerian child for the first nine years of schooling. In reality, parents are charged registration fees, parent-teacher association (PTA) dues, "chalk money," "broom costs," and a host of other levies. When asked what it would take to increase girls' transition from primary to secondary school, many parents mentioned a reduction of secondary school registration fees and increasing opportunities for their daughters to learn to read, write, and do basic math within the current educational system. The core CGE program components—reduction in school levies and mentored girls' clubs to help strengthen learning—took shape in response to these suggestions and concerns.

In 2008 the Bixby Center and PRHI launched the CGE program, an educational enrichment program for girls that complements government secondary schooling by (1) reducing economic and social barriers to secondary school enrollment and completion by facilitating an enabling community environment and reducing registration fees; (2) improving core academic competencies via extended learning opportunities in mentored girls' groups; and (3) providing opportunities to acquire critical life skills, such as social and economic competency, not currently offered in government secondary schools.

Core Components

CGE's core components evolved over six years of careful community-based research with girls based in rural northwest Nigeria and their mothers, fathers, community members, and religious leaders.

Community engagement: The CGE team begins in a new community by meeting first with traditional leaders and then with groups of mothers, fathers, teachers, informal leaders, and other key stakeholders to discuss girls' education and social and economic barriers to access. (People often feel more comfortable expressing their thoughts and concerns in socially homogenous groups). To date, fifty-two communities have participated in the CGE programs. Religious leaders are invited to a one-day workshop to examine support in the Qur'an and Hadith for girls' education. Once the implementation team feels a consensus is near, they organize a larger community meeting to review the key conclusions from the smaller group discussions.

Reduction of school fees: School fees are one of the most cited reason for primary school graduates failing to transition to secondary school in developing countries.[24,25] Studies consistently find that reductions in educational costs boost school participation, often dramatically.[26] Furthermore, reducing school fees typically leads to a greater increase in girls' enrollment than in boys' enrollment.[27] Despite Nigeria's enormous oil wealth, poverty is severe and widespread in the targeted region. Nearly all participants are from farming families with cumulative incomes below a dollar a day.[28] As one pillar of the program, CGE pays girls' registration fees directly to the schools (roughly $24 a year). Parents are more willing to pay for the variety of other periodic expenses throughout the year once the school fees are taken care of, because miscellaneous fees require smaller expenditures per payment.

Mentored girls' clubs: Girls' clubs, led by experienced female teachers, are the cornerstone of the CGE program. Participation in the clubs is meant to enhance the girls' literacy and numeracy skills and provide opportunities to gain crucial life skills not offered in secondary school. The clubs provide opportunities to improve financial literacy skills and meet successful women traders, teachers, health extension workers, and midwives. In the confidential groups, girls are able to discuss their reproductive health concerns, visit local health services, develop relationships of trust, and build social networks. Each club, including approximately fifteen primary school graduates, meets for two hours each week. The clubs meet in quiet rooms in the homes of trusted community members.

Girls in senior secondary who attended clubs when they were younger serve as apprentice mentors and will lead clubs of their own in the future.

The club curriculum is based on research suggesting that girls in many societies require a range of competencies if they are to overcome the multiple disadvantages they face.[29] School curricula are often not relevant to the successful acquisition of these individual, social, and economic competencies.[30,31,32,33,34,35] The use of interactive and nonformal educational strategies within the clubs are particularly suited to girls from rural environments because of their emphasis on practical skills and learning by doing.[36,37]

METHODS

CGE has carried out routine monitoring and evaluation activities continuously from 2008 to 2012. CGE's monitoring and evaluation (M & E) procedures combine (1) traditional anthropological methods of participant observation and in-depth interviewing with (2) quantitative data collection, including the tracking of school and marital status. We also use and report data here from a more in-depth evaluation conducted with only the 2010–2011 CGE cohort to assess more detailed changes in participants' knowledge and skills, including literacy and numeracy as well as reproductive health knowledge.

Monitoring and evaluation is carried out by four full-time ethnographic researchers under the direction of a senior researcher from the Bixby Center. The research assistants spend three days per week in the community attending mentored girls' clubs, having informal conversations with the girls, interviewing parents and community members, and observing life in the community. The monitoring and evaluation piece of the program was approved by the institutional review boards of both Ahmadu Bello University and the University of California, Berkeley.

Ethnographic Research Methods

The major analytical approach was thematic and qualitative. The evaluation team looked for recurring themes as we read and reread field notes and interview transcriptions. This led to the refinement, abandonment, or redevelopment of research questions and to the next series of interviews and observations. We continued this process until a category that had been tentatively labeled appeared to remain stable with additional data.

Quantitative Research Methods

In order to assess the impact of the CGE program in keeping girls in school and delaying marriage, we used data on 2010–2011 CGE program participants from the routine M&E activities and compared them to the results for adolescent girls from a baseline household demographic and reproductive health survey (DRHS) conducted in 2007 by PRHI in three of the original CGE communities. This comparison enabled the program to estimate the proportion of women still in school and unmarried by age as well as the increased probability of getting married at any given point in time. Because primary school completion is a prerequisite to join the CGE program, the comparison group from 2007 included only primary school graduates. These analyses included 400 current CGE program participants and 59 DRHS respondents. Additionally, in 2010, we implemented a more in-depth evaluation with 230 girls to assess changes in knowledge and skills, including literacy and numeracy skills as well as reproductive health knowledge.

RESULTS

Ethnographic Findings

> My father came back home after work and saw the gifts brought by my suitor. He flung the gifts into the courtyard and asked his brothers to return them to my suitor's house. My father wanted me to marry but not into this particular family. My uncles called me and asked if I wanted to marry the man. I said yes, but when I was asked again in my father's presence, I couldn't say a word and just turned my face away. My uncles spoke with my father and he finally accepted the marriage because this is what I wanted. He could not say no to his brothers, especially his oldest, as he was like his father. (A young woman from one of the CGE communities describing her marriage)

The girls participating in the CGE program see education, marriage, childbearing, child rearing, and livelihood as the most critical life events facing them in the coming years. Yet few of the girls interviewed when they entered the program felt they had significant decision-making power over these choices. An adolescent girl would risk alienating those around her if she were to insist on making important decisions regarding her life course herself. Her father will usually decide on school enrollment, while her mother will decide whether she can spare her daughter's labor in order for her to attend school on a particular day. Her uncles, grandparents, and traditional and religious leaders may also wield influence over the timing and selection of her husband-to-be. Once married, decision making shifts to her husband and mother-in-law. "The only thing that could get in the way of my daughter's schooling is marriage," one father of a CGE participant said. "It will be discussed with her suitor, and I hope that he will be someone who will favor education. But if her husband doesn't permit her to continue her education, there is not a lot I can do about it." The girl's mother added, "It isn't easy for a young woman to look after her children, cater to her husband, and see to the running of her home and still be in school at the same time."

With strategic decision making a communal process shaped by conservative gender norms in the region, one way to facilitate expansion of girls' ability to make strategic choices is to emphasize the acquisition of self-expression and negotiation skills. CGE's girls' clubs expose the girls to a variety of pathways potentially available for women in their society besides those restricted to the home. The club mentors—like the girls they serve—cherish Islam and the life it prescribes. However, mentors—often unlike the girls' mothers, aunts, and grandmothers—mostly practice an interpretation of seclusion that permits them to work outside the home. The girls meet women from a variety of trades and professions in the clubs. The girls are also given time and space with their peers and mentors to talk about their current lives and the lives to which they aspire, using discussion, art, games, and role-play. The sessions that encourage girls to express themselves in front of their peers and defend their points of view are designed to help them practice expression and negotiation skills.

The results of the process are often profound. "The girls in the program are different," said one mother. "They speak up for themselves. They might not get what they want, but they express themselves well, and people appreciate that." Virtually all the mentors report that there are girls in their groups who have persuaded parents to delay marriage until they have completed their schooling or coaxed their new husband or mother-in-law, or both, to let them remain in school after marriage. The girls report that they utilize strategies practiced in the girls' clubs, such as speaking with sympathetic family members such as an uncle or grandfather, to help them in their negotiations.

Community Response to CGE

The CGE program has been met with both acceptance and resistance in the community based on our ethnographic research. As an example of resistance, during the first weeks of the program, a man ripped up a program flyer offered by the CGE outreach coordinator. The man said nothing and just walked on. As a further example of resistance, one girl waited for an hour outside the registration room for the program. She asked the CGE staff repeatedly for her books and uniform but refused to come into the room to be registered. Upon further questioning, it was revealed that her father didn't want her to enroll.

As an illustrative example of acceptance, one father who enrolled his daughter into the program said,

> Some people saw me as someone who didn't know what he was doing. They thought that I should marry my daughter off rather than keeping her in school. They said the program is not religiously acceptable. But our religion isn't like that. Islam does not disallow a child from getting an education. I insisted, because it is my right to allow her to go to school and become someone. Now even the *liman* (the head of religious leaders in the community) has two of his daughters in the program.

Despite some evidence of resistance, 97% of the parents of each graduating primary school class in participating communities have enrolled their daughters in secondary school since 2008.

Quantitative Findings

Literacy and numeracy skills: The girls come with a strong desire to build up academic skills and knowledge. Many report that they come to the clubs to learn to read and write, "to become someone," and "to assist my family and community." Becoming "someone" in this context usually refers to becoming a teacher or midwife, as these are the professional women with whom the girls have most often had contact. However, few of the girls learned to read and write competently during their primary school years. Of the 2010–2011 cohort, 74% were unable to read a single Hausa word upon program entrance. The girls demonstrated significant gains in basic reading skills (as measured by the ability to read familiar words, sentences, and simple passages in Hausa) after eight months of participation in the mentored girls' clubs.

Numeracy skills were also weak, as measured at baseline in the same year's cohort, but eight months after entering the CGE program, the percentage of girls assessed with high-level numeracy skills (as assessed by correctly answering at least three out of the four simple computations) increased to 52% on average from 24% at baseline.

Health knowledge: At the conclusion of the mentored girls' clubs, the groups were able to recall much of the health content that they covered

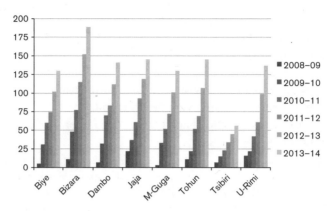

FIGURE 3.1. Number of girls enrolled in secondary school in CGE project communities by school year.

during the prior eight months. On topics related to safe motherhood, 93% of the 2010–2011 groups correctly recalled at least four danger signs during pregnancy, labor, and after birth; 79% recalled at least four benefits of antenatal care; and 93% recalled at least three benefits of hospital delivery. Ninety-eight percent were able to state the key lessons from the sessions on malaria prevention, fever treatment, diarrhea prevention and treatment, puberty, and menstruation. Seventy-three percent of the participants were able to correctly recall key messages about HIV/AIDS.

Secondary school enrollment and retention: When combined, the CGE program components proved to be extremely effective in enrolling and retaining girls in secondary school for a modest investment (figure 3.1). The 2007 DRHS found that only 36% of female rural primary school graduates enrolled in secondary school whereas almost all female primary school graduates in CGE communities (97%) subsequently enrolled.

Kaplan-Meier estimates additionally reveal that 95.6% of all girls from the CGE program remain enrolled in school at the end of the first year of junior secondary school (JSS1). At the end of JSS2, 84.9% of the CGE girls from this year were still enrolled, and 81.6% are projected to graduate from junior secondary school.

Age of marriage: Kaplan-Meier modeling suggests that participation in the CGE program is associated with an average delay of marriage of 2.5 years. Figure 3.2 presents the Kaplan-Meier estimates of the proportion of women unmarried by age for both CGE girls (enrolled in the

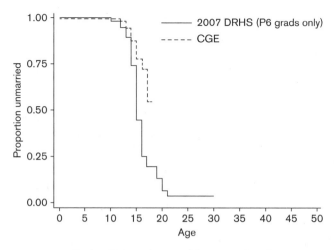

FIGURE 3.2. Kaplan-Meier estimates of the proportion of women unmarried by age.

2008–09, 2009–10, and 2010–11 cohorts) and 2007 DRHS respondents. By age 15 years, only 22.9% of CGE girls since the inception of the program have married compared to 55.1% of the comparison group. *Participating in CGE reduced the probability of being married by 64%* (hazard ratio [HR]: 0.36 [95% CI: 0.23–0.55, $p<0.0001$]) when comparing the marriage ages of CGE participants to the 2007 comparison group.

DISCUSSION

"The girls that attend the mentored girls' clubs are different than other girls," said one mother. "They are composed and can speak up for themselves. My daughter reads at home and helps the younger ones with their homework. She has learned to cook, to cut her nails, and take a bath more often. She taught all the women in the compound to make a sugar, water, and salt drink for diarrhea and how to store food and wash our hands to avoid cholera and dysentery."

Her husband added, "You could say the girls are being reeducated in the fundamentals that they were taught in school but never learned. The CGE mentors sit them down and teach the girls in a practical way, and when they get back home, they share what they learn with their siblings."

Direct advocacy to delay marriage in rural northern Nigeria is seen by some as outside interference in local ways of life. Efforts to discuss the adverse consequences of early marriage often fall on deaf ears or are even met with resistance. CGE has found that working with communities to create socially valued and viable alternatives to early marriage is a far more promising approach. The program's community engagement process and registration fee subsidies aim to reduce barriers to girls' enrollment rather than to convince parents to delay the age of marriage. The mentored safe space clubs result in the quick enhancement of basic academic core competencies and improve school achievement and retention. The girls build relationships of trust with their mentors and each other, enhance social networks, and acquire key social and vocational skills. The clubs are popular with parents and serve as "billboards" for girls' education. Parents see tangible evidence of learning and growth and are more willing to pay education-related expenses and let their daughters proceed further in their studies before marriage. "We are seeing remarkable changes in the girls," one father reported. "They now know the importance of going to school, and they attend school daily without anyone prompting."

It is unlikely that CGE would have experienced the same success had it begun a decade earlier. Parents' attitudes about girls' education appear to be at a tipping point in the region, making this an opportune time to increase school enrollment through strategies that address parental concerns such as enhancing learning outcomes and reducing school fees. Many parents now see education as having value for their daughters and want them to attend school, gain employment if possible, and help the family financially, all goals which are advanced by the described intervention. This is a win-win strategy in which rural parents find common ground with health workers and educators and together build a more promising future for adolescent girls and for the region as a whole.

Our data suggests that participation in the CGE program is associated with a delay of marriage of 2.5 years. Although temporal trends in the region regarding marital age could be contributing to these findings, the enhanced educational opportunities provided by this program are likely to substantially contribute to this finding. Other studies have demonstrated that girls with secondary schooling are six times less likely to marry under the age of 18 compared to girls who have little or no education.[38] Even a delay of two years in marital age could reduce a country's total fertility rate and improve human and environmental health outcomes. Increasing the average marital age and onset of childbearing by five years could directly reduce 15–20% of future population growth in the country, with an even greater reduction in northern Nigeria, where birth rates are higher than the rest of the country.[39]

CGE's fee subsidies reduce the economic burden of secondary school education. However, outside assistance with school fees is not economically sustainable. The long-term solution is for states to honor their legal responsibility to make primary and secondary school education available without hidden costs for all children. Over the next two years, CGE will join with other members of the Consortium to Delay Marriage in Northern Nigeria in a campaign to improve public education and reduce or eliminate school fees. CGE will offer advocacy training to 130 graduates of the program and then mentor them as they travel in teams to state capitals to speak with legislators, ministry officials, and governors about the crises facing public education and the ways in which the myriad school-related fees limit access to education for rural and poor children.

LESSONS LEARNED

Typically, mentored girls' clubs, or safe spaces, are used as an alternative, nonformal approach to educating adolescent girls who are not in—nor likely to return to—school. The Population Council, which has led the development of safe spaces in Africa, Asia, and Latin America, views "a safe place, friends, and a mentor" as the backbone of strong adolescent girls' clubs.[40,41,42,43,44] CGE has adapted the safe space methodology to meet schoolgirls' need for strengthened core academic competencies and mentored support as it actively addresses the challenges encountered in secondary school. The clubs have proven to be an ideal environment in which to offer instruction in literacy and numeracy. Without the accelerated gains in reading, writing, and math skills associated with the clubs, it is likely that many parents would decide against making the financial sacrifices and taking on the opportunity costs that come with educating their daughters.

Public education in Nigeria is in crisis.[45] The Independent Commission for Aid Impact (ICAI)[46] recently reviewed two large-scale UK-funded programs in Nigeria that attempted "to improve the overall education system so that benefits filter down to schools and pupils." After an expenditure of £119.2 million from 2005 to 2012 in ten states (mostly in the north), the ICAI report found "no major improvement in pupil learning." The report concludes that the political and economic barriers to comprehensive educational reform in the region are still so profound that UK aid should focus on "interventions that are proven to improve basic literacy and numeracy" and encourage enrollment by demonstrating to parents that effective learning is taking place. CGE's focused strategy and the results presented above would seem to represent exactly the type of intervention proposed by this commission.[47]

Supporting girls as they make the transition from primary to junior secondary school and from junior secondary to senior secondary—critical risk periods for school withdrawal—has proven to be an effective means for in-school girls to delay their age of marriage. However, there are girls in the same communities in far more vulnerable situations. These include out-of-school girls, disabled girls, and adolescent girls who are married. CGE has received funding to open new girls' clubs to serve these subpopulations. The clubs will focus on functional literacy and numeracy, income generation, and other life skills to help enhance outcomes for these girls.

CONCLUSION

> We were sitting with the girl in her mother's room. It was decorated with flowers from a calendar cut and pasted on the wall and some drawings painted in green and red. The girls' club mentor was sitting across from the girl, who was 16 years old and about to get married.
>   "Will you stay in school after you get married?" asked the mentor.
>   "It's up to my husband to decide," said the girl.
>   "What would you like?"
>   "Whatever he says, I'll do."
>   "But what do you want?"
>   "I want to stay in school."
>   "Then you need to be talking to people about this."

Most of the girls in the CGE program want to marry after graduating from secondary school. They will be 18 years old and better able to express themselves and negotiate with husbands and other family members. They will have learned how to cook healthy meals and about reproductive and child health. Those enrolled in 2008 have now graduated from senior secondary school and are working as apprentice mentors. Within a year or two, many will open new groups in their own communities. People will call them *mallama,* or teacher, a title of respect in Hausa society, and younger girls in the community will see that someone just like them can ultimately achieve such a position. Some girls will choose to continue their education and become teachers, midwives, and community health extension workers. CGE's goal is for all to reach their self-defined goal of "becoming somebody and helping their family and community."

Bina Agarwal writes "any strategy that seeks women's empowerment should have as a central component the enhancement of women's ability to function collectively in their own interest."[48] The girls come together in safe spaces to learn of a wider world, acquire life skills, and express themselves within the group. Even when building individual assets, the girls do so collectively. When one girl expands her ability to participate in decisions about her schooling, marriage, livelihood, and childbearing, she simultaneously expands the possibility for the other girls in the community to do so. Community norms are changing as the number of girls in secondary school grows from ten to twenty to fifty per rural community and increasing numbers of adolescent girls are seen in school uniforms. As these girls become mentors, teachers, and health workers, they will expand the potential of other girls in their region to redefine and expand the social limits of what is possible.[49,50]

Box 3.1. Summary

Geographic area: Northern Nigeria

Global importance of the health condition: Adolescent marriage and childbearing are considerable barriers to the social and economic development of Nigeria and a major concern for women's health and the health of the children born to adolescent mothers. This includes a significantly increased risk of maternal and infant mortality and morbidities.*

Intervention or program: Since 2008, the Centre for Girls Education (CGE)—a joint program of Ahmadu Bello University's Population and Reproductive Health Initiative and the UC Berkeley Bixby Center for Population, Health, and Sustainability—has worked to delay marriage in northern Nigeria by improving girls' access to and retention in secondary school.

Impact: By reducing the social and economic barriers to education and by offering mentoring and support groups to build core academic competencies and life skills, the program reduced cost, improved quality, and enhanced girls' retention in secondary school. Participation in girls' clubs led to improvements in literacy and numeracy and provided opportunities for girls to articulate their aspirations about education and marriage to their parents and strategic members of their extended family. A formative

evaluation of CGE found participation in the program to be associated with up to a 2.5-year delay in the age of marriage.

Lessons learned: Individual empowerment is most effectively
cultivated through a process of collective empowerment. Within
their clubs, the girls reflect on their lives, acquire core academic
competencies and life skills, define their goals, and practice exercising them before the group. The girls discover that they can do
things collectively that they had found difficult to do individually.
Social norms about girls' education and age of marriage change as
the girls become mentors and leaders and increasing numbers of
unmarried adolescent girls in school uniforms make school-going
more visible and acceptable.

Link between empowerment and health: Girls' programs that
intervene during the critical preadolescent years enable girls to
acquire human and social resources and to improve their ability
to define their life goals. In this program, many girls chose to stay
in school and delay marriage, thereby increasing their chances
of living the lives they want while decreasing their risk of averse
health outcomes.

*Adhikari RK. 2003. Early marriage and childbearing: risks and consequences.
In: Bott S, Jejeebhoy S, Shah I, Puri C, editors. *Towards adulthood: exploring the
sexual and reproductive health of adolescents in South Asia*. Geneva: World Health
Organization, pp. 62–66.

Box 3.2. Factors behind the Success of the Centre for Girls Education Program in Nigeria

The CGE program has had a positive impact on participants' lives.
Girls in the program are 65% less likely to be married than their pre-
intervention counterparts. A number of girls have been able to delay
marriage until the completion of school by speaking with sympathetic
extended family members and using other strategies learned and practiced in the girls' clubs. Others have persuaded future husbands to let
them continue attending school after marriage.

Key factors that have contributed to the program's success include
the following:

- *Basing program design on research*: The CGE program
  components were based on patient formative ethnographic
  research (participant observation, in-depth interviews, and
  informal group discussions) and extensive discussions with
  adolescent girls, community members, religious leaders, and

key stakeholders. Early discussions revealed parental concerns regarding school's high cost, low quality, and irrelevance. The program components were subsequently adapted to directly address such concerns.

- *Participatory community discussions*: CGE continually engages with the participants, parents, community members, religious leaders, and other key stakeholders to improve program design.

- *The ten-year partnership between Ahmadu Bello University and the University of California has allowed for the recruitment of a talented and well-trained team* that only time can build. Every CGE staff member speaks fluent Hausa. All but one of the twenty-two staff and mentors are women. The outcome has been high-quality programming and the building of close relationships with parents, teachers, traditional and religious leaders, and local government.

NOTES

1. Raj A, Boehmer U. 2013. Girl child marriage and its association with national rates of HIV, maternal health, and infant mortality across 97 countries. Violence Against Women. 19(4) April:536–51.

2. Raj A, Saqqurti N, Winter M, Labonte A, Decker MR, Balaiah D, Silverman JG. 2010. The effect of maternal child marriage on morbidity and mortality of children under 5 in India: cross-sectional study of a nationally representative sample. BMJ. 21(340) January:b4258.

3. Ityavar D, Jalingo I. 2006. The state of married adolescents in northern Nigeria. Lagos: Action Health Incorporated.

4. Kabeer N. 1999. Resources, agency, achievements: reflections on the measurement of women's empowerment. Dev Change. 30(3):435–464.

5. Kabeer 1999.

6. The 2007 baseline included intensive exploratory ethnographic research and a complete cross-sectional demographic and reproductive health survey modeled after the 2003 NDHS. The ethnographic research employed participant-observation, in-depth interviews, and informal group discussions. The survey included 1,408 women of reproductive age (15–49) and 501 male heads of household, allocated among the communities proportionate to population size.

7. Adiri F, Ibrahim H, Ajayi V, Sulayman H, Yafeh A, Ejembi C. 2010. Fertility behaviour of men and women in three communities in Kaduna State, Nigeria. Afr J Reprod Health. 14:43–51.

8. Ityavar, Jalingo 2006.

9. Smith R, Ashford L, Gribble J, Clifton D. 2009. Family planning saves lives. 4th ed. Washington, DC: Population Reference Bureau.

10. Adiri et al. 2010.

11. Avidime S, Aku-Akai L, Mohammed A, Adaji S, Shittu O, Ejembi C. 2010. Fertility intentions, contraceptive awareness and contraceptive use among women in three communities in northern Nigeria. Afr J Reprod Health. 14(3):65–70.

12. Idris H, Tyoden C, Ejembi C, Taylor K. 2010. Estimation of maternal mortality using the indirect sisterhood method in three communities in Kaduna State, northern Nigeria. Afr J Reprod Health. 14:29–34.

13. Butawa N, Tukur B, Idris H, Adiri F, Taylor K. 2010. Knowledge and perceptions of maternal health in Kaduna State, northern Nigeria. Afr J Reprod Health. 14:7–13.

14. Adiri et al. 2010.

15. Wall L. 1998. Dead mothers and injured wives: the social context of maternal morbidity and mortality among the Hausa in Northern Nigeria. Stud Fam Plann. 29:341–359; Mair L. 1969. African marriage and social change. London: Routledge.

16. Mair 1969.

17. Erulkar A, Bello MV. 2007. The experience of married adolescents in Nigeria. New York: Population Council.

18. Yusuf B. 2005. Sexuality and the marriage institution in Islam: an appraisal. Lagos, Nigeria: African Regional Sexuality Resource Centre.

19. Renne E. 2004. Gender roles and women's status: what they mean to Hausa Muslim women in northern Nigeria. In: Szreter S, Dharmalingam A, Sholkamy H, editors. Qualitative demography: categories and contexts in population studies. Oxford: Oxford University Press. p. 276–94.

20. National Population Commission (NPC) [Nigeria] and ICF Macro. 2009. Nigeria demographic and health survey 2008. Abuja, Nigeria: NPC and ICF Macro.

21. NPC and ICF Macro 2009.

22. Independent Commission for Aid Impact (ICAI). 2012. DfID's education programmes in Nigeria. Report 16. London: ICAI. http://icai.independent.gov .uk/wp-content/uploads/ICAI-Nigeria-Education-report.pdf.

23. RTI International. 2011. Northern Nigeria Initiative (NEI): results of the Early Grade Reading Assessment (EGRA) in Hausa. Durham, NC: RTI International. Prepared for U.S. Agency for International Development, Nigeria.

24. Kremer M, Holla A. 2009. Improving education in the developing world: what have we learned from randomized evaluations? Annual Rev Econ. 1: 513–542

25. Banerjee A, Glewwe P, Powers S, Wasserman M. 2013. Expanding access and increasing student learning in post-primary education in developing countries: a review of the evidence. Cambridge, MA: MIT.

26. Kremer, Holla 2009.

27. Oxfam. Girls' education in Africa. 2005. Education and gender equality series, programme insights. www.ungei.org/resources/files/oxfam_edPaper8% 281%29.pdf.

28. World Bank. 2008. Nigeria: country brief. www.worldbank.org/en /country/nigeria.

29. Lloyd CB. 2013. Education for girls: alternative pathways to girls' empowerment. Issue paper series. GirlEffect.org.

30. Murphy-Graham E. 2010. And when she comes home? education and women's empowerment in intimate relationships. Int J Educ Dev 30(3):320–331.

31. LeVine R, LeVine S, Richman A, Uribe F, Correa C, Miller P. 1991. Women's schooling and child care in the demographic transition: a Mexican case study. Popul Dev Rev. 17(3):459–496.

32. Kumar A, Vlassoff C. 1997. Gender relations and education of girls in two Indian communities: implications for decisions about childbearing. Reprod Health Matters. 10 (November):139–150.

33. Lloyd, CB 2013.

34. Warner A, Malhotra A, McGonagle A. 2012. Girls' education, empowerment and transitions to adulthood: the case for a shared agenda. Washington, DC: International Center for Research on Women (ICRW). www.icrw.org /publications/girls-education-empowerment-and-transitions-adulthood.

35. Mahmud S. 2011. Social and financial empowerment of adolescent girls in Bangladesh: Alternative strategies beyond school. Presented at: Adding It Up: Expert Consultation on Leveraging Education to Empower Girls and Improve Their Transitions to Adulthood; ICRW, Washington, DC.

36. Murphy-Graham E. 2012. Opening minds, improving lives: education and women's empowerment in Honduras. Nashville, TN: Vanderbilt University Press.

37. Lloyd CB 2013.

38. Lloyd CB, editor. 2005. Growing up global: the changing transitions to adulthood in developing countries. Committee on Population and Board on Children, Youth and Families, Division of Behavioral and Social Sciences and Education, National Research Council and Institute of Medicine. National Academies Press: Washington, DC.

39. Bruce J, Bongaarts J. 2009. The new population challenge. In: Mazur LA, editor. A pivotal moment: population, justice, and the environmental challenge. Washington, DC: Island Press. p. 260–275.

40. Austrian K, Ghati D. 2010. Girl-centered program design: a toolkit to develop, strengthen and expand adolescent girls programs. New York: Population Council. www.ungei.org/files/2010PGY_AdolGirlToolkitComplete.pdf.

41. Erulkar AS, Muthengi E. 2009. Evaluation of Berhane Hewan: a program to delay child marriage in rural Ethiopia. Int Perspect Sex Reprod Health.

42. Zibani N, Brady M. 2011. Scaling up asset-building programs for marginalized adolescent girls in socially conservative settings: the Ishraq program in rural upper Egypt. New York: Population Council.

43. Catino J, Colom A, Ruiz MJ. 2011. Equipping Mayan girls to improve their lives. New York: Population Council.

44. Acharya R, Kalyanwala S, Jejeebhoy SJ, Nathani V. 2009. Broadening girls' horizons: Effects of a life skills education programme in rural Uttar Pradesh. New Delhi: Population Council.

45. ICAI 2012.

46. The Independent Commission for Aid Impact (ICAI) is the body responsible for monitoring aid provided by the United Kingdom.

47. ICAI 2012.

48. Agarwal B. 2001. Poverty in a globalizing world at different stages of women's life cycle. Presented at: UN Expert Group Meeting on Gender and Poverty, Institute of Economic Growth.

49. Murphy-Graham, Erin 2012.

50. Mosedale S. 2005. Assessing women's empowerment: towards a conceptual framework. J Int Dev 7(2):243–257.

4

Early Empowerment

The Evolution and Practice of Girls'
"Boot Camps" in Kenya and Haiti

KAREN AUSTRIAN, JUDITH BRUCE, AND
M. CATHERINE MATERNOWSKA

Worldwide, adolescent girls are disadvantaged both by age and gender. During this vital life phase—which can span from 10 to 18 years— many girls are denied the skills and resources they need to protect themselves and ensure their futures. Without access to basic health care, social networks, and economic opportunities, girls' vulnerability early in life can set a precedent for multiple types of violence, the effects of which extend well into adulthood. One in five people in the world (1.2 billion) are 10- to 19-year-olds. Of these 1.2 billion adolescents, 90% live in developing countries (including China) and approximately 510 million are girls.[1] Over 200 million of these adolescent girls (nearly 40%) are at seriously high risk of poor health outcomes and long-term poverty. Numerous structural forces—including ongoing political and social conflict, environmental destruction from climate change,[2] as well as the cycle of poverty—are eroding girls' traditional safety nets, leading to significant health impacts over the lifespan of women.

In this chapter we highlight adolescent girls' programming boot camps, the informal name for a nearly decade-long effort to train organizations working with adolescent girls in the poorest communities. The program encourages organizations to reach girls with asset-building activities to prevent or mitigate the negative critical life events that girls face, such as dropping out of school or having an unwanted pregnancy. Boot camps emphasize prevention—as opposed to responding after such problems occur. An interdisciplinary, data-driven, and participatory approach helps girls develop and strengthen their social, health, and economic assets, which can protect them into adulthood. Building social assets helps girls acquire critical social networks, friendships, mentoring relationships, and self–esteem. Health assets include relevant knowledge, information, and access to services. Economic assets include a range of age-appropriate economic-strengthening activities, from financial education to savings to entrepreneurship.

During boot camps, high- and medium-level program staff are matched with Girl Experts who together (1) work to develop, strengthen, or expand a plan for an adolescent girls' program, emphasizing social, health, and economic asset building; (2) participate in workshops with over a dozen organizations to discuss and learn about best practices in developing culturally relevant girl-focused programs; and (3) finalize program plans and seek funding for implementation. While this approach has gained momentum globally, the focus here is on two programs—in the country where it was first developed, Kenya, and in the country where work on girls in emergencies was initiated, Haiti. The girls at risk, though divided by thousands of miles, share the common disadvantage of gender in the midst of ongoing political and environmental crises. In this chapter, we show how, even when mired in deep poverty, boot camps in each country strengthen social processes (networks, friendships, safe spaces, and participatory platforms) in order to enhance health and economic empowerment for poor girls in their communities. While asset-building programs—the outcomes of the process—have been evaluated, the method of transferring knowledge through boot camps has not yet been measured. This chapter describes the methodology applied and the number of girls reached by girls' programs in Kenya and Haiti to date.

CONTEXT: COMMON VULNERABILITIES ON COMMON GROUND—THE BIRTH OF GIRLS' BOOT CAMPS

In 2006, like-minded researchers from the United States, Kenya, Nigeria, Zimbabwe, Tanzania, and the Democratic Republic of Congo, working with girls at the intersection of health and livelihoods, convened in Nairobi, Kenya, for a conference on data-driven approaches to transform the lives of marginalized girls.[3] Facilitated by the Population Council and the University of California, San Francisco (UCSF), participants from numerous eastern and southern African countries agreed to "confess" program failures and successes in order to design more effective approaches, to transform and evolve current programs, and to bench-mark successes.[4] Common themes surfaced around violence, early marriage, transactional sex, migration, and early school-leaving, all of which systematically exclude adolescent girls from asset-building opportunities. Existing programs for "youth" were not reaching many girls, and programs that targeted girls directly were few.

Themes that emerged in Kenya in 2006 generated an almost identical list of vulnerabilities on the other side of the world, during a boot camp workshop in 2010 in Haiti:

- Girls' human rights are threatened by harmful traditional practices (such as female genital mutilation [FGM] and child marriage), and as economies modernize, the exclusion of girls from full and safe participation in society persists, with rising pressures for poverty-driven sex-for-money exchanges to meet economic and education needs.

- Adolescent girls' morbidity and mortality remain unacceptably high. Rates of some communicable illnesses (e.g., HIV/AIDS) in girls are persistently, and shockingly, higher than those among boys in the same age group.[5]

- Adolescent girls are twice as mobile as adolescent boys, often connected to their gendered disadvantage, "pushed" from rural areas with few opportunities and threats of child marriage and "pulled" to perceived better opportunities in urban areas. Migration does not mitigate exposure to violence, HIV acquisition, and poor reproductive health outcomes. Many migrant girls living apart from one or both parents are out of school and may be engaged in unsafe, exploitative work.[6]

- Political and resulting economic turmoil, as well as environmental catastrophes, heightened civic insecurity, eroding the rights of society's most vulnerable citizens, including young girls.

- Restricted access to existing services is related to girls' relative social isolation and lack of safety, which tends to increase around puberty.[7]

- Much of the infrastructure, entitlements, and approaches (e.g., child health initiatives, civic participation programs, conventionally configured youth initiatives, youth media programs, schooling systems, maternal-child health services such as "safe motherhood" programs, and livelihood programs) do not effectively reach girls in need. When available, they are often culturally inappropriate for girls and/or inaccessible to younger adolescents.[8]

Reflections from the Kenya workshop and emerging research at the time pointed to universal challenges around how to address girls' specific needs to affect change throughout the life cycle. It was from this discussion that the "boot camp" concept was born—a process by which adolescent girls' programs could be developed and strengthened while creating a forum for national cross-learning.

The first official Adolescent Girls Programming Workshop—or boot camp—in Kenya in 2008 was largely founded upon evaluations of the Population Council's global body of adolescent girls' programs. The work of Binti Pamoja (Daughters United)—a program dedicated to strengthening girls' social, health, and economic assets in Kibera, a slum community in Nairobi—also informed the program structure. The Haitian Adolescent Girl Network, referred to locally as Espas Pa Mwen (My Space), rose from the rubble of the catastrophic 2010 earthquake. Some of this learning has since informed the formation of a Girls in Emergencies collaborative,[9] expanding evidence-based, targeted approaches to reaching girls under threat in emergencies arising from conflict, climate change, and infectious diseases such as Ebola. The following sections provide context to girls' struggles in each distinct setting prior to describing the programs that were developed to address them.

Kenya

Kenya has long been considered a generally stable East African country, but indices that define stability have much to do with economic prospects and little to do with the girls and women trapped in inequitable growth.[10] Large-scale national surveys show a country riddled by violence against women and children: the 2008–09 Kenya Demographic and Health Survey described almost half (45%) of 15-to 49-year-old women reporting a lifetime experience with either physical or sexual violence.[11] A review of interpersonal violence in ten developing countries ranked Kenya among the countries with the highest prevalence of reported sexual violence in current relationships (15%),[12] corroborated by a survey concluding that the most common human rights violation in Kenya is domestic violence.[13] The potential for violence begins early in life, with 26% of Kenyan girls marrying before the age of 18, most often to an older man.[14] This is hazardous to the best interests of the girl child, given the health risks of premature pregnancy and foregone education; moreover, early marriages are often arranged contrary to or without the girl's consent. In Kenya, girls who marry early are likely to be at a higher risk of contracting HIV than their unmarried sexually active counterparts. Studies in Kenya and Zambia show that HIV infection rates among married girls are 48–65% higher than among sexually active unmarried girls.[15]

A recent nationally representative study on violence against children shows that one in three girls is likely to suffer some form of sexual violence before the age of 18 years.[16] However, nationally representative studies, such as the Demographic and Health Survey (DHS), can "hide" the true picture of most vulnerable girls as survey data is collected from populations with defined income levels in the country or province. Special studies of subpopulations (i.e., slum communities, out-of-school girls, or married adolescents) are needed to identify geographic and demographic "hot spots" of vulnerability for programmatic targeting.

Haiti

As a failed state, Haiti ranks number 12 behind such countries as Sierra Leone and North Korea, making the general environment far from kind for children.[17] The 2006–2007 Demographic and Health Survey found that 5% of girls (and 3.9% of boys) aged 10–14 were not in school and not living with either parent. Further, it was estimated that up to half a million children lived with nonrelatives as unpaid domestic servants.[18,19] A recent survey estimates that over one-fourth of females (25.7%) and over one-fifth of all males (21.2%) between 18 and 24 years old experienced some form of sexual abuse prior to age 18. Physical abuse is even higher, with 60.5% of females and 57.2% of males between 18 and 24 years old reporting physical violence prior to age 18.[20,21] As in Kenya, early marriage is common, with 30% of girls wed before the age of 18. As many as 74% of girls think wife beating is justified.[22] Not surprisingly, Haiti has the region's highest recorded rates of violence against women and ranks among the highest in the world.[23] One study (2004–2005) found that more than half of the estimated 35,000 sexual assaults in the Port-au-Prince area were of girls under 18,[24] while another study found that among victims of sexual violence seeking help in a Port-au-Prince clinic from 2000 to 2008, 42% were under 18 years old and nearly half of these were 12–14 years old.[25,26] Young people from a vast Port-au-Prince slum reported that violence was a driving force in their lives.[27]

While the situation in Haiti was already critical, the earthquake heightened the issues of violence and children's vulnerability.[28] Estimates made in 2010 suggested 1.5 million Haitian children were affected by the earthquake, with approximately 500,000 children living in extremely vulnerable circumstances.[29] Prior to the earthquake, an estimated 42% of Haitian girls in urban areas lived without parents, many as unpaid domestic servants. After the earthquake, even more girls were living alone or with strangers in dangerous camps, subject to sexual violence, hunger, and lack of access to education or any means of livelihood. At the time, a stark increase in survival-based sexual activity among very young girls, for money or food, was reported. Rape was widespread.[30]

METHODS: "BOOT CAMPS"—AN EVIDENCE-BASED, GIRL-FRIENDLY, AND SEQUENTIAL APPROACH TO PROGRAMMING

In the midst of crises—political, economic, or climatic—boot camps have effectively established girl-centered learning communities, creating a network of organizations developing programs to reach the most vulnerable girls. The basis of boot camps is twofold: first, to use existing national data sequentially to guide programs,[31,32] and second, to build in-country organizational capacity to implement programs that help vulnerable girls build protective assets.

Boot camps are designed to help organizations improve their ability to locate pockets where vulnerable girls reside and to determine which social, health, and economic assets they need as they progress into and through adolescence. Early in life, girls may benefit from birth registration campaigns, immunization outreach, and school enrolment programs, but these interventions typically cease after the age of 6, leading to girls' increasing invisibility. Worldwide, national studies gathering data on children between the ages of 6 and 15 years are few. In response, beginning on the late 1990s, the Population Council created Adolescent Data Guides,[33] drawing principally on data from the Demographic and Health Surveys (DHS), reconfigured and reanalyzed in graphs, tables, and maps (wherever possible) to highlight the situation for males and females ages 10–18 plus young women ages 19–24.[34] A second generation of the guide is even more granular in disaggregating data within smaller geographic areas as well as providing relevant comparisons between and among males and females.[35] The guides, combined with in-country research, inform programs, provoke discussion, and ensure that interventions are based on evidence (see figure 4.1).

Policies and programs that are not data driven ignore large neglected and pivotal subgroups of adolescents, such as 10- to14-year-olds who are out of school. Thus, segmenting vulnerable girls is a critical step in improving reach and tailoring services for youth. During boot camps, participants use the guides to identify high-risk groups of girls by age and location, making it possible to target vulnerable populations and also work with parents and community leaders to establish programs that are likely to make a difference.

For example, the research done in Kenya identified the following segments of girls for the programs:

- Girls (10–14), both in and out of school, who are living in areas where child marriage is prevalent;
- Girls (10–14) who are out of school and not living with parents, facing multiple risks to their health and well-being, including HIV infection;
- Girls who are out of school and engaged in unsafe work;
- Girls and young women (10–24) who are married; and
- Girls (10–19) who have migrated from rural to peri-urban environments

While nearly all girls in Kenya are at risk according to one or more of these criteria, the primary focus was on girls at risk of being married in childhood, acquiring HIV, or both. The segmentation of girls' subpopulations in the list above provides an example of how programs serving girls can use demographic targeting to reach the most vulnerable girls.

In Haiti, the boot camp initiated a similar process. Five months after the earthquake, boot camp program participants were concerned that there were no dedicated programs for girls. They identified five subgroups of girls of special interest:

- Girls who were out of school;
- Girls who had become heads of households due to the loss of a parent or other household head;
- Girls who were disabled;

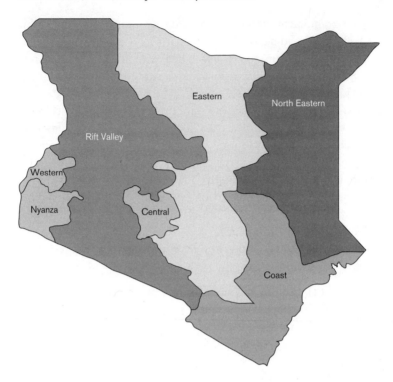

Percentage of 6- to 17-year-old females
who are not in school, by province

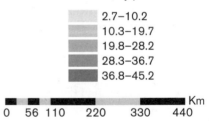

2.7–10.2
10.3–19.7
19.8–28.2
28.3–36.7
36.8–45.2

━━━━━━━━━━━━━━━━━━━━ Km
0   56 110   220   330   440

FIGURE 4.1. Adolescent Data Guide, 6- to 17-year-old females not in school, Kenya, 2007–2008

- Girls who were survivors of sexual assault; and
- Girls who had babies.

This list illustrates how demographic targeting can be used by girls' programs in the context of humanitarian emergencies or other sudden changes in context. Through this exercise, for example, it became clear that Haitian girls with babies were extremely socially isolated and required intensive focused efforts in order to reach them.

In all boot camps, organizations are encouraged to look first to the data to determine where to locate programs—ideally, where there are high concentrations (segments) of girls who are at higher risk because of their age and/or socioeconomic situation. This is a critically important point for program design. These data enable program staff to tailor content, mentorship, and other strategic decisions to the needs of these specific segments of girls.

Once key subgroups are identified by location, risk level, and age, the focus of the boot camp programs is on assisting the organizations to develop segment-specific plans. This includes selecting the meeting venues for girls' groups, choosing appropriate mentors, and building a series of interlinked activities designed to build girls' assets. These assets include social assets (friends, supportive adults, and a safe place for girls' groups to meet), health assets (health knowledge and access to healthcare services), and economic assets (financial literacy, savings, and, ultimately, micro-credit loans). During the boot camps, participants also discuss the evolving capacity of adolescent girls and how they can adjust the asset-building focus as girls increase in age, knowledge, and skill level or as new threats arise in girls' lives. Central to this process is an exercise in which boot camp participants imagine an average 10-year-old girl and decide what assets she needs,[36] progressing in intervals up to the age of 22. Programs with the best results, as we have seen in Kenya and Haiti, are not only practical and relevant to girls' needs but are fun, focused, and engaging.

The Binti Pamoja Center

The Binti Pamoja (Daughters United) Center in Kenya is one example of a program that benefited from its involvement in the initial boot camp in Kenya. Binti Pamoja provides safe spaces and programming for adolescent girls, with a focus on integrated reproductive health information, personal skills and self-esteem development, and financial literacy training. The center started in May 2002 as a women's rights and reproductive health program for adolescent girls in the Kibera slum of Nairobi. Girls and families in Kibera greatly appreciated the provision of services for girls in the midst of this poor community challenged by chronic violence and recurrent ethnic and political clashes. In fact, the staff struggled to retain a reasonable group size given increasing demand by girls to join the program.

In Binti Pamoja's Safe Spaces program, the staff trained and supported alumni to become mentors of younger girls, including supervision, a monthly stipend, and a program budget to run their own girls' groups. Over time, special subgroups were formed for girls who were young mothers, who had disabilities, and who were HIV positive.

While Binti Pamoja provided a forum for intensive health education and personal growth for the members, it was *not* addressing the girls' economic circumstances or the fact that transactional sex was a pervasive activity for adolescent girls in Kibera. At the time, the Global Financial Education Program offered Binti Pamoja an opportunity to develop a financial literacy curriculum for girls and a partnership with the Population Council, and K-Rep Bank enabled the organization to start offering its members girl-friendly savings accounts. Programs addressing poverty often recommend income-generating activities without giving participants the requisite skills they need to understand and manage money smartly and safely; Binti Pamoja's Safe Spaces Program provided both. The spin-off effect of this model has been remarkable.

While the direct reach of Binti Pamoja is relatively small in terms of numbers, it has informed best practices in adolescent girls' programming in Kenya and beyond. Dozens of similar organizations that participated in the Kenyan boot camps benefited from a concrete example of how girl-centered programming can be achieved. In addition, several larger programs modeled after Binti Pamoja now reach large numbers of girls. Critical learnings from Binti Pamoja on combining safe spaces and financial education and on the need for savings accounts led to the development of the Safe and Smart Savings Program for Vulnerable Adolescent Girls, which has engaged four financial institutions in Kenya and Uganda and now reaches over 12,000 girls. The program was also replicated with over 10,000 girls in both urban and rural areas of Zambia through the Adolescent Girls Empowerment Program. In addition, the best practices documented by Binti Pamoja have made their way into the mainstream adolescent girls' programming language, shaping the work of bilateral, multilateral, and private donors related to adolescent girls, ultimately affecting over a million girls.[37]

The Haitian Adolescent Girl Network: Espas Pa Mwen

The Haiti Adolescent Girl Network (HAGN),[38] locally referred to as Espas Pa Mwen (My Space), is a coalition of humanitarian organizations launched in 2010 in response to the alarming situation of young girls in post-earthquake Haiti, especially in internally displaced persons' camps. HAGN focused on addressing sexual violence and the immediate need for safe spaces within and outside camps, as well as education, skills-building, and girls' empowerment programs.

Without basic infrastructure and bereft of a safe, private space adolescent girls could not build much-needed social capital and economic assets. To remedy this, Espas Pa Mwen established programs in seventeen sites, with over forty participating organizations. It currently serves over 1,000 adolescent girls who meet at least once a week to share experiences, learn and play.

Mentors serve as bridges to help adolescent girls access services, negotiate family challenges, and navigate school settings and unsafe communities. A month into the programming, the network distributed dignity kits (small kits with basic hygiene supplies) to 450 adolescents. It also delivered core program content, including thirty hours of materials in Haitian Creole in sexual and reproductive health, leadership, community engagement, preventing and addressing violence, psychosocial support, financial literacy,[39] and water and sanitation.

The "spaces" that first emerged in Haiti were often around therapeutic services since girls had lost so much: their homes, their parents, and, hence, their sense of direction. The curriculum addresses health and developmental rights through photography, theatre, and art. With young teenage girls serving as mentors, the curriculum for very young girls was adapted to the age group and taught through music and storytelling, strong cultural traditions in Haiti. In subsequent generations of the program, the emphasis changed, distinguishing the needs of in-school girls from the more vulnerable out-of-school girls. Community mapping helped recruit the most socially isolated girls, such as those with babies. An important addition was the integration of an age-graded, Haitian Creole financial literacy program developed by a consortium of Making Cents, Save the Children, FONKOZE (a large Haitian microfinance institution), and Espas Pa Mwen.

An Espas Pa Mwen leader identified these priorities for a strong network:

- A collaborative and carefully built learning environment, as organizations in emergency contexts may not come together with a sense of shared trust.

- An effective process for defining catchment areas—often requiring house-to-house surveys using GPS for targeted recruitment—because demand-led recruitment may bypass invisible segments of adolescent girl populations.

- An articulate voice for participating organizations so they can advocate for creating girl-only spaces. This signals a transformation for girls and a transformation in the organizational culture of traditional NGOs.

- A network coordinator who can connect actors and organizations at various levels and share adaptable, open-source materials.

- A defined meeting space reserved for use by adolescent girls during specific periods of time. This guarantees both physical security and aural privacy.[40]

- Engaging and participatory pedagogical tools and approaches that enable girls to build health, social, and economic skills.

- Giving mentors basic financial security through small stipends in recognition of their value and of the fact that mentors often face the same pressures as the adolescent girls they serve. This has provoked some resistance from traditional NGOs, who are accustomed to volunteer mentors.

HAGN fosters the practice of creating girl-only spaces, with gender-specific and age-graded programming to replace "child-friendly" spaces that can overlook the particular needs of young adolesecent girls or "women's programs" that tend to attract adult women rather than girls. Further, it expanded conventionally configured content for girls to go beyond the risks of violence and other health issues to include financial literacy.

It also inspired the Sierra Leone Adolescent Girls Network, which has over thirty member organizations and is in the process of rolling out 240 girls' clubs. Plans were set in place before the Ebola outbreak, but the initiative took on a particular salience when Ebola cut off entire communities. Developing local capacity, particularly of adolescent girl caregivers at risk of transmission, was crucial. Clubs now reach different segments of girls, including once-quarantined households. With the support of a local communications program, the network offers mentored girls' groups nonformal education and financial literacy and has introduced protective and productive technologies such as solar-powered lanterns.

RESULTS: BUILDING GIRLS' MOVEMENTS, ONE COUNTRY AT A TIME

Binti Pamoja and HAGN/Espas Pa Mwen have contributed to building girls' movements in their respective countries in very different ways. Binti Pamoja's focused work in one community allowed for experimentation and the testing of various girl-friendly methodologies. The work of Binti Pamoja gave birth to the boot camp trainings, providing many of the formative lessons for how to work with girls. The program also recognized the importance of working with adults (particularly parents) in the community to support girls through innovative parent-oriented activities. Tools developed by Binti Pamoja, captured in a multilingual toolkit available online, make it possible for girls' programming staff across the world to learn about strategies for early empowerment.[41]

Haiti's catastrophic earthquake not only proved to be a trigger bringing global attention to Haiti's poor but also provided a strong rationale to introduce new resources to help girls. When donor interest turned to Haiti, HAGN/Espas Pa Mwen provided the justification for girl-only platforms, given the huge increase in sexual violence resulting from severe social disruption in an already fragile society. Today twenty-five different organizations, including international and local NGOs, grassroots groups, and technical organizations are collaborating to create a network of girl-only spaces as a permanent feature in Haiti. This has inspired girls' programs in other countries where emergencies are all too common.

Combined, the work in Kenya and Haiti has been a catalyst for change on a larger scale, applied in at least twenty countries—including Burkina Faso, Niger, Sierra Leone, Benin, Nigeria, Uganda, Tanzania, Mozambique, Zambia, Guatemala, Mexico, Belize, El Salvador, and Nicaragua.

Evaluation of Adolescent Girls' Programming

Years of experience with adolescent girls' programming has yielded many important findings, but among these are three pillars essential to sustainable gains for girls. We review them here.[42]

1. Expanding girls' access to *safe and supportive spaces* that girls can rely on at home, in schools and in the community is the first

pillar of programming. Program planners need to create girl-only spaces because public spaces are often dominated by men, and, as noted, youth centers are often frequented by older adolescent males and even men in their twenties.[43] Potential locations identified by girls' groups include under trees and in community halls, village homes, churches, schools, and even empty shipping containers.[44,45] Identifying an appropriate space is a participatory exercise taught during boot camp sessions, using community mapping of locations where girls feel safe. This is often followed by exercises to identify key community stakeholders and gate-keepers, so that obtaining permission to use the space is a calculated part of the community-wide awareness of girls' empowerment processes.

2. Building *female mentors* into program structures is the second pillar essential to girls' empowerment. Practice shows that the best mentors are young women from the community with whom the girls can identify.[46] Mentors are ideally "on call" for girl participants, serving as critical role models and helping to adapt and implement the curriculum. In contrast to peer educators, mentors are always slightly older than the girls for whom the program is designed. Local girls who have managed to beat the odds and remain in school are often ideal mentors because they have a solid understanding of the local context and are often eager to serve in a leadership capacity.

3. Creating safe spaces inevitably leads to establishing *social networks*, the third pillar of successful adolescent girl programming. Many studies point to the importance of social networks for good health,[47,48,49] but social isolation is a common phenomenon among young girls worldwide.[50] In poor communities, sisters, mothers, aunts and grandmothers, traditionally key figures of social support, are often missing or earning income for the family away from home. The arrival of puberty decreases a girl's access to friends and curtails her freedom to move around the community. Puberty often coincides with school-leaving, increased domestic chores, or preparations for marriage. All of these events lead to precariously thin friendships and social networks, leaving girls without places to stay when they are in danger and without friends from whom they can borrow money in the event of an emergency.[51,52]

The boot camp process and accompanying follow-on mentorship has catalyzed change at three levels: (1) the level of the girl, (2) the level of the organization, and (3) ultimately, the level of the community. Local organizations have benefited from boot camps with exposure to best practices in girls programming, including sound monitoring and evaluation practices, and from attending workshops and receiving one-on-one mentoring. Community-based platforms anchor this approach. Programming helps engage girls in strong networks that enable them to individually and collectively capture the resources they deserve. Finally, the momentum achieved by the large number of programs, networks, and working groups focused on adolescent girls has created a change in orientation at the national level and among key donors. Altering perspectives within the development world is no easy task. Yet, key decision makers are now realizing the importance of investing in adolescent girls by shifting resource allocations and facing the challenges of building capacity. Documentation on the impact of these programs worldwide shows that without dedicated efforts, adolescent girls in the poorest communities will be left behind. The unlearning agenda is sometimes larger than the learning agenda.

LESSONS LEARNED: MONITORING (AND MAINTAINING) GAINS FOR GIRLS

Country-Level Challenges

Assessing the impact of these programs is not simple because many effects may not be seen until years later—and translating prevention into evidence is always difficult.[53] However, many asset-building programs for adolescent girls have had measurable impacts on widely validated benchmarks such as delays in the age of marriage,[54] more realistic HIV risk perception, better reproductive health practices,[55] and improved social capital among socially isolated girls.[56] A recent review of the costs of such programs examined five diverse examples.[57] A longitudinal, randomized cluster design study that will assess the impact of an asset-building program for vulnerable girls ages 10 to 19 in Zambia on HIV and human simplex virus (HSV)-2 prevalence, age at marriage, age at first birth, age at first sex, and educational attainment started in 2013. This study will provide unprecedented, rigorous data on the impact of such programs. In the meantime, keeping programs funded and sustainable is likely to be difficult without evidence. In Haiti and Kenya, funding, and in some cases follow-up programming, had to be supported by a network of forward-thinking individuals, agencies, and foundations.[58]

Where girls' programs have been established, structural barriers persist. High levels of interest among girls to participate in programs often lead to waiting lists and overcrowding. In opposition to this keen interest, girls worldwide wrestle with the demands of other obligations. Shifting these structural burdens of household work will remain an ongoing challenge for girls living in poverty.

Continent- and Global-Level Challenges

There is growing recognition of the critical role that adolescent girls play in development. This is evidenced by recent initiatives of the World Bank, the United Nations, and global partners such as the Adolescent Girls Initiative, the Sahel Women's Empowerment and Demographic Dividend Project, The Girls in Emergencies Collaborative, and Together for Girls. These global consortiums are working to coordinate efforts by harnessing the latest data on girls, putting knowledge into practice, and making it clear that sustainable development will be difficult without a prioritization of girls' needs. Girl-centered work, at the global level, is often criticized as discriminating against the "boy-child" even though there is evidence that for certain periods of time, girls need girl-only spaces to flourish.

Where girl-centered policies are taking hold, there is still a gap in programming with little international commitment for needed capacity and funding on the ground. This is complicated by the fact that girls' needs, and often the services required to ensure their safety, are multisectoral (i.e., social, health, and economic), but typically these fields of development are separated by funding streams, policy, and even expertise.

CONCLUSION: MAKING GIRLS VISIBLE

Compared to boys, girls experience more gender-based violence and social isolation, weaker social networks, and greater financial responsibilities in the household.[59] Girls with the weakest social networks are at highest risk. Strikingly, they are also the least likely to benefit from conventionally configured youth programs and policies. Reversing these troubling trends requires commitment to building the protective assets of adolescent girls through developing the capacity of those who design and implement programs for them.

Boot camps, and the evolution of the organizations that participate in them, explicitly fill the gap between shifting global policy and advocacy efforts that have increased recognition of the needs of adolescent girls but lack the ground capacity and programs to directly reach those girls. In Kenya and Haiti, boot camps provided the first important step of early empowerment—providing training, support, and in some cases, funding to participating organizations. This enables programs to reach girls who are at the height of risk but who are also the most likely to be their own agents for change. In the end, this is what early empowerment is all about.

Box 4.1. Summary

Geographic area: Kenya and Haiti.

Global importance of the health condition: With over 600 million girls in the developing world, wise investments are needed to reach the most vulnerable. The best advocacy for adolescent girls is successful on-the-ground programs supported by local champions, but youth programs need to be reoriented by age and gender to engage marginalized subgroups of adolescent girls.

Intervention or program: Adolescent girls' programming "boot camps" are a three-part process designed to protect and empower adolescent girls through developing the capacity of those who design and implement programs for them. Participating organizations (1) work with a "girl expert" to draft an initial program plan for new or existing programs, (2) attend a workshop to improve their plan after learning about best practices in girls' programming, and (3) finalize their plan and implement the program. Boot camps enhance national cross-learning by inviting organizations from different regions to learn together and build their network.

Impact: The boot camp approach has achieved impact at three levels: (1) individual, (2) organizational, and (3) national. Nearly 5,000 Kenyan girls benefited from girl-centered programming implemented by the organizations that participated in the first Kenyan boot camp in 2006. Half of these girls have received small subgrants from the Kenya Brain Trust. In Haiti, 1,270 girls benefited from girl-centered programming through twenty-six organizations that were influenced by the 2010 and 2011 boot camps. Over time, these and other outcomes will also be measurable at the national level through emerging evidence to shift policies and practice to squarely address girls' needs.*

Lessons learned: Prevailing programmatic paradigms not only fail to include girls, but they can in some cases intensify their exclusion, discourage them, and even render them more vulnerable. A good program plan is a start, but it is not enough. Organizations need capacity building and funding to effectively target vulnerable girls and to make lasting impact. This requires buy-in from the heads of organizations. Finally, better evaluations are needed to show which type of girl-centered programs work best and how.

Link between empowerment and health: Intergenerational poverty; high, unwanted fertility; and poor health have common roots in the early adolescence of poor girls. Developing the capacity of stakeholders to build the health, social, and economic assets of vulnerable subgroups of adolescents as an empowerment strategy is critical.

*In addition to the boot camps described in detail in the chapter, five others have been held (four in sub-Saharan Africa) reaching over sixty additional organizations.

Box 4.2. Challenges for Girls' Programming Boot Camps in Kenya and Haiti and How to Overcome Them

CONSTRAINTS TO GIRLS' PROGRAMMING SUCCESS

Gender inclusion: Allowing boys to dominate youth programs versus maintaining girl-only spaces.

Organizational change: Traditional peer programming dominates girl-led, participatory methods.

Funding: Challenge of securing funding for programs following the boot camps.

Lack of evidence: Inadequate organizational capacity to build strong prevention evaluations.

Technical assistance: Challenge of providing ongoing technical assistance to support novel participatory processes.

HOW THESE CONSTRAINTS WERE OVERCOME

Gender inclusion: Determine program's "typical client" through a careful review of girls' vulnerability in the area, using data to shed light on the program's actual reach.

Organizational change: Invite two participants per organization— at management and field levels.

Funding: This has not been overcome and remains a challenge.

Lack of evidence: Investing in up-front funding for evaluation as part of the program.

Technical assistance: Funding staff time to provide technical support (which remains a challenge) and training local girl experts in order to leave expertise at the country level after the boot camp "faculty" go home.

WHAT NEEDS TO HAPPEN FOR SIMILAR GIRLS' PROGRAMMING TO SCALE UP?

Gender inclusion: Support organizations to make a strong, evidence-based case for girls-only spaces. However, concerns that we are neglecting the boys will continue.

Organizational change: Ensure top-level commitment to make investments in girls' programs (including staff) prior to starting the boot camp process.

Funding: Programs that come to boot camps with funding appear more likely to succeed.

Lack of evidence: Program design must be as evidence-based as possible; thus, encouraging at least basic evaluation at a level that the program can handle is essential.

Technical assistance: Funding for boot camps must include faculty time before, during, and after the boot camp.

NOTES

1. Calculated by John Bongaarts, Population Council, based on United Nations Department of Economic and Social Affairs, Population Division, 2013, *World Population Prospects: The 2012 Revision,* New York: United Nations, http://esa.un.org/wpp/documentation/pdf/wpp2012_%20key%20findings.pdf.

2. Atkinson, Holly G., and Judith Bruce. 2015. "Adolescent Girls, Human Rights, and the Expanding Climate Emergency." *Annals of Global Health Press* 81 (3): 323–330.

3. Boot camps were and continue to be implemented around the world. The first prototype was in Guatemala (2004), followed by Kenya (2008); Liberia (2009); Zambia, Burkina Faso, and Haiti (2010); Tanzania (2011); Nicaragua (2012); and Kenya (2013).

4. These countries included Ethiopia, Kenya, Tanzania, South Africa, and Zimbabwe. See Summary document from 2006. Adolescent Girls' Social Support and Livelihood Program Design Workshop, Nairobi, Kenya, sponsored by Population Council and University of California, San Francisco, March 22–23. www.popcouncil.org/pdfs/2006AdolGirlsWorkshopReport.pdf.

5. Bruce, Judith, and Kelly Hallman. 2008. "Reaching the Girls Left Behind." *Gender and Development* 16 (2) July 1: 227–245. www.popcouncil.org/pdfs/JournalArticles/GD_16_2.pdf

6. Temin, Miriam, Mark R. Montgomery, Sarah Engebretsen, and Kathryn M. Barker. 2013. *Girls on the Move: Adolescent Girls and Migration in the Developing World.* New York: Population Council. www.popcouncil.org/research/girls-on-the-move-adolescent-girls-migration-in-the-developing-world.

7. Hallman, Kelly K., Nora J. Kenworthy, Judith Diers, Nick Swan, and Bashi Devnarain. 2015. The Shrinking World of Girls at Puberty: Violence and Gender-Divergent Access to the Public Sphere among Adolescents in South Africa. *Global Public Health: An International Journal for Research Policy and Practice* 10 (3): 1–17. www.tandfonline.com/doi/abs/10.1080/17441692.2014.964746#.Vb-Q36bB9ek. (published online October 10, 2014)

8. Bruce and Hallman, "Reaching the Girls Left Behind," 2008.

9. The Girls in Emergencies (GIE) Working Group grew out of the GIE workshop of the Adolescent Girls Learning Circle led by the Population Council and its steering committee, which includes representatives from major organizations such as the International Rescue Committee, Mercy Corps, Plan International, USAID, the Women's Refugee Commission, and the Human Rights Program, Arnhold Institute for Global Health at Mount Sinai. See GIE Collaborative. 2015. "Statement and Action Agenda from the Girls in Emergencies Collaborative." *Annals of Global Health* 81 (3) May–June: 331–332. www.sciencedirect.com/science/article/pii/S2214999615012205?np=y

10. Blanchard, Lauren. 2013. "U.S.-Kenya Relations: Current Political and Security Issues." *CRS Report for Congress.* Washington, DC: Congressional Research Service 7-5700 R42967, September 23. https://www.fas.org/sgp/crs/row/R42967.pdf.

11. Kenya National Bureau of Statistics (KNBS) and ICF Macro. 2010. "Kenya: Demographic and Health Survey 2008–09." Calverton, MD: KNBS and ICF Macro. www.measuredhs.com/pubs/pdf/FR229/FR229.pdf.

12. Hindin, Michelle, Kishor Sunita, and Donna L. Ansara. 2008. *Intimate Partner Violence among Couples in 10 DHS Countries: Predictors and Health Outcomes.* DHS Analytical Studies No. 18, December. Calverton, MD: Macro International. www.measuredhs.com/pubs/pdf/AS18/AS18.pdf.

13. Kimuna, Sitawa, and Yanyi K. Djamba. 2008. "Gender Based Violence: Correlates of Physical and Sexual Wife Abuse in Kenya." *Journal of Family Violence* 23 (5) July: 333–342.

14. UNICEF. 2013. "Child Protection: Child Marriage." UNICEF Data: Monitoring the Situation of Women and Children. www.childinfo.org/marriage_countrydata.php.

15. Longmans, Carine, and Wendy Graham. 2006. "Maternal Mortality: Who, When, Where And Why." *Lancet* 368 (9542) September 30: 1189–1200. www.thelancet.com/journals/lancet/article/PIIS0140-6736(06)69380-X/abstract.

16. UNICEF Kenya Country Office, U.S. Centers for Disease Control and Prevention, National Center for Injury Prevention and Control, Division of Violence Prevention, and the Kenya National Bureau of Statistics. 2012. *Violence against Children in Kenya: Findings from a 2010 National Survey.* Nairobi, Kenya: UNICEF. www.unicef.org/esaro/VAC_in_Kenya.pdf.

17. "2009 Failed States Index-Interactive Map and Rankings." 2009. *Foreign Policy,* June 21. http://foreignpolicy.com/2009/06/22/2009-failed-states-index-interactive-map-and-rankings/.

18. UNICEF. Updated December 27, 2013. "Statistics." At a glance: Haiti. www.unicef.org/infobycountry/haiti_statistics.html.

19. *The Adolescent Experience In-depth: Using Data to Identify and Reach the Most Vulnerable Young People: Haiti 2005/06.* 2009. New York: Population Council. www.popcouncil.org/uploads/pdfs/PGY_AdolDataGuides/Haiti2005–06.pdf.

20. Interuniversity Institute for Research and Development, Comité de Coordination. 2014. *Violence against Children in Haiti: Findings from a National Survey, 2012.* Port-au-Prince, Haiti: Centers for Disease Control and Prevention. www.cdc.gov/violenceprevention/pdf/violence-haiti.pdf.

21. UNICEF. 2013.

22. *Haiti Demographic and Health Survey 2005–2006.* 2006. Global Health Data Exchange. Seattle, WA: Institute for Health Metrics and Evaluation, University of Washington. http://ghdx.healthdata.org/record/haiti-demographic-and-health-survey-2005–2006.

23. Kambou, Sarah D. 2010. "Rebuilding Efforts Should Focus on Women to Make a Difference." Commentary: Women Are the Epicenter of Haiti's Renewal. Washington, DC: International Center for Research on Women. www.icrw.org/media/news/commentary-women-are-epicenter-haiti's-renewal.

24. Kolbe, Athena, and Royce Hutson. 2006. "Human Rights Abuse and Other Criminal Violations in Port-au-Prince, Haiti: A Random Survey of Households." *Lancet* 368 (9538): 1189–1199. www.ijdh.org/pdf/Lancet%20Article%208-06.pdf.

25. GHESKIO (Groupe Haitien d'Étude du Sarcome de Kaposi et des Infections Opportunistes). 2010. "Sexual Violence in Haiti: GHESKIO's Response and Recommendations." Report produced for USAID Haiti, January 31. Port-au-Prince, Haiti: Les Centres Gheskio, Institut National de Laboratoire et de Recherches (INLR).

26. Reza, Avid, Matthew Breiding, Curtis Blanton, et al. 2007. *A National Study on Violence against Children and Young Women in Swaziland,* October. Mbabane, Swaziland: Swaziland UNICEF and U.D. Centers for Disease Control and Prevention. www.unicef.org/swaziland/Violence_study_report.pdf.

27. Wilman, Ania, and Louis Herns Marceling. 2010. "'If they could make us disappear, they would!'—Youth and Violence in Cité Soleil, Haiti." *Journal of Community Psychology* 38: 515–31. http://hdl.handle.net/10986/5391.

28. U.S. Department of State, Office of the Haiti Special Coordinator. 2012. "State Department Fact Sheet on Gender-Based Violence in Haiti." IIP Digital. November 26. http://iipdigital.usembassy.gov/st/english/texttrans/2012/11/20121126139127.html#axzz2puC4YF1s.

29. UNICEF Haiti. 2010. *Children of Haiti: Milestones and Looking Forward Six Months.* Port-au-Prince, Haiti: UNICEF, July. www.unicef.org/emerg/files/UNICEF_Haiti_-_Six_Months_Report_Final.pdf.

30. Amnesty International, International Secretariat. 2011. *Haiti: Aftershocks—Women Speak Out against Sexual Violence in Haiti's Camps.* London, UK: Amnesty International. AMR 36/001/2011, January. www.amnesty.org/en/library/asset/AMR36/001/2011/en/57237fad-f97b-45ce-8fdb-68cb457a304c/amr3600120011en.pdf.

31. Engebretsen, Sarah. 2012. *Using Data to See and Select the Most Vulnerable Adolescent Girls.* New York: Population Council. July. www.popcouncil.org/uploads/pdfs/2012PGY_GirlsFirst_Data.pdf

32. Austrian, Karen, and Dennitah Ghati. 2010. *Girl-Centered Program Design: A Toolkit to Develop, Strengthen, and Expand Adolescent Girls Programs.* New York: Population Council. www.popcouncil.org/research/girl-centered-program-design-a-toolkit-to-develop-strengthen-and-expand-ado.

33. The Population Council series *The Adolescent Experience In-Depth: Using Data to Identify and Reach the Most Vulnerable Young People* can be accessed at www.popcouncil.org/research/the-adolescent-experience-in-depth-using-data-to-identify-and-reach-th.

34. Population Council. 2009. *The Adolescent Experience In-Depth: Using Data to Identify and Reach the Most Vulnerable Young People: Haiti 2005/06.* New York: Population Council. www.popcouncil.org/pdfs/PGY_AdolDataGuides/Haiti2005–06.pdf.

35. Hallman, Kelly, Ilan Cerna-Turoff, and Neema Matee. 2015. *Participatory Research Results from Training with the Mabinti Tushike Hatamu Out-of-School Girls Program: Tanzania 2015.* New York: Population Council. www.popcouncil.org/uploads/pdfs/2015PGY_TanzaniaParticipatoryResults.pdf.

36. *Building Assets Toolkit: Developing Positive Benchmarks for Adolescent Girls.* 2015. New York: Population Council, July. www.popcouncil.org/research/building-assets-toolkit-developing-positive-benchmarks-for-adolescent-girls.

37. Some of the notable bilateral and multilateral agencies affected by the Binti Pamoja program include the Nike Foundation, the World Bank's Adolescent Girls' Initiative, the United Kingdom's Department for International Development, the NoVo Foundation, and UNICEF.

38. More information about the Haitian Adolescent Girls Network can be found at http://haitigirlsnetwork.org/.

39. The financial education module was developed by Making Cents International to help educate girls around money matters, especially in the absence of banks for the poor and disenfranchised.

40. Siddiqi, Anooradha. 2012. *Missing the Emergency: Shifting the Paradigm for Relief to Adolescent Girls*. Washington, DC: Coalition for Adolescent Girls and United Nations Foundation. May. http://humanitarianlibrary.org /sites/default/files/2014/02/2012-05-23-Missing-the-Emergency-FINAL1%20 %281%29.pdf.

41. *The Girl-Centered Program Design: A Toolkit to Develop, Strengthen & Expand Adolescent Girls Programs* (www.popcouncil.org/publications/books /2010_AdolGirlsToolkit.asp) is targeted towards those working with adolescent girls ages 10–24.

42. Bruce, Judith. 2015. "Commentary: Investing in the Poorest Girls in the Poorest Communities Early Enough to Make a Difference." *Global Public Health: An International Journal for Research, Policy, and Practice* 10 (22): 225–227.

43. Youth centers typically define youth as 15 to 30 (or even 35). Males may join "youth" programs as younger adolescents but often a core of regulars remain well into their later years. Most youth center directors are male as well, and unless special efforts are made, these male spaces become unsafe for females.

44. Austrian, Karen. 2012. *Girl's Leadership and Mentoring*. New York: Population Council and UN Adolescent Girls Task Force. www.popcouncil.org /pdfs/2012PGY_GirlsFirst_Leadership.pdf.

45. Catino, Jennifer, Alejandra Colom, and Marta Julia Ruiz. 2011. "Equipping Mayan Girls to Improve Their Lives." *Promoting Healthy, Safe, and Productive Transition to Adulthood*. Brief no. 5, March. www.popcouncil.org /pdfs/TABriefs/05_MayanGirls.pdf.

46. Austrian, Karen. 2007. "Expanding Safe Spaces and Developing Skills for Adolescent Girls." *Promoting Healthy, Safe, and Productive Transitions to Adulthood*, Brief no. 29, October. New York: Population Council. http://citeseerx.ist .psu.edu/viewdoc/download?rep=rep1&type=pdf&doi=10.1.1.175.8209.

47. Bruce, Judith. 2007. "Reaching the Girls Left Behind: Targeting Adolescent Programming for Equity, Social Inclusion, Health, and Poverty Alleviation." Prepared for Financing Gender Equality: A Commonwealth Perspective, at Commonwealth Women's Affairs Ministers' Meeting, Kampala, Uganda, June 11–14. www.epfweb.org/userfiles/gallery/globalconferences/G8/Paris/Bruce .pdf. (accessed January 6, 2013)

48. Erulkar, Annabel, Semunegus Belaynesh, and Gebeyehu Mekonnen. 2010. "Biruh Tesfa Program Provides Domestic Workers, Orphans and Migrants in Urban Ethiopia with Social Support, HIV Education, and Skills." *Promoting Healthy, Safe, and Productive Transitions to Adulthood*, Brief no. 21. New York: Population Council. www.popcouncil.org/pdfs/TABriefs/21_ BiruhTesfa.pdf.

49. Erulkar, Annabel, and Eunice Muthengi. 2007. *Evaluation of Berhane Hewan: A Pilot Program to Promote Education and Delay Marriage in Rural Ethiopia*. New York: Population Council. http://dspace.cigilibrary.org/jspui /handle/123456789/24798.

50. Hallman, Kelly, Nora Kenworthy, Judith Diers, Nick Swan, Bashi Devnarain, and Nonkululeko Mthembu. 2013. "The Contracting World of

Girls at Puberty: Violence and Gender-Divergent Access to the Public Sphere among Adolescents in South Africa." *Poverty, Gender and Youth Working Paper* no. 25. New York: Population Council. http://popcouncil.org/pdfs/wp/pgy/025.pdf.

51. Erulkar, Annabel, Tekle-Ab Mekbib, Negussie Simie, and Tsehai Gulema. 2004. *Adolescent Life in Low Income and Slum Areas of Addis Ababa, Ethiopia.* New York: Population Council. www.popcouncil.org/uploads/pdfs/AdolescentLife.pdf.

52. Hallman, Kelly. 2008. "Researching the Determinants of Vulnerability to HIV among Adolescents." *IDS Bulletin* 39 (5) January 26: 36–44. http://onlinelibrary.wiley.com/.

53. Chong, Erica, Kelly Hallman, and Martha Brady. 2006. *Investing When It Counts: Generating the Evidence Base for Policies and Programmes for Very Young Adolescents.* New York: UNFPA and Population Council. https://www.unfpa.org/public/global/publications/pid/363.

54. Erulkar and Muthengi, *Evaluation of Berhane Hewan,* 2007.

55. Hallman, Kelly. 2005. "Gendered Socioeconomic Conditions and HIV Risk Behaviours among Young People in South Africa." *African Journal of AIDS Research* 4(1): 37–50. www.tandfonline.com/doi/abs/10.2989/16085900509490340.

56. Erulkar, Annabel, Abebaw Ferede, Woldemariam Girma, and Worku Ambelu. 2013. "Evaluation of 'Biruh Tesfa' (Bright Future) Program for Vulnerable Girls in Ethiopia." *Vulnerable Children and Youth Studies* 8 (2): 182–192. www.tandfonline.com/doi/full/10.1080/17450128.2012.736645.

57. Sewall-Menon, Jessica, Judith Bruce, Karen Austrian, Raven Brown, Jennifer Catino, Alejandra Colom, Angel Del Valle, Habtamu Demele, Annabel Erulkar, Kelly Hallman, Eva Roca, and Nadia Zibani. 2012. *The Cost of Reaching the Most Disadvantaged Girls: Programmatic Evidence from Egypt, Ethiopia, Guatemala, Kenya, South Africa, and Uganda.* New York: Population Council. www.popcouncil.org/pdfs/2012PGY_CostOfReachingGirls.pdf.

58. Haiti support: Nike Foundation, Population Council, AmeriCares, Abundance Foundation, NoVo Foundation, Procter & Gamble, Partridge Foundation, American Jewish World Service, Benenson Family Foundation, United Nations Foundation, Elissa Epstein, Soroptimist, EarthSpark International, Cindy Simon, and Anonymous. Kenya support: Nike Foundation, NoVo Foundation, Unbound Philanthropy, Anonymous, and the Packard Foundation.

59. Bruce, "Reaching the Girls Left Behind" 2007.

5

Empowerment and HIV Risk Reduction among Sex Workers in Bangladesh

VICTOR ROBINSON, THERESA Y. HWANG,
AND ELISA MARTÍNEZ

Empowerment processes are highly context dependent. Empowerment takes place in the context of individual lives embedded in relationships, institutional structures and cultural constructs. To understand the empowerment of sex workers and its relationship to HIV risk reduction, one must understand the environment in which sex workers live and work.

The international development organization, CARE, defines women's empowerment as "the sum total of changes needed for a woman to realize her full human rights."[1] The CARE model emphasizes three dimensions of empowerment: agency (a woman's aspirations and capabilities), structure (the environment that surrounds and conditions a woman's choices), and relations (the power relations through which she negotiates her path).[2] Research in 2007–2008 under CARE's Strategic Impact Inquiry (SII) on Women's Empowerment applied this framework in examining CARE Bangladesh's HIV prevention work with sex workers between 1995 and 2005. The research focused on developing a deeper understanding of the nature of empowerment and the role of empowerment processes in HIV prevention. In this chapter, CARE's intervention with sex workers in Bangladesh will be examined through the lens of the SII research.

The first case of HIV in Bangladesh was identified in 1989. Although HIV prevalence in Bangladesh is low in the general population, a concentrated epidemic was first identified in 2006 among male injecting drug users (IDU). Like IDUs, commercial sex workers are highly vulnerable to HIV infection. There are an estimated 100,000 to 150,000 commercial sex workers in Bangladesh, and their risk of contracting HIV is heightened due to economic insecurity and limited power in negotiating condom use with concurrent sexual partners.

In 1995, CARE's SHAKTI (Stopping HIV/AIDS through Knowledge and Training Initiative) project became the first nationwide HIV program in Bangladesh to work with brothel-based sex workers. Most SHAKTI staff had no prior experience working in a brothel environment. They planned to implement a traditional array of HIV prevention strategies (behavior change, condom distribution, educational programming, STI services, etc.) but soon realized the sex workers faced so many challenges in their lives that they were not going to attend to HIV messages unless the intervention also spoke to more immediate concerns. Over the next ten years, CARE developed a more holistic approach, drawing on lessons learned from the innovative Sonagachi project, SHIP.

The Sonagachi project, widely regarded as a model intervention with sex workers, was initiated in Kolkata, India, in 1991 under the name SHIP (Sexually Transmitted Disease/HIV Intervention Project). A 2004 journal article coauthored by the leader of SHIP, Dr. Samarajit Jana, identified the core innovation emerging from Sonagachi:

> By redefining sex work as employment, and increasingly engaging sex workers in roles of power and decision making within the program, a set of principles emerged that assisted in reframing the problem of HIV from an issue of individual motivation, will, or behavioral commitment to a problem of community disenfranchisement.[3]

Dr. Jana brought this experience with him to work with CARE on the SHAKTI project in Bangladesh.

SHAKTI's first major intervention was a response to sex worker reports that they were not using mainstream health services because health workers' interactions with them made them feel "disgrace" and "shame."[4] SHAKTI helped the sex workers develop an on-site clinic in the brothel, training sex workers to manage clinic activities while training health care workers in nondiscriminatory care. Within eighteen months of opening, management and all nonmedical activities of the clinic were run by the sex workers themselves.

In 1997, SHAKTI extended its work to street-based sex workers in Dhaka, establishing outreach centers to provide clinical services, educational materials, and safe spaces where street-based sex workers could bathe, rest, sleep, connect with their peers, and obtain meals. Fifty-two of these drop-in centers were established and are now managed by the sex workers themselves.

As social stigma and violence against sex workers emerged as critical issues, SHAKTI began to focus on advocacy training, coalition-building, public education through media, and direct interaction with police.[5] In 1998, the project facilitated the formation of two self-help groups: Durjoy Nari Sangha (DNS; Invincible Women's Organization), which represented street-based sex workers in Dhaka, and Nari Mukti Sangha (NMS; Women's Liberation Organization), which represented brothel-based sex workers in Tangail. In subsequent years, the project implemented many of its activities through these two organizations.[6]

In this chapter, we will seek to answer these questions:

- What is the context for street-based sex work in Dhaka and for brothel-based sex work in Tangail?
- What challenges do sex workers face in each of those environments?
- How do the women engaged in SHAKTI define empowerment?
- How did SHAKTI contribute to women's empowerment?
- What links between changing levels of women's empowerment and women's vulnerabilities to HIV were suggested by the research?

METHODS

This study is one of six country studies in the final phase of CARE's 2005–2009 global Strategic Impact Inquiry (SII) focused on women's empowerment and its relationship to HIV vulnerability.

The global research design emphasized using women's own views of empowerment in the local context to ground the research framework and guide data analysis. Specifically, this study focused on the context of power, which both reinforces and limits the empowerment of sex workers in Bangladesh, and the context of women's lives and aspirations that gives meaning to the empowerment process. This was consistent with CARE's commitment to rights-based principles of participation, voice, and accountability. It also reflected methodological considerations: contextualized information across varying population groups in six different countries about how respondents themselves understood empowerment was essential for valid interpretation of women's responses.

Local context was a central concern of the research design. This can best be understood in terms of grounded theory. In the spirit of "discovering" that is central to grounded theory,[7] the study's central methodological tenets were (a) suspending theoretical assumptions to truly discover and engage with local realities and knowledge and (b) sampling for theoretical, as opposed to statistical, representativeness. Further, taking a critical and feminist standpoint on the production of knowledge about sex workers' lives,[8] the study team developed the design, data collection, and analysis in close collaboration with local sex workers.

What emerged was a mixed-methods assessment in three stages:

Stage 1: Context analysis and focus groups. Formative research involving a preliminary context analysis[9] and nine focus group discussions (FGDs) with sex workers, former SHAKTI staff, and other key informants.[10]

Stage 2: Survey. A semistructured questionnaire administered to 342 sex workers.[11] Areas of inquiry included personal and household demographics, personal and collective empowerment, the context of sex work, and HIV risk reduction.

Stage 3: In-depth interviews. Twenty-six in-depth interviews with former project staff, sex workers, and others in the sex work community.

The survey research was conducted by a consultant from the Bangladesh Institute for Development Studies. Survey responses were tabulated and disaggregated by workplace and respondents' level of prior involvement with SHAKTI activities. Interviews and FGDs were conducted by CARE Bangladesh's Social Development Unit. Data analysis was a collaborative effort among research teams. Field researchers met daily during data collection to debrief. These meetings produced coded matrices, which were synthesized by the lead consultant and served as the basis for further analysis by an advisory team in Dhaka. A final workshop with a wider group of stakeholders reviewed the synthesized findings and explored remaining questions.

A combination of purposive and snowball sampling was used in all three stages. Focus group participants and survey respondents were selected to represent a range of levels of participation in project activities, and interview respondents were selected for their ability to provide perspective on specific issues. The field researchers worked closely with the two sex worker organizations to identify and elicit the cooperation of respondents.

Although the involvement of the self-help groups DNS and NMS introduces potential biases in our sample, it would have been difficult to conduct research in these locations on this scale without their cooperation. The power of these organizations to mediate access to sex workers is itself a topic deserving of further critical inquiry. While limiting the generalizability of results, the sampling strategy brought out important differences across the program populations. Given the challenges of developing a probabilistic sample in hidden and vulnerable populations,[12] this approach was deemed appropriate to the theoretical nature of our inquiry.

One significant shortcoming in our sample was our inability to gain direct access to *chukris* (bonded sex workers). Chukris' contacts outside the brothel are tightly controlled by the *sardanis* (madams) who hold their contracts. Some insight on their perspective was provided by in-depth interviews with sex workers recently released from bonded status.

FINDINGS

1. The Context of Sex Work in Bangladesh

Both the legal status of brothel-based and street-based sex workers and social attitudes towards them were investigated. Lack of legal protection coupled with social stigma framed the lives of sex workers.

Legal Context

The legal status of sex work in Bangladesh can best be described as ambiguous. The Bangladesh High Court ruled in 2000 that commercial sex work was protected by the constitutional right "to enter into any lawful profession or occupation."[13] However, in 2010, another constitutional clause, which states that "the state shall adopt effective measures to prevent prostitution and gambling," was cited in the reversal of a decision by the Bangladesh Election Commissioner to recognize prostitution as a profession on voter ID cards.[14]

The Suppression of Immoral Traffic Act of 1933 makes it illegal to manage a brothel or live off the earnings of a sex worker. Nevertheless, there are over a dozen highly visible brothels in Bangladesh and a

well-established system under which brothel-based sex workers are registered with a magistrate's court and lists of registered sex workers are
maintained by local police. While this procedure does not confer legal
status, it does bring brothel-based sex work into a quasi-institutional
framework that seems to provide some protection for brothel-based sex
workers.

Street-based sex workers have no such protection. Street-based sex
work is not covered under the 1933 Act or by any other national legislation. Public solicitation for purposes of prostitution is illegal by local
statute in some cities, including Dhaka. In past years, sex workers in
Dhaka were also frequently taken into custody under the Vagrancy Act
and in some cases remanded to vagrancy homes for years.[15] Human
Rights Watch reports that arrests of sex workers in Bangladesh rarely
lead to legal procedures but are instead often a pretext for extortion and
violence, including rape.[16]

In our survey, 67% of street-based respondents reported experiencing
physical or sexual violence by police in the past twelve months. Sex
workers seem to have little recourse to legal protection against violence
by any perpetrators. Fewer than 1% of street-based and 9% of brothel-
based sex workers indicated that recent perpetrators of violence were
arrested. In the majority of cases (80% of street-based and 56% of
brothel-based sex workers), no action was taken against the perpetrator.

Social Context

Legal status is linked to social attitudes about sex work, both reflecting
and influencing them. Negative attitudes towards sex work surface in
recurring attempts to close down brothels and in sex workers' accounts
of daily struggles against humiliation and exploitation. When asked
about obstacles to their empowerment, street-based sex workers listed
(among other responses): "Society does not recognize the work" and
"Sex work is neglected." Another group declared: "*Samaj* [the social
leadership] hates us" and "We are untouchables."

Internalization of negative social attitudes was common. In response
to a series of questions about their attitudes towards sex work, responses
of 55% of sex workers indicated a high level of stigma associated with
sex work, 25% a medium level, and 20% a low level of stigma. The
strongest indicator was in response to the statement "I feel that sex
work is shameful and undignified and I have always wanted to leave it,"
with 72% agreeing or strongly agreeing.[17]

Social stigma no doubt plays a role in the level of violence and exploitation in the sex trade. It also disrupts family relations. In our survey, 67% of sex workers said they would not be welcome at a relative's home, and 58% said they would not be welcome in their home village. Two-thirds were providing financial support for their children, but over half who have children were not currently living with them. Family members or the children themselves may refuse contact, or the sex workers avoid contact to hide their profession or avoid stigmatizing their children through association.

2. Power and Relationships in Sex Workers' Lives

Information about the key actors in a large brothel in Tangail and among sex workers in Dhaka was first collected informally as part of the research design process. Data collected by more formal methods was later used to verify these initial findings.[18]

Kandapara Brothel

Kandapara brothel is situated on three acres of land in the city of Tangail. At the time of this research (2007), 718 sex workers lived in the brothel community. There were sixty houses there with 666 rooms owned by forty-five *bariwalas* (landladies). There were three categories of sex workers here: chukris (28% of the sex worker population), independent sex workers (68%), and inactive sex workers (4%).

Key actors in the brothel community include the following:

Chukris, sardanis, and dalals (middlemen): Chukris are in bonded service to sardanis, who provide food and shelter while exercising nearly complete control over all aspects of the chukri's life. Chukris are recruited by dalals, who often use deception to bring women to the brothel. Sardanis are traditional leaders in the brothel. They pay dalals to recruit chukris, and they interact with police and public authorities to register them. Relationships with clients and influence in the brothel also bring them into contact with powerful actors in the wider community.

Independent sex workers and bariwalas (landladies): Most independent sex workers entered the brothel as chukris. They now control their own income, working conditions, and choice of clients and sexual practices. Their primary constraint is the need to maintain good relations with the bariwala, to whom they pay rent on a daily basis. Bariwalas maintain relationships with sardanis and pay extortion money to local youth, political figures, and party cadres to ensure a stable environment for the sex business. Despite the sardanis' traditional leadership role, sex workers repeatedly identified bariwalas as the most powerful women in the brothel.

Nari Mukti Sangh: NMS's elected leaders represent the collective power of independent sex workers in the brothel. Since its creation in 1998, NMS has played a key role in supporting the brothel community, including improving access to health services and preventing an eviction attempt in 2006. NMS's leaders sometimes intervene with sardanis who are excessively violent with a chukri or who tries to involve a minor in sex work, and they have worked to impose limits on the length of time a chukri is in bonded service to a sardani.

Other key actors in brothel life include *babus* (lovers), police, *mastans* ("gangsters," often with political affiliations), and local political figures who can have a significant impact on the daily lives of sex workers.

Street-Based Sex Workers in Dhaka

The street-based sex trade is less structured than life in the brothel. Sexual transactions are negotiated in public places. Because street-based sex work takes place in no fixed location and over a wide geographic area, there is less of a coherent community among the sex workers. Although those working in a given location will sometimes loosely organize for mutual support and protection, generally street-based sex workers must be more self-reliant than brothel workers.

Consistent with other research,[19] violence in the lives of the street-based sex workers in our study is astonishingly high. In our survey, 81% of street-based sex workers reported having been slapped, pushed, kicked, beaten, or threatened by a weapon in the last twelve months by someone other than their intimate partner. The most frequent perpetrators were police, mastans, and customers.

The key actors in street-based sex work are the following:

Dalals: In this context, the word *dalal* is sometimes translated as "pimp." These relationships are frequently exploitative. Dalals sometimes demand free sex, cheat sex workers financially, or sell vulnerable sex workers into bonded service in a brothel.

Clients: Interactions with customers in street-based sex work are more dangerous than in the brothel. While brothel-based sex work takes place in close proximity to colleagues, street-based sex workers have to find a private area hidden from view to conduct their business. Street-based sex workers report that, in addition to committing violence against them, customers cheat them in various ways: stealing, refusing payment, or insisting that the sex worker service more customers than agreed.

Durjoy Nari Sangho (DNS): The sex workers' organizations in Dhaka and Tangail have similar structures but evolved differently. Like NMS, DNS has organized protests around specific incidents and engaged in outreach to police. However, DNS tends to focus more on service provision and less on the type of collective negotiation and relationship-building in which NMS has been involved. DNS partners with other NGOs to provide services to sex workers and has been the direct recipient of a large contract from the Global Fund.

Other influential actors in the lives of street-based sex workers include husbands (street-based sex workers are more likely to be married than brothel-based ones) as well as babus, police, and mastans. Rickshaw pullers are particularly ubiquitous in the narratives of street-based sex workers as clients, acting as dalals, and sometimes intervening with abusive customers.

3. A Demographic Profile

Table 5.1 presents a profile of the respondents in our survey research.[20] As noted earlier, we cannot reliably generalize from this data. However, the basic demographic profile is consistent with other studies of the population in the same time period.[21]

Survey responses highlighted two important demographic differences between brothel-based and street-based sex workers: All brothel-based respondents reported having a home within or outside the brothel, but almost 40% of street-based sex workers were homeless. Street-based respondents were also more likely than brothel-based ones to be currently married (38% compared to 10%) and living with their husband (31% compared to 7%). This may account for differences in responses around issues of mobility, decision making, and violence in intimate relationships.

All groups reported similar levels of condom use with clients, with 57–66% indicating that they "always" used condoms with clients. With lovers, 49% reported "always" using condoms while 21% reported "never" using condoms. Condom use with husbands was in almost

TABLE 5.1   DEMOGRAPHICS OF SEX WORKERS IN THE STAGE 2 SURVEY

	Tangail	Dhaka		All
	Brothel-based (n = 69)	Street-based (n = 207)	Hotel-based (n = 40)	(N = 316)
Age				
mean years	29.4	26.1	24.2	26.6
Religion				
% Muslim (all others Hindu)	95.7%	99.5%	100%	98.7%
Marital status				
% currently married	10.1%	37.7%	37.5%	31.6%
Children				
% with one or more children	47.8%	45.9%	52.5%	47.1%
Education				
% no school	55.0%	62.3%	59.4%	60.8%
% 5+ years school	17.5%	15.0%	10.1%	14.2%
Income				
average total personal monthly income, in takas (Tk)	11,877 Tk	7,725 Tk	9,945 Tk	8,913 Tk

reverse proportion, with 23% reporting "always" and 44% reporting "never." The most commonly reported reason for sex without a condom was "client did not want to" (55%). However, 86% reported that they "always" or "most of the time" felt confident discussing condom use with a partner, and 72% felt that they could "always" or "most of the time" convince a partner who did not want to wear a condom that it was necessary to do so.

4. Perspectives on Empowerment

What do you understand by empowerment in your life?

I was weak in the past. A fear always haunted me that if I do not go with him, he will beat me. I was bound to go with him whether I was paid or not. I was bound to go with him whenever he called. At that time, I used to find myself helpless and weak. I used to find myself very inferior. But I am not weak any more. Now I understand that I also have rights and deserve the fulfillment of my wishes. I also deserve liberty. I can protest against any injustice now. (25-year-old street-based sex worker in Dhaka)

Empowerment of the sex workers means being courageous to raise their voices; to be economically solvent, as everybody shows deference to solvent people. If a person shows deference to another, it proves the empowerment of that person. Here "money is *the* power." (36-year-old brothel-based sex worker in Tangail)

To facilitate a contextualized understanding of empowerment *from the sex workers' perspective*, the research team took a deliberately skeptical stance towards CARE's own definitions and frameworks while asking sex workers in FGDs a series of questions designed to elicit their views. The analysis that followed data collection was then consciously developed as a dialogue between the views of the sex workers and CARE's own conceptual frameworks.[22]

Responses to these formative questions were first coded and organized into four categories that emerged from the data:

1. *Personal attributes:* Education, intelligence, and self-confidence were the personal attributes most commonly associated with empowerment. Courage, patience, and honor were also mentioned by more than one group.

2. *Interpersonal influence:* Interpersonal influence was sometimes explicitly identified as an ability to negotiate or to influence others. More often, it was implied as a consequence of appropriate conduct ("behaves well with others," "can talk in a nice manner") or effective communication skills ("can talk with group in an organized way," "can make people understand").

3. *Achieving personal goals:* Economic issues were central to most sex workers' aspirations. Wealth or financial security was seen as a goal or signifier of empowerment as well as a means for achieving other goals. It was frequently associated with aspirations for one's children, which had an economic aspect but was also linked to issues such as social acceptance and education.

4. *Collective identity and group leadership:* Street-based sex workers raised issues of collective identity and unity in relation to empowerment and, when asked about the characteristics of empowered women, discussed capabilities related to group leadership ("can solve problems" and "[deal with] complex issues") and project management ("can manage projects" and "can manage funds"). Brothel-based groups also spoke about leadership, and one group

spoke at great length about social acceptance of sex workers collectively.

Even the simple categorization above obscures the richness and complexity of the sex workers' perspectives on empowerment. We tried to recapture some of that complexity by first identifying a set of cross-cutting themes in the FGDs: protest and resistance; confidence, courage, and self-esteem; acceptance; and presentation and identity. We next looked for differences in perspective among different groups and found significant variations between street and brothel-based sex workers and between those who had been in leadership roles (in one of the sex workers' organizations or project activities) and those who had not.

Street-based sex workers tended to identify individuals as the locus of empowerment while brothel-based sex workers tended to focus on groups and relationships. Those in leadership roles tended, not surprisingly, to frame empowerment around leadership and the well-being of groups but also tended to have broader conceptions of empowerment more generally. While nonleaders framed empowerment largely in terms of individual agency, perspectives of those in leadership roles ranged across all three dimensions of CARE's empowerment framework: agency, structure, and relationship. Responses of the leadership suggested that their contact with NGOs strongly influenced their conception of empowerment.[23]

5. Program Impacts

This research was not intended to be a rigorous impact evaluation.[24] We were interested in casting a wide net to understand multiple outcomes and possible interactions between these outcomes in order to deepen our understanding of empowerment processes. That said, program impacts were assessed in FGDs, interviews, and survey results, including assessment of varying participation, exposure, and utilization of program components.

With respect to issues directly related to HIV prevention, the data indicated the following:

- *SHAKTI played a significant role in raising awareness about HIV and AIDS among sex workers* and contributed to increased availability of health services for sex workers. Among street-based sex workers, those who participated in program activities were more likely to have been tested for HIV than those who had not.[25]

- *SHAKTI participation was associated with higher levels of individual and relational confidence and greater negotiating power related to condom use.* Those who actively participated in SHAKTI were more confident in their ability to purchase condoms, discuss condom use with sexual partners, convince partners to use a condom, and negotiate services with clients.

- *Participation in SHAKTI was associated with increased condom use with husbands and lovers among both street- and brothel-based sex workers.* However, project participation increased condom use *with clients* among brothel-based sex workers only. This may be because street-based sex workers have more limited access to condoms and more limited negotiating power with clients.

On more general empowerment issues, the following outcomes were identified:

- *Participation in SHAKTI activities was associated with increased confidence among individual sex workers about their own personal agency.* Respondents associated with SHAKTI reported higher confidence in their ability to solve "common problems faced in their everyday lives," to "influence community decision making," and to resist violence and exploitation.

- *They also reported increased confidence and demonstrated signs of personal agency within intimate relationships* (ability to influence decision making in relationships with husbands and lovers).

In almost every area in which we identified project impacts, *the positive impact among brothel-based sex workers was stronger than among street-based sex workers.* A number of contextual factors make intervention with street-based sex workers more challenging, including more acute poverty, less social support, a weaker sense of community, and differences related to the circumstances of sex work in these different contexts.

With respect to the sex-work environment, the self-help groups DNS and NMS were central to many changes in structure and power relations within the sex-worker communities and in their relations with the wider community. CARE facilitated the formation of the two groups and worked closely with them over the ten years. In many cases, it is impossible to separately attribute specific outcomes to the CARE project, as opposed to effects attributable to either DNS or NMS.

Among the major changes in the brothel- and street-based sex-work environment (a key aspect of the structural dimension of empowerment), including those that followed the establishment of DNS and MNS, were the following:

- *Changes in governance and power relations within the brothel in Tangail.* Kandapara brothel had a long-standing tradition of governance under the leadership of sardanis and bariwalas. NMS did not supplant this traditional power structure but inserted a more democratic element into it. The elected officers of NMS now play key roles, along with sardanis and bariwalas, in decision making within the brothel, in conducting *shalish* (arbitration of internal disputes), and negotiating relationships with external actors. They sometimes intervene in relationships between sardanis and chukris.

- *Structural change in the community of street-based sex workers.* DNS represents 2,500 sex workers in Dhaka (compared to 650 in the Kandapara brothel) spread over a wide geographic area. DNS found a role for itself mediating access to the sex-worker community for other organizations.[26] Sex workers tended to describe DNS as a service provider rather than a union or governing body. However, as there was no preexisting formal structure linking the community of street-based sex workers, DNS has provided some level of organization and representation. When asked about changes in the lives of sex workers, "greater unity" was among the five most common responses of both street- and brothel-based respondents.

- *Improved relationships with external power holders.* CARE provided support to help sex-worker organizations build relationships with external parties, particularly with the police but also with local political actors and businesses in the surrounding communities. Successful interventions built confidence among the organizations' leaders in their ability to negotiate improved relationships on behalf of their constituents.

- *Reduced stigma about sex work perceived by respondents.* There was widespread agreement among the sex workers that community attitudes towards sex workers had changed positively in the previous ten years.[27] Such changes were attributed less to any direct action in the communities than to changes in the sex workers themselves—changes in self-image, how they present themselves, and their willingness (and will) to resist exploitation.

CONCLUSIONS

Our research suggests that the basic HIV prevention strategies—enhancing HIV awareness, knowledge of risk reduction strategies, condom availability, and accessibility of testing and health care services—are necessary but not sufficient for sustainable reduction of HIV risk among vulnerable populations such as the sex workers in Bangladesh. A comprehensive women's empowerment approach addresses the whole woman, not just sex work. In order to sustainably impact prevention of sexual transmission of HIV, efforts must respond to women's own aspirations in the context of various relationships of power that are influenced by institutional and cultural constructs in both public and private spheres of their lives. We must be willing to challenge assumptions about who these women are, what they seek, and how to support them.

The Tangail brothel is an example of a "mature" HIV intervention in this respect. In the brothel 100% of sex workers report they are aware of HIV, 100% know where they can be tested, there is a fairly high level of knowledge about HIV transmission and risk reduction, and condoms and health services are accessible. Still, 34% of brothel-based sex workers report they don't always use condoms with clients, including 23% who say they only sometimes do and 3% who report they rarely or never do.

Our research suggested four key behavioral and contextual factors in this persistence of high-risk behaviors: client preference, financial needs and incentives, use of force or threat of violence, and, with respect to husbands and lovers, the desire to please a loved one. Each of these can be linked to specific aspects of the disempowerment of sex workers. The fact that sex workers identify client preference as a justification for high-risk behaviors reflects, in part, sex workers' lack of negotiating power in their relationships with clients. Financial need, at least for those at the extreme end, can be associated with the marginalization of sex work and sex workers. Force or coercion is a clear manifestation of the lack of esteem in which sex workers are held by the wider society, normalization of violence against women, and lack of protections available to them.

Strategies involving all three aspects of empowerment in the CARE model were at work in the program intervention. Improving sex workers' ability to negotiate services with clients and to protest or resist exploitation are issues of personal agency. Building or improving relationships with outside agencies, service providers, police, and members of the wider community may have been a factor in reducing violence in the brothel and contributing more generally to improved community attitudes towards sex workers. Structural changes, in addition to creating a mechanism for sex workers' self-governance, provided a sustainable institutional structure for disseminating HIV information and services and, in the brothel, limited the worst excesses of the bonded sex-work system.

At the start of this chapter, we suggested that SHAKTI's empowerment approach was simply a response to the challenge of attempting to get sex workers to pay more attention to HIV messages. The research helps us understand that the program probably would not have had the success it did if it had not adopted this more holistic empowerment approach to HIV risk reduction, addressing the vulnerabilities that women face. The clearest finding to emerge from this study was that empowerment processes are extremely context dependent. At every step of the research we found salient contextual differences between the brothel and the street, which contributed to differences in the nature and impact of empowerment strategies and, ultimately, to differences in impact on HIV risk reduction.

In the end, HIV risk reduction comes down to specific choices and decisions made by individual women and men. Those choices are made in the context of individual lives but are shaped, directed, and constrained by a complex interplay of institutional structures, socioeconomic factors, and cultural factors. The better we understand the specific contextual constraints that influence personal choices, the better positioned researchers and practitioners will be to implement strategies that expand the range of choices and opportunities available to sex workers and their clients. This is the goal of empowerment and the means by which empowerment strategies can contribute to reducing HIV vulnerability among sex workers and ultimately in the larger community.

Box 5.1. Summary

Geographic area: Two sites in Bangladesh: the capital city of Dhaka (street-based sex workers) and Kandapara brothel in the town of Tangail (brothel-based sex workers).

Global importance of the health condition: Because HIV prevalence is relatively low in the general population, it is critical that prevention efforts in Bangladesh target high-risk groups. Poverty and extreme social marginalization make sex workers in Bangladesh a particularly vulnerable population.

Intervention or program: A ten-year HIV intervention with sex workers began under the name SHAKTI (Stopping HIV/AIDS through Knowledge and Training Initiative) and was later brought under the umbrella of CARE's integrated HIV program in Bangladesh. Key aspects of the program included establishing a self-managed health clinic for brothel-based sex workers in Tangail, developing a network of fifty-two drop-in centers in Dhaka for accessing and training street-based sex workers as peer educators for HIV/STI prevention, and facilitating the formation of sex-worker self-help groups in both locations.

Impact: SHAKTI resulted in higher utilization of STI and HIV services and higher levels of self-confidence to (a) purchase condoms, (b) negotiate services with clients, and (c) convince partners to use condoms. Program participants also reported increased confidence in solving common problems in their lives and in influencing community decision making, and they reported increased ability to resist violence and exploitation. There were positive changes (less exploitation and more democratic governance) in power relations within the sex-worker communities and improved relationships with external power holders.

Lessons learned: Empowerment efforts must respond to women's own definitions of empowerment and women's aspirations while taking into account the complex interplay of institutional, interpersonal, and cultural constructs in public and private life.

Link between empowerment and health: Interventions that shift individual sex workers' own sense of self-esteem and personal agency and reduce the stigma associated with sex work improve sex workers' ability to negotiate condom use and reduce other high-risk behaviors, thereby potentially reducing vulnerability to HIV.

Box 5.2. Evaluating the Needs of Sex Workers to Increase Their Empowerment

Sex workers have long been objectified in research as "high-risk vectors" for the spread of both physical and social ills, while their voices and experiences are overlooked. By focusing attention on the experiences and priorities of women involved in sex work, the current study challenges the traditional focus on solving the problems sex work causes while emphasizing how women in sex work can overcome the problems that society causes them.

Research and development programs are often asked to produce "the numbers" to demonstrate impact and to contribute to building generalizable evidence about what works. While such research has strong policy appeal and deserves a place in the analysis of social change, researchers in the current program deliberately put aside preconceived notions to listen to sex workers' own views on empowerment and their opinions on its relationship to HIV vulnerability. The data that emerged shed light on the degree to which meanings, relationships, and processes vary, even within one community. These data also introduce questions about the challenge of accurately reflecting local realities when seeking to produce generalizable, quantitative data about complex social dynamics.

ACKNOWLEDGMENTS

We would like to acknowledge the contributions to the chapter or the original research, or both, of CARE Bangladesh, Madhu Deshmukh, Leah Berkowitz, and Nadia Shadravan.

NOTES

1. CARE n.d.
2. Ibid.
3. Jana et al. 2004, 407.
4. Magar and Jana 2006, 8.
5. The most commonly identified perpetrators of violence against sex workers in Bangladesh were police and *mastans* (usually translated as "criminals" or "gangsters" often affiliated with political parties).
6. As this abbreviated history of the project may suggest, SHAKTI maintained a flexible approach to intervention design throughout the project. Specific activities were developed in dynamic response to the evolving needs of the sex worker communities (identified in collaboration with the sex workers themselves).
7. Glaser and Strauss 1967.

8. Ghose, Swendeman, and George 2011.

9. Context analysis involved informal on-site observation and key informant interviews to better understand the context of sex workers' lives, focusing particularly on relationships and power dynamics at both individual and institutional levels. For more structured discussion of approaches to context analysis, see UNDP 2012.

10. Six focus groups were held with sex workers grouped by levels of prior involvement with the CARE intervention. Three additional focus groups were held with others closely associated with the sex work community.

11. The sample was later reduced to 316, removing respondents who were not currently active sex workers.

12. For a concise review of methodological issues in research with sex workers, see Seib 2007, 42–56.

13. Godwin 2012, 61; Constitution of the People's Republic of Bangladesh 1972, section 40.

14. UN Office for the Coordination of Humanitarian Affairs 2010; Constitution of the People's Republic of Bangladesh 1972, section 18.

15. This practice has been greatly reduced in recent years in part due to advocacy and interventions by DNS.

16. Maru 2003, 29.

17. The survey data does indicate that the CARE intervention reduced internalized stigma about sex work to some degree. Respondents with greater exposure to the CARE intervention were less likely to hold these negative views.

18. The contextual information in this section was initially framed by a preliminary study of power relations in the sex worker communities during the formative research. This was an informal study drawing on interviews and observations in the two sex worker communities and was intended to provide a basic contextual framework for guiding the research design. The information was later verified and supplemented with data gathered in the more formal stages of data collection.

19. Miller 1993; Pyett and Warr 1997; Lowman 2007; Church et al. 2001.

20. The original research design involved only street- and brothel-based sex workers, but 40 of 247 respondents in Dhaka identified themselves as hotel-based in response to an open-ended survey question. Disaggregated data about hotel-based sex workers was included in the basic demographic analyses but, because a contextual framework for hotel-based sex work hadn't been established, data from these respondents was not included in later in-depth analysis.

21. For example, National AIDS/STD Programme 2007, 17.

22. Analysis in this section is based on qualitative data from FGDs in the formative stage of research. All direct quotes are from those FGDs.

23. A challenging translation issue came up early in the research design process as the research team was preparing interview questions. CARE staff in Bangladesh characterized the Bengali word for "empowerment" (khomotayon) as an "NGO word"—one not commonly used except in NGO circles or among educated elites. Even the word for empowerment carries connotations of external influence in Bangladesh.

24. The findings reported in this section draw primarily on analysis of the survey data. An initial report on the survey research was prepared by an external

consultant (Mannan 2008). The survey data was submitted to further analysis and integrated with findings from interviews and focus groups for the final research report on which the analysis here is based (Robinson 2009). The final research report can be accessed through the CARE web site at http://gender .care2share.wikispaces.net/file/view/SII+Women%27s+Empowerment+and+HI V+Bangladesh+Final+Report+2008.pdf.

25. In the brothel, however, the reverse was true. This may be due to the fact that active project participants were, on average, older than those with less participation in project activities. Since HIV testing services are more accessible to brothel-based sex workers (through the on-site clinic), factors other than project exposure (such as age and sexual activity) which might affect use of testing services became more significant.

26. The role and function of DNS and NMS were clearly shaped by the environment in which they were operating. They did not emerge as wholly integral and independent structures, but rather each found a very different function within the context of existing institutional frameworks. Rather than thinking of the creation of a self-help organization as a stand-alone piece of structural engineering, it may be better understood as an evolutionary process, with the goal of inserting a change agent within existing institutional frameworks.

27. The survey data corroborates the perspective expressed in focus groups and interviews: 87% of sex workers in the semi-structured interviews agreed or strongly agreed with the statement "During the last ten years community attitudes towards sex workers have changed positively." Ten percent disagreed or strongly disagreed. Street and brothel-based respondents were similar in their responses to this question.

REFERENCES

CARE. n.d. "Women's Empowerment SII Framework." Strategic Impact Inquiries. http://pqdl.care.org/sii/Pages/Women's%20Empowerment%20SII%20 Framework.aspx.

Church, Stephanie, Marion Henderson, Marina Barnard, and Graham Hart. 2001. "Violence by Clients towards Female Prostitutes in Different Work Settings." *British Medical Journal* 322: 524–525.

Constitution of the People's Republic of Bangladesh. 1972. Laws of Bangladesh, Government of the People's Republic of Bangladesh. http://bdlaws .minlaw.gov.bd/pdf_part.php?id=367.

George, A. 2010. Negotiating Contradictory Expectations: Stories from "Secret" Sex Workers in Andhra Pradesh, India." *Wagadu, Journal of Transnational Women's and Gender Studies,* 8: 258–272.

Ghose, Toorjo, Dallas T. Swendeman, and Sheba M. George. 2011. The Role of Brothels in Reducing HIV Risk in Sonagachi, India. *Qualitative Health Research,* 21(5) May.

Glaser, Barney, and Anselm Strauss. 1967. *The Discovery of Grounded Theory: Strategies for Qualitative Research.* New York: Aldine de Gruyter.

Godwin, John. 2012. *Sex Work and the Law in Asia and the Pacific: Laws, HIV and Human Rights in the Context of Sex Work*. Bangkok: UNDP Asia-Pacific Regional Centre.

International Union for Conservation of Nature and Natural Resources (IUCN). n.d. IUCN's *Situation Analysis: An Approach and Method for Analyzing the Context of Projects and Programme*. http://cmsdata.iucn.org/downloads /approach_and_method.pdf

Jana, Samarajit, Ishika Basu, Mary J. Rotheram-Boru, and Peter A. Newman. 2004. "The Sonagachi Project: A Sustainable Community Intervention Program." *AIDS Education and Prevention* 16(5): 405–414.

Jenkins, C., and Rahman, H. 2002. Rapidly Changing Conditions in the Brothels of Bangladesh: Impact on HIV/STD. *AIDS Education and Prevention* 14 (Supplement A): 97–106.

Lowman, John. 2007. "Violence and the Outlaw Status of (Street) Prostitution in Canada." *Violence Against Women* 6(9): 987–1011.

Magar, Veronica, and Samarajit Jana. 2006. "Now They Look at Us as Normal: Stigma, Violence, Sex Worker Resistance and HIV/AIDS in Bangladesh." (Unpublished manuscript). Microsoft Word file.

Mannan, M. A. 2008. "Strategic Impact Inquiry Study (SII)." (Unpublished manuscript).

Maru, Vivek. 2003. Ravaging the Vulnerable: Abuses against Persons at High Risk of HIV Infection in Bangladesh. New York: Human Rights Watch, August 19. www.hrw.org/report/2003/08/19/ravaging-vulnerable/abuses-against-persons-high-risk-hiv-infection-bangladesh.

Miller, Jody. 1993. "Your Life Is on the Line Every Night You're on the Streets: Victimization and Resistance among Street Prostitutes." *Humanity & Society* 17(4): 422–445.

National AIDS/STD Programme, Ministry of Health and Family Welfare, Government of the People's Republic of Bangladesh. 2007. *National HIV Serological Surveillance, 2006 Bangladesh: 7th Round Technical Report*. Dhaka: Government of Bangladesh.

Pyett, Priscilla. and Deborah Warr. 1997. "Vulnerability on the Streets: Female Sex Workers and HIV Risk." *AIDS Care* 9(5): 539–547.

Robinson, Victor. 2009. "Context and Power in Sex Work in Bangladesh: An Inquiry into Empowerment and HIV Risk Reduction among Sex Workers in Dhaka and Tangail." (Unpublished manuscript). Microsoft Word file.

Seib, Charlotte. 2007. "Health, Well-being and Sexual Violence among Female Sex Workers: a Comparative Study." PhD thesis, Queensland University of Technology. http://eprints.qut.edu.au/.

Sprague, Joey. 2005. *Feminist Methodologies for Critical Researchers: Bridging Differences*. Walnut Creek, CA: Rowman Altamira.

UN Development Program (UNDP). 2012. *Institutional and Context Analysis—Guidance Note*. Oslo: Oslo Governance Center.

UN Office for the Coordination of Humanitarian Affairs. 2010, October 12. "Mixed Messages on Sex Work Undermine HIV Prevention." *IRIN Humanitarian News and Analysis*. www.irinnews.org/fr/node/249447.

6

Gender Roles in U.S. Women with HIV

Intersection with Psychological and Physical Health Outcomes

LESLIE R. BRODY, SANNISHA K. DALE, GWENDOLYN
A. KELSO, RUTH C. CRUISE, KATHLEEN M. WEBER,
LYNISSA R. STOKES, AND MARDGE H. COHEN

Women with or at risk for HIV infection often experience gender ine-quality, tend to be African American or Latina, live in poverty, and have a history of trauma (Amaro and Raj 2000; Centers for Disease Control and Prevention 2016; Gupta 2000). HIV-infected women in the United States, especially African Americans, demonstrate poorer health outcomes, such as lower rates of virologic suppression and higher rates of morbidity and mortality, than their male counterparts (National Center for Health Statistics 2011). Given these outcomes, it is impor-tant to identify the coping strategies that are related to better health outcomes. We are interested in coping strategies that reflect individual agency and empowerment, defined by Kabeer (2001) as the expansion of women's abilities to make strategic life choices in a context where this ability was previously denied to them.

The coping strategies women utilize in their close and sexual relation-ships are of particular interest, since the majority of women are infected with HIV via heterosexual contact. Moreover, the quality of women's relationships with their sexual partners, family members, and care pro-viders affects how they cope with HIV and adhere to HIV treatment recommendations (Demarco 2010; Brody, Stokes, Dale et al. 2014). In particular, traditional gender role behaviors—in which women prioritize care for others over self-care (termed unmitigated communion or care as self-sacrifice), and silence the needs of the self to avoid relational conflict and loss (termed self-silencing)—have been found to increase HIV risk

(Dworkin, Beckford, and Erhardt 2007; Exner et al. 2003) and lead to poor health outcomes among infected women (Dale et al. 2011; Grant et al. 2011; Jack and Ali 2010; Kelso et al. 2010; Brody, Stokes, Dale, et al. 2014; Brody, Stokes, Kelso, et al. 2014). Further, the traditional role of having low power in sexual relationships has been found to be related to lower levels of condom use and higher levels of experienced violence than having high power in sexual relationships (Dworkin, Beckford, and Erhardt 2007, Teitelman, Ratcliffe, Morales-Aleman, et al. 2008).

The extent to which women adopt traditional gender role behaviors in their relationships can be viewed as adaptations to inequitable systems that may punish women for stepping outside of gendered expectations, including self-advocacy (Jack and Ali 2010). Women with HIV may adhere to traditional gender role behaviors because of their lower levels of education and employment, inadequate financial resources, the stresses of single parental status, and abuse histories, all characteristics found to be associated with traditional gender role behaviors in seronegative women (Fortin 2005; Teitelman, Ratcliffe, Dichter, et al. 2008; Wingood et al. 2001).

BARRIERS TO EMPOWERMENT IN OLDER WOMEN WITH HIV

Women with HIV who are over 50 years of age have less social support, increased social isolation, fewer financial resources, higher rates of depression, and lower self-efficacy in negotiating condom use than their younger counterparts (Emlet 2006; Engstrom et al. 2011; Grov et al. 2010; Neundorfer et al. 2005). Age-related social norms that dictate discretion in openly discussing topics such as drug use and sexual relations, the physical complications of aging, and age and gender biases of health care providers all contribute to reduced HIV testing rates and delayed diagnoses in older women (Akers et al. 2007; Grant and Ragsdale 2008; Plach, Stevens, and Keigher 2005; Theall et al. 2003).

Gender role behaviors may play an especially important role in the lives of older women with HIV. Older women often perceive a loss of "currency" in sexual relationships, which places them at higher risk for a sense of reduced power in these relationships (Auerbach and Coates 2000). Older women who adhere to traditional gender roles report experiencing greater feelings of HIV stigma than those with less traditional gender roles, and in turn, a sense of stigma is related to nondisclosure of HIV status, depression, and social isolation (Jacobs and Thomlinson 2009; Jacobs and Kane 2010).

This chapter describes a survey study and a peer advocacy program. The study identifies (1) how gender role behaviors are related to coping strategies reflecting individual agency (or agentic strategies) utilized by at-risk and HIV-infected women and (2) how gender role behaviors and agentic coping strategies are related to women's depression, experiences of physical violence, quality of life, and resilience, with a special emphasis on older women. The peer advocacy program utilizes empowerment-based strategies to optimize health outcomes among HIV-infected women.

COPING

Managing the multiple stressors that are risk factors for and consequences of HIV infection—including limited economic resources and educational and job opportunities; history of trauma; exposure to violence, racism and sexism; substance abuse; depression and fatigue; medication and health-care management; and potential stigma and social isolation—requires adaptive coping strategies (Cohen et al. 2000; Machtinger, Haberer, et al. 2012; Machtinger, Wilson, et al. 2012; Tufts, Wessell, and Kearney 2010; Wingood et al. 2007; Wingood and DiClemente 2000; Brief et al. 2004). In particular, physical and sexual abuse histories (experienced by 67% of HIV-positive women in one large cohort; Cohen et al. 2000) are associated with inconsistent condom use, high-risk partners, lower rates of self-efficacy, and poor communication regarding safe sex practices (Amaro and Raj 2000; Sareen, Pagura, and Grant 2009).

Coping can be defined as a set of cognitive, affective, behavioral, and physiological processes that are consciously and/or unconsciously employed to deal with stressors (Lazarus and Folkman 1984). Active coping strategies (such as exercise), problem-focused coping strategies (employing a plan of action aimed at altering the stressor, such as advocating for social change), and positive cognitive and emotion focused strategies aimed at changing feelings and thoughts about the stressor (such as optimism or acceptance of HIV diagnosis) result in positive health consequences, including decreases in HIV disease progression, lower rates of morbidity and psychological distress, and improved quality of life (Hansen et al. 2006; Ironson et al. 2008; Kelso et al. 2013; Konkle-Parker, Erlen, and Dubbert 2008; O'Cleirigh et al. 2003; O'Cleirigh et al. 2008; Plach, Stevens, and Keigher 2005; Prado et al. 2004). Other examples of active and positive cognitive and emotion-focused coping strategies include persistence, self-reliance, meaning making (the ability to recognize or create some positive outcome or value resulting from traumatic experiences), generativity (concern for establishing and guiding the next generation), and insightfulness about previous behaviors and social inequities that may have contributed to HIV acquisition. In general, coping strategies and their effects and enhancers have not been extensively studied in women with HIV.

GENDER ROLES AND COPING STUDY

Our sample for the survey study consisted of a subset of participants in the Chicago Women's Interagency HIV Study (WIHS), a National Institutes of Health-funded, longitudinal, multicenter cohort study of HIV positive women and women at risk for HIV. Details of the study have been previously reported (Barkan et al. 1998). Women with and at risk for HIV are matched for age, race/ethnicity, level of education, injection drug use histories, and total number of sexual partners. WIHS participants attend semiannual study visits comprised of a battery of psychosocial, medical history, and demographic surveys; a physical and pelvic examination; and collection of blood and gynecologic specimens.

We enrolled 83 women (50 HIV-seropositive and 33 HIV-seronegative) from the Chicago WIHS site for this study. Informed consent was obtained for all enrolled women. Participants received a financial honorarium, transportation support, and child-care provision for their time and effort. The study protocol was approved by the Stroger Hospital of Cook County (Chicago) and Boston University Institutional Review Boards and the overall WIHS Executive Committee.

Table 6.1 shows that the participants were between the ages of 25 and 72, with a mean age of 43 years (SD = 8.96). Just over 90% of the sample identified as Black and non-Hispanic, and almost half of the participants reported that they had never been married. Previous work with this sample indicated that the HIV-positive and HIV-negative participants did not differ in age, race, marital status, smoking, drinking, drug use, or number of sexual partners, either from each other or from comparable groups in the larger WIHS cohort (Kelso et al. 2010). In the current study, data from the two groups of women (HIV-positive and HIV-negative) were pooled to investigate gender roles and coping strategies because all participants originated from demographically similar disenfranchised communities that face a myriad of structural challenges such as poverty, limited educational opportunities, homelessness, violence, abuse, and

TABLE 6.1 DEMOGRAPHIC INFORMATION FOR HIV-POSITIVE AND HIV-NEGATIVE
WOMEN AND DIFFERENCES BETWEEN GROUPS

Characteristic	HIV-positive women (n = 50)		HIV-negative women (n = 33)		Group difference
	Mean	SD	Mean	SD	t
Age	43.78	7.82	41.18	10.39	−1.51
	n	%	n	%	χ^2
Education					4.48
Grades 1 to 6	22	44	8	24.2	
Grades 7 to 11	17	34	12	36.4	
Completed high school	10	20	11	33.3	
Some college	1	2	2	6.1	
Income					11.07*
$ 0–6,000	15	30	13	39.4	
$ 6,000–12,000	23	46	4	12.1	
$ 12,001+	12	24	16	48.5	
Marital status					1.06
Married (legally or common-law)	8	16	6	18.2	
Living with partner	3	6	3	9.1	
Divorced	8	16	3	9.1	
Separated	6	12	4	12.1	
Widowed	4	8	3	9.6	
Race/ethnicity					3.01
African American	46	92	30	90.9	
Hispanic	2	4	3	9.1	
White	1	2	0	0	
Other	1	2	0	0	
Unemployed	42	84	19	57.6	7.13*

NOTE: * $p < .05$.

substance abuse—all factors that place women at risk for HIV across ethnic groups (CDC 2012; Cohen et al. 2000). However, since previous work (Kelso et al. 2010) had shown that the seronegative and seropositive women in the sample differed from each other and the larger Chicago cohort in terms of educational attainment and income, the variables of education and income were treated as independent covariates in all analyses. Of note, education level and income were only moderately correlated with each other ($r = .34$, $p < .002$)

A subsample of 67 women (43 HIV-seropositive and 24 HIV-seronegative) provided autobiographical narratives that were analyzed for types of coping and resilience. This subsample did not differ significantly from the larger group of 84 women in age, income, education, employment, or race. Measures for the study included self-reported standardized instruments, interview questions, and autobiographical narratives. Measures of gender role behaviors included the following:

1. the *Silencing the Self Scale* (*STSS;* Jack and Dill 1992), a 31-item scale measuring the degree to which participants silence their own needs to avoid relational loss and conflict (Cronbach's alpha = .88), with four subscales, including *Silencing the Self (SS)*, inhibiting self-expression and behaviors in order to avoid conflict or loss of relationship; *Divided Self (DS)*, behaving in ways that do not reflect inner feelings in order to conform to gendered expectations; *Care as Self-Sacrifice (CS)*, placing the needs of others before the needs of the self; and *Externalized Self-Perception (EXP)*, judging the self by external standards;

2. the *Revised Unmitigated Communion Scale (RUCS;* Fritz and Helgeson 1998), a 9-item self-reported scale assessing the degree to which participants' care for others at the expense of their own needs (Cronbach's alpha = .47; the relatively low reliability is consistent with previous literature [see Brody et al. 2014]); and

3. the *Sexual Relationship Power Scale (SRPS;* Pulerwitz, Gortmaker, and DeJong 2000), a 23-item questionnaire with two subscales measuring participants' perceptions of (1) the degree to which they experience relationship control from male partners (partners monitoring their behavior, such as dress) and (2) how much decision-making power they have relative to their partner (Cronbach's alpha = .90).

Measures of health included the following:

1. the *Center for Epidemiological Studies Depressive Symptoms Scale (CES-D Scale;* Radloff 1977), a 20-item self-report measure to assess depressive symptoms (Cronbach's alpha = .90) and

2. the *Medical Outcome Study (MOS-HIV;* Bozzette et al. 1995), a 21-item short form of MOS-HIV, a widely used disease specific instrument to assess quality of life; with four subscales: *physical functioning* (Cronbach's alpha = .81), *role functioning*

(Cronbach's alpha = .75), *emotional well-being* (Cronbach's alpha = .71), and *health perception* (Cronbach's alpha = .60).

3. *Experiences of Physical Violence* were gathered in interviews and categorized as 0 = never experienced any violence, 1 = experienced violence in the past from anyone, and 2 = currently experiencing violence in a relationship.

Coping strategies were assessed with the *Guided Autobiography Task* (McAdams et al. 2006), in which participants were asked to narrate three significant turning points in their lives. Narratives were coded for resilience and agentic coping strategies, which are listed and defined in table 6.2. Each was assessed using a four-point scale: 0 = no evidence of use, 1 = minor use/level, 2 = moderate use/level, and 3 = high use/level, as adapted from Vaschenko, Lambidoni and Brody (2007), with interrater reliability levels ranging from moderate to high (Cohen's kappa = .43–.80). Resilience was defined as thinking or behaving adaptively and competently, recovering from trauma, and/or achieving positive outcomes (including better health, improved relationships, higher self-esteem, or employment) despite experiencing acute stressors or being in high-risk environments.

Data were analyzed using partial correlations (controlling for income and education), two-tailed *t* tests, and hierarchical linear multiple regression equations. All analyses were conducted using SPSS version 19.00.

RESULTS

Relationships between Gender Roles, Coping Strategies, and Mental Health

Partial correlations controlling for income and education level revealed several significant relationships between coping strategies and scores on traditional gender role scales. Less traditional (or more egalitarian) gender role behaviors, such as lower rates of self-silencing, lower unmitigated communion (caring for others at the expense of self-care), lower levels of violence, and higher sexual relationship power were related to higher levels of agentic coping strategies, including seeking formal or informal education, generativity, insight, meaning making, persistence, self-reliance, and social activism. Specific correlations are presented in tables 6.3 and 6.4.

TABLE 6.2 DEFINITIONS OF COPING STRATEGIES CODED FROM NARRATIVES

Coping strategy	Definition
Active steps	Taking active steps to resolve an identified problem in order to improve one's self, one's situation, or one's circumstances.
Generativity	Concern for and commitment to promoting the well-being of future generations through parenting, teaching, mentoring, or leaving a positive legacy.
Insight	Understanding or awareness of one's thoughts, motives, feelings, or behaviors and the family/social contributors to those processes.
Leaving abusive situations	Physically removing one's self from environments and relationships that are harmful and/or dysfunctional.
Meaning making	Having a positive perspective or identifying a positive outcome as a result of an illness or trauma.
Mindfulness	A mental state characterized by the awareness of one's body functions, feelings, or thoughts.
Optimism	Having a positive attitude or outlook about current and/or future circumstances whether or not they are overtly favorable.
Persistence	Sustained pattern of attitudes and behaviors that serve to reach a goal despite obstacles and adverse circumstances.
Seeking education	Learning or gathering more information in formal or informal settings.
Self-reliance	Taking care of one's self in an appropriately independent way; turning to one's self first when attempting endeavors of which one is capable.
Setting realistic goals	Setting goals that are feasible and attainable given one's current situation.
Social activism	Empowering and/or making changes in others' lives or within the social/political sphere by providing education, aid, or advocacy.

Table 6.5 shows results of partial correlations indicating that many agentic coping strategies are significantly associated with lower levels of depression and higher levels of resilience, although not to quality-of-life measures. Specifically, women who sought fewer formal or informal educational experiences were more depressed, and women who were more insightful; who used more meaning making, mindfulness, and persistence; and who left abusive situations more often were more resilient.

TABLE 6.3   PARTIAL CORRELATIONS BETWEEN COPING STRATEGIES AND GENDER
ROLES, CONTROLLING FOR EDUCATION AND INCOME ($n = 67$)

Coping strategy	STSS EXP	STSS CS	STSS SS	STS DS	RUCS
Active steps	−0.17	−0.07	−0.02	0.01	−0.10
Seeking education	−0.29*	−0.01	−0.29*	−0.21ᵗ	−0.22ᵗ
Generativity	−0.05	−0.09	−0.10	−0.11	0.00
Insight	−0.21ᵗ	−0.13	−0.34**	−0.14	−0.04
Leaving abusive situations	0.07	−0.06	0.08	0.08	−0.12
Meaning making	−0.14	−0.15	−0.29*	−0.12	0.05
Mindfulness	−0.01	−0.05	0.03	−0.03	−0.02
Optimism	−0.15	−0.13	−0.05	−0.08	0.07
Persistence	−0.27*	−0.03	−0.26*	−0.21ᵗ	0.03
Self-reliance	−0.23ᵗ	−0.11	−0.20	0.01	−0.27*
Setting realistic goals	−0.16	−0.04	−0.06	−0.10	−0.12
Social activism	−0.04	−0.05	0.11	0.13	0.04

NOTES: STSS = Silencing the Self Total Scale. STSS EXP = Externalized Self-Perception subscale of STSS. STSS CS = Care as Self-Sacrifice subscale of STSS. STSS SS = Silencing the Self subscale of STSS. STSS DS = Divided Self subscale of STSS. RUCS = Revised Unmitigated Communion Scale.

ᵗ$p < .10$, *$p < .05$, **$p < .01$.

TABLE 6.4   PARTIAL CORRELATIONS BETWEEN COPING STRATEGIES, PHYSICAL
VIOLENCE, AND SEXUAL RELATIONSHIP POWER, CONTROLLING FOR EDUCATION
AND INCOME ($n = 67$)

Coping strategy	Physical violence	SRPS decision making	SRPS relationship dominance
Active steps	−0.15	0.06	−0.06
Seeking education	−0.34**	−0.04	0.25*
Generativity	0.05	0.27*	0.23ᵗ
Insight	0.10	0.06	0.22ᵗ
Leaving abusive situations	0.25*	−0.05	-0.11
Making meaning	0.13	−0.17	0.16
Mindfulness	0.02	−0.21	−0.02
Optimism	0.04	−0.90	−0.04
Persistence	−0.09	0.04	0.20
Self-reliance	−0.25*	0.02	0.24ᵗ
Setting realistic goals	−0.29*	0.02	-0.11
Social activism	0.12	0.22ᵗ	-0.10

NOTES: SRPS = Sexual Relationship Power Scale.

ᵗ$p < .10$, *$p < .05$, **$p < .01$.

TABLE 6.5 PARTIAL CORRELATIONS BETWEEN COPING STRATEGIES AND
PSYCHOLOGICAL OUTCOMES, CONTROLLING FOR INCOME AND EDUCATION

Coping strategy	CES-D	MOS HIV	Resilience
Active steps	−.12	−.18	.06
Seeks education	−.30*	.19	.26*
Generativity	.06	−.17	−.02
Insight	−.03	.05	.54**
Leaves abusive situations	.06	.05	.35**
Meaning making	.14	−.02	.50**
Mindfulness	−.01	.05	.26*
Optimism	.08	.01	−.09
Persistence	.11	−.15	.36**
Self-reliance	−.08	.05	.24^t
Sets realistic goals	−.21^t	.15	−.01
Social activism	−.04	−.00	.13

NOTES: CES-D = Center for Epidemiological Studies Depressive Symptoms Scale. MOS HIV = The Medical Outcome Study assessing quality of life.

^{t} p < .10; * p < .05; ** p < .01.

Age in Relation to Coping, Gender Roles, Depression, and Quality of Life

As displayed in the partial correlations in table 6.6, older women in our sample tended to be less optimistic, use less meaning making, and to be less self-reliant than younger women. They also tended to have a higher degree of self-silencing, a lower quality of life, and less resilience than younger women. There were no relationships between age and depression, sexual relationship power and control, or levels of experienced violence.

Multiple regression analyses also revealed that age significantly moderated relationships between quality of life and gender role behaviors. For older women, more traditional gender role behavior (in the form of prioritizing the needs of others over the needs of the self) was significantly related to lower quality of life ($\beta = -.35$, $t = -2.46$, $p < 0.05$), and greater use of meaning making was related to greater resilience ($\beta = .35$, $t = 3.11$, $p < 0.01$).

DISCUSSION

Traditional gender role behaviors are related to lower levels of agentic coping strategies among HIV-positive women. Higher levels of self-silencing, in which women silence themselves to avoid relational loss

TABLE 6.6 PARTIAL CORRELATIONS OF AGE WITH COPING STRATEGIES, RESILIENCE, GENDER ROLES, DEPRESSION, QUALITY OF LIFE, AND PHYSICAL VIOLENCE FOR HIV+ AND HIV− WOMEN AND TOTAL SAMPLE, CONTROLLING FOR EDUCATION AND INCOME

	Partial correlations with age		
	HIV-positive (n = 43)	HIV-negative (n = 24)	Entire sample (N = 67)
Coping strategy			
Active steps	0.29^t	−0.14	0.04
Seeking education	0.16	0.02	0.00
Generativity	0.21	−0.26	0.03
Insight	0.10	−0.34	−0.12
Leaving abusive situations	0.21	−0.36	0.00
Making meaning	−0.17	−0.20	−0.22^t
Mindfulness	−0.12	−0.04	−0.03
Optimism	−0.12	−0.42^t	−0.21^t
Persistence	0.25	0.00	0.08
Self-reliance	−0.02	−0.33	−0.22^t
Setting realistic goals	0.29^t	−0.41^t	−0.05
Social activism	0.23	0.04	0.17
Resilience	−0.10	−0.29	−0.22^t

	HIV-positive (n = 50)	HIV-negative (n = 33)	Entire sample (N = 83)
Gender roles			
STSS Care as self-sacrifice	−0.08	−0.22	−0.08
STSS Divided self	0.14	−0.11	0.08
STSS Externalized self-perception	0.05	0.09	0.13
STSS Self-silencing	0.22	0.06	0.20^t
SRPS Decision-making dominance	0.29^t	−0.21	0.02
SRPS Relationship power	0.01	−0.23	−0.11
Unmitigated communion	−0.2	−0.05	−0.09
CES-D	−0.13	0.12	−0.03
MOS HIV	−0.10	−0.01	−0.21^t
Physical violence	0.15	0.07	0.12

NOTES: STSS = Silencing the Self Scale. SRPS = Sexual Relationship Power Scale. CES-D = Center for Epidemiological Studies Depressive Symptoms Scale. MOS HIV = The Medical Outcome Study.

$^t p < .10.$

and conflict, as well as higher unmitigated communion, in which women prioritize care for others over self-care, were related to lower levels of seeking formal or informal education, generativity, insight, meaning making, persistence, self-reliance, and social activism.

This study also demonstrates that women with higher levels of agentic coping strategies and lower levels of traditional gender role behaviors in sexual relationships (characterized by higher relationship power and lower violence rates) had higher levels of resilience and lower levels of depression. Because our results present cross-sectional associations and not multivariate or longitudinal analyses, it is impossible to assert the directionality of these effects, although literature on psychological trauma indicates that being a victim of violence is associated with subsequent consequences such as self-blame and feelings of helplessness and worthlessness (Herma 1992), all of which reflect disempowered and nonagentic coping strategies. The question remains whether women who are in relationships in which they have more decision-making power have come by this power by virtue of utilizing more agentic coping strategies and less traditional gender roles, or alternatively, whether their relatively egalitarian relationships provide the support and shared decision-making power that they need to ultimately employ more agentic coping strategies.

Finally, our results show that older women with and at risk for HIV were more likely to report traditional gender role behaviors than younger women, especially in prioritizing the care of others over self-care, that place them at risk for low quality of life and low resilience. For older women, meaning making was especially related to higher resilience, while prioritizing care for others over self-care was especially related to lower quality of life when compared to younger women. It may be that older women are less able to physically and emotionally cope with the multiple challenges faced by this cohort. Given the demands of the aging process, self-care may become even more important in maintaining quality of life at older ages. Further, meaning making may be an especially important coping strategy for older women because of their developmental life stage. Being able to make meaning from their many years of past experience may be especially important to them as compared to younger women, for whom it is more developmentally appropriate to be looking ahead to the future.

In sum, agentic coping strategies, such as persistence and making meaning by finding the positive value in traumatic experiences, are related to more egalitarian gender role behaviors, and both agentic coping strategies and egalitarian behaviors are related to higher resilience in women with and at risk for HIV. These coping strategies and behaviors are good examples of Kabeer's (2001) "strategic life choices previously denied." Designing interventions to teach these coping skills and behaviors has the potential to improve the functioning and health of women with and at risk for HIV and to prevent new infections.

WOMEN ORGANIZED TO RESPOND TO LIFE-THREATENING DISEASES (WORLD)

WORLD is a grassroots organization designed to support HIV-positive women in Oakland, California, and incorporates support for many of the agentic coping strategies delineated in the WIHS study described above. WORLD was founded in 1991 by a small group of HIV-positive women, led by Rebecca Denison, in response to the paucity of specific support-services geared towards HIV positive women. It now provides direct services, including education, peer advocacy, and support, to 800 women living with HIV, mostly in the Oakland–San Francisco Bay Area, some of whom are participants in the San Francisco–area WIHS study, as well as to other demographically similar HIV-infected women. Services are also provided through website resources, national trainings, and direct support to international groups setting up similar organizations for HIV-infected women. WORLD is an example of an intervention program designed to positively impact empowering coping strategies in HIV-infected women with likely beneficial and sustainable effects on their health and the health of the community.

Table 6.7 links each service that WORLD provides to one or more of the coping strategies coded from the narratives above and summarized in table 6.2. Theoretical reasoning and examples from other women's empowerment interventions support the imputed impacts of each WORLD service on the coping strategies identified by the survey above. Further program evaluation is ongoing to assess the impact of WORLD services on specific health outcomes. The results of our survey study may be able to inform future programmatic interventions at WORLD and other organizations designed to support HIV-positive women in terms of empowerment strategies and gender roles.

LESSONS LEARNED

This study demonstrates that, within a context of gender inequality, traditional gender role behaviors are associated with lower levels of

Coping strategy	WORLD program
Active steps	Peer advocacy, support groups, HIV University, Lotus Project[1], retreats, HIV Speakers' Bureau[2], POWERR[3]
Generativity	Peer advocacy (for advocates), support groups, HIV University, Lotus Project, newsletters, HIV Speakers' Bureau, Phoenix Project[4]
Insight	Peer advocacy, support groups, HIV University, Lotus Project retreats, newsletters, HIV Speakers' Bureau, POWERR
Leaving abusive situations	Support groups, retreats
Meaning making	Peer advocacy, support groups, HIV University, Lotus Project, retreats, newsletters, HIV Speakers' Bureau, POWERR
Mindfulness	Peer advocacy, support groups, HIV University, retreats, newsletters
Optimism	Peer advocacy, support groups, retreats, newsletters, POWERR
Persistence	Peer advocacy, support groups, retreats, Phoenix Project, POWERR
Seeking education	Peer advocacy, support groups, HIV University, Lotus Project, retreats, newsletters, HIV Speakers' Bureau, POWERR
Self-reliance	Support groups, HIV University, Lotus Project, retreats, newsletters, HIV Speakers' Bureau, POWERR
Setting realistic goals	Peer advocacy, support groups, retreats, Phoenix Project
Social activism	Peer advocacy (for advocates), support groups, Lotus Project, newsletters, HIV Speakers' Bureau, Phoenix Project

[1] Lotus Project: National skills building training for women living with HIV that trained over 200 women to become peer educators. The program also provided technical assistance and capacity building to over 10 organizations throughout the US developing peer programs for women in their communities.

[2] HIV Speakers' Bureau: A cadre of HIV-positive educators at WORLD trained in delivering lectures on HIV and its impact on women to policy groups and peers.

[3] POWERR (Prevention Outreach with Women Empowering Risk Reduction) was a program developed by WORLD for African American girls based on principles of gender empowerment and social network theories.

[4] Phoenix Project: An initiative to locate women who have fallen out of care and connect them back to health and wellness. This joint pilot project between WORLD and the East Bay AIDS Center combined the efforts of medical providers and WORLD peer advocates.

agentic coping strategies. Moreover, traditional gender role behaviors and lower levels of agentic coping strategies are associated with higher levels of depression and lower levels of resilience in women with and at risk for HIV. When compared to younger women, older women with HIV are more likely to report traditional gender role behaviors and have a poorer quality of life, although the coping strategy of meaning making minimizes this risk. These findings should inform the design of clinical interventions to educate women about gender role behaviors and teach them self-advocacy and self-care skills to increase their power within sexual relationships. Coping skills of seeking education, persistence, self-reliance, generativity, insight, and meaning making are especially important to emphasize. WORLD, an organization in Oakland, California, is highlighted as an intervention program designed to positively impact these coping strategies in HIV-infected women and can serve as a model for the development of similar programs for at-risk and infected women worldwide.

Box 6.1. Summary

Geographic area: Chicago and the San Francisco–Oakland Bay Area, United States

Global importance of the health condition: Women represent a significant percentage of all HIV cases in the United States, with heterosexual contact being the primary means of HIV acquisition in this group. Investigating women's coping strategies, gender role behaviors, and sexual power and violence in their relationships can be critical for preventing further spread of the disease and reducing morbidity rates for those infected.

Intervention or program: A survey was carried out with eighty-three women with HIV and at risk for HIV, participants in the National Institutes of Health–funded Chicago Women's Interagency HIV Study (WIHS). Relationships among gender role behaviors, depression, quality of life, resilience, and coping strategies were investigated with a special emphasis on older women. A nonprofit organization in Oakland, California, Women Organized to Respond to Life-Threatening Diseases (WORLD), provides a set of interventions including peer advocacy, health education, and support to HIV-infected women, designed to positively impact coping strategies, resilience, and health outcomes in this population.

Impact: Lower levels of traditional gender role behaviors (including higher power and less violence in sexual relationships) and higher levels of coping strategies reflecting individual agency, such as persistence, meaning making (the ability to recognize or create positive outcome or value resulting from traumatic experiences), generativity (concern for establishing and guiding the next generation), insight (awareness of thoughts, motives, feelings, or behaviors and the family and social contributors to those processes), seeking formal or informal education, and self-reliance were related to lower levels of depression and higher resilience in the survey study. For older women, more traditional gender role behaviors (especially prioritizing the needs of others over the needs of the self) were related to lower quality of life, and greater use of meaning making was related to higher resilience. WORLD's services are highlighted since they include programs to enhance the coping strategies identified in the survey study to improve participants' sense of community, self-efficacy, and mental and physical health.

Lessons learned: Clinical interventions should be developed to educate women with HIV about the relationship between gender roles and coping skills and teach them self-advocacy and self-care skills to increase their power within sexual relationships. Coping skills of education seeking, persistence, self-reliance, generativity, insight, and meaning making, especially for older women, are important to emphasize. WORLD is a model of one such interventional program.

Link between empowerment and health: Egalitarian gender roles and active, problem-focused coping strategies for women with and at risk for HIV constitute a form of individual empowerment (the ability to make strategic life choices) that may likely improve health outcomes and decrease HIV acquisition rates in these groups, respectively. Interventions to improve individual empowerment in HIV-infected women will be likely to improve health outcomes.

For a video about Women Organized to Respond to Life-Threatening Disease (WORLD), see https://youtu.be/FgYzjR3VfUY

Box 6.2. Shifts in Organizational and Educational Strategies to Lower Depressive Symptoms and Assist Quality of Life and Resilience in U.S. Women Living with HIV

OLDER PERSPECTIVES

- Minimize the importance of how internalized gender roles (on a continuum from traditional to egalitarian) impact health outcomes in women with HIV.

- Focus on avoidant and passive coping strategies that are maladaptive for health, rather than on active coping strategies that are adaptive and foster resilient functioning.

- Fail to differentiate between the psychological and health needs of younger and middle-aged women with HIV.

NEWER PERSPECTIVES

- View HIV-positive and at-risk women as positive agents of change who can employ more egalitarian gender roles and active coping strategies to increase personal power and satisfaction in relationships.

- Perceive that egalitarian gender roles, positive attributes, and proactive coping strategies such as persistence, meaning making, generativity, insight, seeking formal or informal education, and self-reliance can improve health outcomes and engagement in care.

- Understand that it is critical to include middle-aged women's needs in program content; programs need to teach a balance between self-care and care for others; and making meaning from previous experiences has a positive impact on women's health and empowerment.

REFERENCES

Akers, A, L Bernstein, S Henderson, J Doyle, and G Corbie-Smith. 2007. Factors associated with lack of interest in HIV testing in older at-risk women. *J Womens Health (Larchmt)* 16 (6):842–858.

Amaro, H, and A Raj. 2000. On the margin: Power and women's HIV risk reduction strategies *Sex Roles* 42:723–749.

Auerbach, JD, and TJ Coates. 2000. HIV prevention research: accomplishments and challenges for the third decade of AIDS. *Am J Public Health* 90 (7):1029–1032.

Barkan, SE, SL Melnick, S Preston-Martin, K Weber, LA Kalish, P Miotti, M Young, R Greenblatt, H Sacks, and J Feldman. 1998. The Women's

Interagency HIV Study. WIHS Collaborative Study Group. *Epidemiology* 9 (2):117–215.

Bozzette, SA, RD Hays, SH Berry, DE Kanouse, and AW Wu. 1995. Derivation and properties of a brief health status assessment instrument for use in HIV disease. *J Acquir Immune Defic Syndr Hum Retrovirol* 8 (3): 253–265.

Brief, DJ, AR Bollinger, MJ Vielhauer, JA Berger-Greenstein, EE Morgan, SM Brady, LM Buondonno, and TM Keane. 2004. Understanding the interface of HIV, trauma, post-traumatic stress disorder, and substance use and its implications for health outcomes. *AIDS Care* 16 Suppl 1:S97–120.

Brody, LR, LR Stokes, SK Dale, GA Kelso, RC Cruise, KM Weber, JK Burke-Miller, and MH Cohen. 2014. Gender roles and mental health in women with and at risk for HIV. *Psychol Women Q* 38:311–326.doi:10.1177/0361684314525579.

Brody, LR, LR Stokes, GA Kelso, SK Dale, RC Cruise, KA Weber, JK Burke-Miller, and MH Cohen. 2014. Gender role behaviors of high affiliation and low self-silencing predict better adherence to antiretroviral therapy in women with HIV. *AIDS Patient Care and STDs.* 28(9):459–461.

Carver, CS, MF Scheier, and JK Weintraub. 1989. Assessing coping strategies: A theoretically based approach. *J Pers Soc Psychol* 56 (2):267–283.

Centers for Disease Control and Prevention. 2016. *HIV among Women.* [accessed June 3 2016]. www.cdc.gov/hiv/group/gender/women/.

Cohen, M, C Deamant, S Barkan, J Richardson, M Young, S Holman, K Anastos, J Cohen, and S Melnick. 2000. Domestic violence and childhood sexual abuse in women with HIV infection and women at risk for HIV. *Am J of Pub Health* 90:560–565.

Dale, SK, G Kelso, C Watson, K Weber, J David, V Linh-Phuong, M Cohen, and LR Brody. 2011. Trauma history, resilience and gender roles among women with HIV or at risk for HIV. Presented at 119th Annual APA Convention; Washington, DC.

DeMarco, RF (2010). Supporting voice in women living with HIV/AIDS. In: DC Jack and A Ali, editors. *Silencing the self across cultures: depression and gender in the social world.* New York, NY: Oxford University Press. p. 343–362. doi: 10.1093/acprof:oso/9780195398090.003.0017.

Dworkin, SL, ST Beckford, and AA Ehrhardt. 2007. Sexual scripts of women: a longitudinal analysis of participants in a gender-specific HIV/STD prevention intervention. *Arch Sex Behav* 36 (2):269–279.

Emlet, CA 2006. An examination of the social networks and social isolation in older and younger adults living with HIV/AIDS. *Health Soc Work* 31 (4):299–308.

Engstrom, M, T Shibusawa, N El-Bassel, and L Gilbert 2011. Age and HIV sexual risk among women in methadone treatment. *AIDS Behav* 15 (1): 103–113.

Exner TM, SL Dworkin, S Hoffman, and AA Ehrhardt. 2003. Beyond the male condom: the evolution of gender-specific HIV interventions for women. *Annu Rev Sex Res* 14:114–136.

Fortin, NM. 2005. Gender role attitudes and the labour-market outcomes of women across OECD countries. *Oxf Rev Econ Policy* 21 (3):416–438.

Fritz, HL, and VS Helgeson. 1998. Distinctions of unmitigated communion from communion: self-neglect and overinvolvement with others. *J Pers Soc Psychol* 75 (1):121–140.

Grant, K, and K Ragsdale. 2008. Sex and the "recently single": perceptions of sexuality and HIV risk among mature women and primary care physicians. *Cult Health Sex* 10 (5):495–511.

Grant, TM, DC Jack, AL Fitzpatrick, and CC Ernst. 2011. Carrying the burdens of poverty, parenting, and addiction: depression symptoms and self-silencing among ethnically diverse women. *Community Ment Health J* 47:90–98. doi: 10.1007/s10597-009-9255-y.

Grov, C, SA Golub, JT Parsons, M Brennan, and SE Karpiak. 2010. Loneliness and HIV-related stigma explain depression among older HIV-positive adults. *AIDS Care* 22 (5):630–639.

Gupta, GR. 2000. Gender, sexuality and HIV/AIDS: the what, the why and the how. Paper read at International Conference on AIDS, June 9–14; Durban, South Africa.

Hansen, NB, N Tarakeshwar, M Ghebremichael, H Zhang, A Kochman, and KJ Sikkema. 2006. Longitudinal effects of coping on outcome in a randomized controlled trial of a group intervention for HIV-positive adults with AIDS-related bereavement. *Death Stud* 30 (7):609–636.

Herman, JL. 1992. *Trauma and recovery: the aftermath of violence—from domestic abuse to political terror.* New York, NY: Basic Books.

Ironson, G, E Balbin, E Stieren, K Detz, MA Fletcher, N Schneiderman, and M Kumar. 2008. Perceived stress and norepinephrine predict the effectiveness of response to protease inhibitors in HIV. *Int J Behav Med* 15 (3):221–226.

Jack, DC, and A Ali, editors. 2010. Self-silencing and depression across cultures: depression and gender in the social world. New York, NY: Oxford University Press.

Jack, DC, and D Dill. 1992. The silencing the self scale: schemas of intimacy associated with depression in women. *Psychol Women Q* 16 (1):97–106.

Jacobs, RJ, and B Thomlison. 2009. Self-silencing and age as risk factors for sexually acquired HIV in midlife and older women. *J Aging Health* 21 (1):102–128.

Jacobs, RJ, and MN Kane. 2010. HIV-related stigma in midlife and older women. *Soc Work Health Care* 49 (1):68–89.

Kabeer, N. 2001. Reflections on the measurement of women's empowerment. In: *Discussing women's empowerment—theory and practice.* Sida Studies no. 3. Stockholm, Sweden: Novum Grafiska AB.

Kelso, GA, MH Cohen, KM Weber, SK Dale, RC Cruise, and LR Brody. 2013. Critical consciousness, racial and gender discrimination, and HIV disease markers in African American women with HIV. *AIDS Behav* Sep 28.

Kelso, GA, L Stokes, S Dale, J Kim, L Lombardo, M Cohen, K Weber, and LR Brody. 2010. Self-silencing and quality of life in women as a function of HIV status. Presented at: APS Annual Convention; Boston, MA.

Konkle-Parker, DJ, JA Erlen, and PM Dubbert. 2008. Barriers and facilitators to medication adherence in a southern minority population with HIV disease. *J Assoc Nurses AIDS Care: JANAC* 19 (2):98–104.

Lazarus, RS, and S Folkman. 1984. *Stress, appraisal and coping.* New York: Springer.

Machtinger, EL, JE Haberer, TC Wilson, and DS Weiss. 2012. Recent trauma is associated with antiretroviral failure and HIV transmission risk behavior among HIV-positive women and female-identified transgenders. *AIDS Behav* Nov; 16 (8):2160–2170.

Machtinger, EL, TC Wilson, JE Haberer, and DS Weiss. 2012. Psychological trauma and PTSD in HIV-positive women: a meta-analysis. Review. *AIDS Behav* Nov; 16 (8):2091–2100. doi: 10.1007/s10461-011-0127-4.

McAdams, DP, JJ Bauer, AR Sakaeda, MA Machado, KW White, JL Pals, K Magrino-Failla, and N Akua Anyidoho. 2006. Continuity and change in the life story: a longitudinal study of autobiographical memories in emerging adulthood. *J Pers* 74 (5):1371–1400.

National Center for Health Statistics, Centers for Disease Control. 2011. Deaths: final data for 2009. NVSS. Dec; 60 (3). www.cdc.gov/nchs/deaths .htm.

Neundorfer, MM, PB Harris, PJ Britton, and DA Lynch. 2005. HIV-risk factors for midlife and older women. *Gerontologist* 45 (5):617–625.

O'Cleirigh, C, G Ironson, M Antoni, MA Fletcher, L McGuffey, E Balbin, N Schneiderman, and G Solomon. 2003. Emotional expression and depth processing of trauma and their relation to long-term survival in patients with HIV/AIDS. *J Psychosom Res* 54 (3):225–235.

O'Cleirigh, C, G Ironson, MA Fletcher, and N Schneiderman. 2008. Written emotional disclosure and processing of trauma are associated with protected health status and immunity in people living with HIV/AIDS. *Br J Health Psychol* 13 (Pt 1):81–84.

Parker, JDA, and NS Endler. 1996. Coping and defense: a historical overview. In: Zeidner, M, and Endler, NS, editors. *Handbook of coping: theory, research, applications.* Oxford, England: Wiley.

Plach, SK, PE Stevens, and S Keigher. 2005. Self-care of women growing older with HIV and/or AIDS. *West J Nurs Res* 27 (5):534–553.

Prado, G, DJ Feaster, SJ Schwartz, IA Pratt, L Smith, and J Szapocznik. 2004. Religious Involvement, coping, social support, and psychological distress in HIV-seropositive African American mothers. *AIDS Behav* 8 (3):221–235.

Pulerwitz, J, SL Gortmaker, and W DeJong. 2000. Measuring sexual relationship power in HIV/STD research. *Sex Roles* 42 (7):637–660.

Radloff, LS. 1977. The CES-D scale: A self-report depression scale for research in the general population. *Appl Psychol Meas* 1 (3):385–401.

Sareen, J, J Pagura, and B Grant. 2009. Is intimate partner violence associated with HIV infection among women in the United States? *Gen Hosp Psychiatry* 31 (3):274–278.

Teitelman, AM, SJ Ratcliffe, ME Dichter, and CM Sullivan. 2008. Recent and past intimate partner abuse and HIV risk among young women. *J Obstet Gynecol Neonatal Nurs* 37 (2):219–227.

Teitelman, AM, SJ Ratcliffe, MM Morales-Aleman, and CM Sullivan. 2008. Sexual relationship power, intimate partner violence, and condom use among minority urban girls. *J Interpers Violence* Dec; 23 (12): 1694–1712.

Theall, KP, KW Elifson, CE Sterk, and H Klein. 2003. Perceived susceptibility to HIV among women. *Res Aging* 25 (4):405–432.

Tufts, KA, J Wessell, and T Kearney. 2010. Self-care behaviors of african american women living with HIV: a qualitative perspective. *J Assoc Nurses AIDS Care: JANAC* 21 (1):36–52.

Vashchenko, M, E Lambidioni, and LR Brody. 2007. Late adolescents' coping styles in narratives of interpersonal and intrapersonal conflicts using the narrative disclosure task *Clin Soc Work J* 35 (4): 245–255.

Wingood, GM, and RJ DiClemente. 2000. Application of the theory of gender and power to examine HIV-related exposures, risk factors, and effective interventions for women. *Health Educ Behav* 27 (5):539–565.

Wingood, G.M, RJ DiClemente, DH McCree, K Harrington, and SL Davies. 2001. Dating violence and the sexual health of black adolescent females. *Pediatr* 107 (5): e72.

Wingood, GM, RJ DiClemente, I Mikhail, DH McCree, SL Davies, JW Hardin, S Harris Peterson, EW Hook, and M Saag. 2007. HIV discrimination and the health of women living with HIV. *Women Health* 46 (2–3):99–112.

7

Examining the Impact of a Masculinities-Based HIV Prevention and Antiviolence Program in Limpopo and Eastern Cape, South Africa

SHARI L. DWORKIN, ABIGAIL M. HATCHER,
CHRISTOPHER COLVIN, AND DEAN PEACOCK

Seventy percent of all HIV transmission worldwide is due to heterosexual activity (*UNAIDS Report* 2012). The probability of male-to-female transmission is twice that of female-to-male transmission, given women's greater biological susceptibility to HIV and because men frequently have more sexual partners than women, as well as more economic and sexual negotiating power (Higgins, Hoffman, and Dworkin 2010). Research finds that men who conform to narrow definitions of masculinity emphasizing risk-taking, sex with multiple partners, having sex without a condom, and adversarial and inequitable attitudes towards women are at heightened risk of HIV acquisition and subsequent transmission to women (Exner et al. 2003; Hunter 2005; Jewkes et al. 2010; Shannon et al. 2012). Sexual violence enacted by men has also been shown to increase HIV risk for both women and men (Dunkle et al. 2006; Jewkes et al. 2011), and men who endorse traditional masculine ideologies and/ or inequitable attitudes are more likely to endorse rape-supportive attitudes and to have already committed sexual aggression against women (Jakupcak, Lisak, and Roemer 2002; Kalichman et al. 2007; Shannon et al. 2012). Moreover, in much of the world, women's HIV risks are mainly through their marriages or primary male partner (Hirsch et al. 2007; *UNAIDS Report* 2012). To slow the pace of the global HIV epidemic, work with heterosexually-active men requires more attention.

South Africa has one of the highest rates of HIV prevalence in the world (*UNAIDS Report* 2012). There is a significant gender gap in people living with HIV in South Africa, with fourteen HIV positive women for every ten HIV positive men (*UNAIDS Report* 2012). The difference between women's and men's HIV prevalence rates is even more pronounced in the 15–24 age group: young South African women are reported to have between two and four times the HIV prevalence of men (Rehle et al. 2010; *UNAIDS Report* 2012). This disparity has led to renewed efforts to address gender inequalities in South African society and beyond. HIV prevention interventions that are gender-specific have focused on improving women's economic empowerment, helping women to negotiate safer sex in relationships, and shifting relationship and community-level norms concerning violence against South African women (Jewkes et al. 2009; Pronyk et al. 2006). Heightened attention to gender equality and women's empowerment has also catalyzed non-governmental organizations (NGOs) to focus on challenging norms of masculinity and the role of men in advancing gender equality and achieving improved health outcomes for both men and women (Barker et al. 2010; Kalichman et al. 2009; Peacock and Levack 2004). Here, the emphasis has been on the development of programs that work with men and boys to promote more equitable gender relations, reduce violence against women, and reduce the spread and impact of HIV (Barker et al. 2010; Dworkin, Treves-Kagan, and Lippman 2013).

The current case study is a qualitative impact analysis of one NGO-implemented masculinities and rights-based program in South Africa known as One Man Can (OMC). This research project is an academic/NGO collaboration between the University of California, San Francisco, the University of Cape Town, and Sonke Gender Justice. Sonke Gender Justice is a South African non-governmental organization that was established in 2006 and has the goals of "strengthening civil society, government, and citizen capacity to support men and boys to take action to promote gender equality, reduce violence against women and children, and prevent the spread and impact of HIV and AIDS" (Sonke Gender Justice n.d.), using a broad mix of strategies designed to promote individual and social change. Sonke reaches nearly 25,000 men each year through workshops and community dialogues, as well as ten million listeners a week via community radio shows, and millions more as a result of media coverage of its high-profile advocacy work to effect change in government policies and practice. The current study assesses the impact of the OMC workshops, which include a combination of small-group discussions and community action teams (described below), to discuss and alter norms of masculinity in each setting. The program has been implemented in all provinces in South Africa and by 2013 had expanded to North Sudan, Swaziland, Lesotho, Mozambique, Zambia, and Malawi.

To better understand how the One Man Can program impacts men's attitudes about gender equality, women's empowerment, and relationship power, the researchers conducted sixty qualitative in-depth interviews with men who participated in OMC in rural Limpopo and Eastern Cape, South Africa. The study also sought to examine the impact of OMC on gender-based violence and HIV transmission. This qualitative analysis is part of a broader research project (Dworkin et al. 2013; Dworkin 2015) that seeks to understand the context of changing gender relations in South Africa, including changes at the individual, household, relationship, and community levels, along with the gender- and health-related impacts of gender-transformative programming with heterosexually active men.

CONTEXT

Recent studies suggest that gender inequality fuels the dual epidemics of HIV and violence in South Africa and globally (Dunkle et al. 2006; Jewkes et al. 2009, 2010). Unequal power relations in sexual decision making and experiences (or fears) of violence make it difficult or impossible for women to negotiate condom use and safe partnerships (Dunkle et al. 2006; Jewkes et al. 2009; Pulerwitz et al. 2002). In South Africa, not only are HIV prevalence rates among the highest in the world (*UNAIDS Report* 2012), but rates of domestic and sexual violence are also extremely high (Dunkle et al. 2006; Jewkes et al. 2009; Jewkes, Nduna et al. 2006). Nearly thirty percent of South African men in one study reported having committed an act of rape, and nearly half reported that they have been physically violent to an intimate partner, with fifteen percent reporting that they had perpetrated domestic violence in the last twelve months (Jewkes et al. 2011).

The One Man Can Program

The One Man Can program was launched on the International Day to End Violence Against Women, November 25, 2006, in South Africa and then in Geneva on December 6, 2006, as part of the United Nations High Commissioner for Refugees (UNHCR) 16 Days of Activism to End Violence Against Women campaign. Recognizing the importance of collaboration and the significant contribution made by many organizations across the world in developing and researching concepts relevant to OMC, the initiative was launched as a formal partnership of a wide range of South African and international organizations, including women's rights organizations. OMC is based on the premise that changing deeply held gender- and sexuality-related beliefs and practices requires comprehensive, multifaceted strategies. OMC works with men and boys of all ages and is rooted in the belief that men can become advocates for gender equality and active participants in efforts to respond to violence and HIV and AIDS. The program is implemented in urban, peri-urban, and rural areas and targets a wide range of men and boys, including members of the following groups: religious and traditional leaders; young and adult men in prisons and upon release; farm workers; miners; commercial fishermen; schoolchildren and their parents; health service providers; and policy makers at national, provincial, and local levels.

One Man Can was designed by men and women from relevant organizations working together and then reviewed by many different women's rights activists in South Africa. OMC uses small-group workshops led by male facilitators to actively engage with men and boys in the process of understanding, reflecting on, and reconfiguring gender relations and health outcomes in their relationships and communities. The workshops are designed to (1) examine the links between gender, power, and health-related metrics (alcohol use, violence, HIV/AIDS risk and outcomes); (2) reflect critically upon and achieve change in what it means to be a man in relationships with women, other men, and the broader community; (3) use rights-based concepts (participation, non-discrimination, accountability) to engage men in reducing violence against women and reduce HIV transmission and mitigate the negative impacts of HIV; and (4) encourage men to take action at the community level to promote gender equality and reduce violence and HIV risk.

The program explicitly defines masculinity as constructed, embedded in local contexts, achieved via interaction, strategic, and in flux (Connell 1987, 1995). The OMC workshops recognize how gender relations do not operate in isolation from other relations of inequality, such as race and class. The OMC materials link programmatic work on gender inequalities to the history of racial inequalities and apartheid in South Africa. For example, the program sessions underscore how power relations reinforce continuing mistreatment of subordinated groups, including Black South Africans and women, hindering their access to health care and affecting health outcomes. By highlighting these parallels, the program positively engages men in discussions of gender inequality and draws on South Africa's legacy of social justice activism to promote the idea that men can be positive agents of change in their homes and in their communities.

Many health-related programs utilize small-group workshops to achieve individual-level changes in gender ideologies and health behaviors (Dworkin et al. 2012; Kippax et al. 2013). OMC recognizes that individual-level changes in gender relations are not sufficient for creating sustained changes in health and justice-related outcomes. To counter the limitations of small-group workshops, the program deliberately pairs participatory workshops (that generally have short-term impacts) with Community Action Teams (CATs) efforts that are voluntary, are launched at the close of the workshops, and are designed to promote medium- to long-term change at the community level. Through CATs, men work within their own communities to determine what specific gender equality and health promotion activities they wish to undertake in their communities, with the large majority of these focusing on violence and AIDS prevention. The workshops and CATs activities are facilitated by men who are trained by Sonke, and the program content is delivered over four to eight sessions (one to two months) with groups of fifteen to twenty men.

METHODS

For this particular study, sixty men were recruited from the Eastern Cape Province ($N = 30$) (Mvumelwano, Bhlasi, and Qumbu), and Limpopo Province ($N = 30$) (Thoyandau) from February to September 2010, two of the provinces where Sonke Gender Justice implemented its One Man Can initiative. Inclusion criteria for the current study were as follows: age 18 years or older, completion of One Man Can workshops no more than six months from the date of the interview, and residence in a community where Sonke was carrying out ongoing One Man Can activities. The provinces for the current study, Limpopo and Eastern Cape, were selected because Sonke Gender Justice carried out a needs assessment and determined that these underserved rural areas also experience high rates of poverty, HIV, violence, and gender inequality (Colvin 2011; Pronyk et al. 2006). Participants were recruited by research assistants through Sonke's community partners.

To minimize social-desirability bias, we hired research assistants who were external to Sonke to carry out the interviews with the sixty OMC participants. Interviews focused on topics related to the broader context of change in South African society, such as gender relations and rights, violence, HIV risk, alcohol use, fatherhood, and relationships. Interviewers were trained for three days in qualitative methods and human subjects review principles. The research assistants were already experienced in probing sensitive topics such as gender, masculinities, HIV, and sexuality. Interviews were carried out in the local languages (Venda or Xhosa), transcribed into the local languages, and then translated into English. Each man was interviewed once at the conclusion of a one- to two-month workshop series between February and August 2010, and interviews lasted between one and two hours. This research protocol was approved by the Faculty of Health Sciences Human Research Ethics Committee at the University of Cape Town, South Africa, and at the University of California, San Francisco, United States. In accordance with the rules of South African ethical review boards, participants were offered R100 (about U.S. $12) for their participation in the qualitative study.

To analyze the data, two researchers first extracted excerpts of the translated interviews relating to the health impacts of the OMC workshops. After reviewing these excerpts, we generated a code book and subsequently wrote analytical memos to capture main themes and to lift multiple subcodes to a broader thematic analysis (Lofland and Lofland 1995). We also generated an analytical matrix where we mapped and charted primary and secondary codes across the entire sample, as described by Lofland and Lofland (1995). This process helped to ascertain recurrent themes. Any inconsistencies in the coding were discussed between the two researchers, and decision trails were noted in order to ensure consistency in the analysis.

RESULTS

Topics emerging from the interviews can be grouped into three broad themes. The first theme concerned men's views of women's empowerment and rights in these two provinces of South Africa. The second theme concerned men's perceptions about how participating in OMC had led to shifts in relationship power dynamics in their own households and relationships. The third theme captured men's perceptions that participating in OMC led them to alter their health-related behaviors, such as reducing alcohol use, avoiding violence, and engaging in less risky sexual practices. Each of these three themes is discussed below.

Theme 1: Men's View of Women's Empowerment

Most men reported that gender relations in contemporary South Africa were already changing, with women having more power and rights. One participant explained:

> Women's rights . . . not only in my community, but throughout the country, are something that is said everywhere. Men now know that women have rights and if they do not support them to realize them, they easily face the music of law. The government does not take any nonsense when it comes to women's rights, and that makes everyone change their attitude and respect the fact that women's rights are here to stay, forever. (age 36, married)

Men described their heightened awareness of women's rights, stemming from shifts in broader societal norms and their individual participation in the OMC program, which they generally framed as a promising development. The positive attitude towards women's rights was evident when men discussed the need to reduce violence against women. Views such as the following were not uncommon across both regions:

> There is change that can be credited to the One Man Can training. . . . For example, after a community meeting, men sometimes decide to hold their own meeting to discuss how they can change their behavior and lifestyles. . . . We (the older generation) grew up in disregard of women's rights. To us, women were supposed to be subservient to men, agree with men, and also know that men were the heads of the household. We did not know anything about women's rights. We have come to realize that women have to be treated as equals in the home and in the community and we are not supposed to abuse them. (age 62, single)

Several men expressed willingness to take on new roles in the home and family, as part of a shift towards more equality, which one man described this way:

> I had heard about women's rights but did not fully understand what they meant. For an example, if you have a wife and a child, you will find that the wife is cooking and at the same time taking care of the child while the husband is busy watching TV. OMC made me realize that in such a situation, the man must also be helping her. I now know that household chores are not only for women, but the man should also help. (age 25, single)

While many men embraced these changes and thought that women deserved enhanced rights, a few men felt that improving women's rights disempowered men and took away their power. For example, one participant complained:

> Women's rights takes away men's lives completely and puts it into the hands of women. Women control everything in men's lives, rather than consulting and living their lives together with balance . . . like they say 50-50. Now men are victims, and it has turned to 80-20. (age 56, married)

Theme 2: Shifts in Relationship Power

In the interviews, men also described specific changes in relationship power that had occurred as a result of their participation in the One Man Can program. One man explained these changes in terms of the visibility of women and their decision-making power in relationships:

> A lot has changed, like I said. My childhood observations of man as boss were wrong. Before I attended OMC sessions, I continued to believe that it is the same wrong things that need to be done. But after some sessions and engagement in discussions with various people with various points of view, I then realized that it is wrong to treat women like they do not exist. (age 32, single)

While the above quote is clearly not a strong narrative of gender equality, it does reveal a nuanced understanding of what a change towards more gender equality looks like if men previously held a tight grip on decision-making authority. Without giving up a hold on male authority, it would be impossible to see, hear, and take into account women's needs, inputs, and points of view.

In addition to men articulating that the OMC workshops helped them to increasingly take women's decision-making contributions into account, many men in our sample described a newfound appreciation of why women's rights deserved protection and enhancement. In addition, men in our sample described how OMC translated abstract rights-based principles as relevant to their own lives, such as how men should treat their wives or girlfriends. For example, by participating in OMC, one man explained how he started to challenge his previously held ideas about women's rights and male-dominated decision making:

> Before I joined OMC, I was very critical of women's rights, or more accurately, I did not believe that there was any need for women to be accorded special rights. In one of my frequent drunken states, I would go and look for my girlfriend, and when I wanted her to come along with me, there would be no compromise. My word was the final word and I would not take any input from her. Attending the OMC workshops, I got to understand the wrongs of my past behavior and I started understanding that men should also listen to the women's input. During the workshops I would feel as if the facilitators were talking directly to me or that maybe one of them knew about my life. (age 33, single)

Theme 3: Health Behavior Changes

In addition to seeking to transform men's views of gender relations and women's empowerment, OMC aimed to alter health behaviors and outcomes, such as reducing violence against women and men and HIV risk behaviors for both women and men. Many health behavioral changes were reported by participants in our sample. For example, some men reined in their tendency to use violence in their relationships:

> It [OMC] changed me in a way because it changed my own relationship. If my girlfriend is angry with me, and even if she is the one that is wrong, I calm down and talk to her without fighting. I respect her and I know that I should not beat her up. She even told me that things have changed in the way I act in our relationship and she is happy about it. (age 34, married)

Other men actively reduced their use of alcohol, which they now saw as being directly linked to domestic violence and risky sex. More than one-third of the men indicated that their OMC program participation was responsible for this change.

> OMC changed me for the better. . . . It has made me a better man because now if I feel I have had enough to drink, I go home, as opposed to the earlier habits of going to see girlfriends. That was risky because I was putting myself at risk of unprotected sex and HIV. I have also reduced on the amount of alcohol that I consume. (age 19, single)

In addition to men describing individual-level changes in alcohol use (which were often linked to descriptions of reduced violence and/or HIV risks), some men were members of a community action team (CAT) that focused on reducing alcohol use at the community level. Here, several men stated that they negotiated with local tavern owners to close bars (shebeens) early. These men believed that because so much unsafe sex and violence ensued at taverns (or after their close), cutting back on the hours of the tavern could reduce the volume of alcohol that is consumed and that this could have a major impact on women's and men's health. While we did not carry out long-term follow-up interviews to see if health changes were achieved at the community level over time, it is important to underscore how the workshops clearly sparked, supported, and facilitated community-level mobilization that stimulated health behavior change beyond the individual level. This level of change is often critical in achieving sustained improvements in health (Kippax et al., 2013; Lippman et al., 2013)

Some men also perceived that the OMC program specifically shifted their view of masculinity and thereby lowered their risky sexual behavior. Some noted that OMC program content helped them to realize that being masculine did not necessitate having many girlfriends but could instead involve being loyal to one partner, as one man explained:

> To be honest with you, I was a person who did not admire a man who was loyal to his one girlfriend. I viewed such men as weak, desperate, and being *izishumane* [a man who cannot get a girlfriend]. My view was that to be respected by other men, one should be involved with at least three women. However, since I started OMC, I took the decision to have one partner and be loyal to the partner. . . . I also improved my communication with my partner and I no longer drink as much as I used to, and that makes my partner happy. (age 41, married)

The narrative above is important because it underscores the way that the empowerment of women not only requires changes between women and men but also requires changes in how masculinity is defined and enacted in the presence other men. That is, prior to OMC, it was not simply that having many female sexual partners bolstered masculinity for any given individual man, but it was also the case that masculinity is achieved *collectively* in the eyes of other men (Connell 1995; Messner 1997). As such, it is critical to recall that masculinity is a collective practice and is more than the simple sum of men's individual behaviors.

DISCUSSION

Programs working towards gender equality often begin with recognition that men are frequently the decision makers and arbiters of women's and men's sexual and reproductive health outcomes within individual relationships (Barker 2010; Dworkin et al. 2011; Dudgeon and Inhorn 2004; Dworkin, Fullilove, and Peacock 2009; Kalichman et al. 2007, 2009). However, it is also common for public health interventions to pathologize men, to consider masculinity solely to be a "problem" that needs to be blamed and changed (Barker et al. 2010). Programs may emphasize that men benefit from structures of gender inequality but do not often recognize that men can and do fight for gains in equality and against oppression at the individual and community level (Dworkin et al. 2011, 2013; Peacock and Levack 2004).

While Sonke is best recognized for its work to transform harmful norms of masculinity and to mobilize men for gender justice, it deliberately rejects the term "men's organization" because of the ways this can easily be misconstrued to mean that Sonke focuses on advancement of men's rights. Instead, Sonke defines itself as a feminist organization working to achieve gender transformation (i.e., recognizing gendered power inequalities and shifting narrow and constraining definitions of what it means to be a man) as one of its principal strategies through the engagement, education, and mobilization of men. Sonke's campaigns and many workshops often explicitly portray men and women working together for gender justice. This collaboration demonstrates that gender inequalities are also men's issues and that men and women can and should work together to achieve a gender-equitable and healthy world.

Mobilizing men and boys in the effort to achieve greater gender equality can be difficult and time-consuming. A few scholars have noted that some men can feel blamed for women's poor health outcomes when they are treated as being a monolithic group or are the sole target of programming, and that this can impact engagement in health programs (Dworkin et al. 2013; Peacock et al. 2009). In addition, programs that work with men have tended to rely on small-group approaches to transforming gender relations by focusing on personal reflection to achieve interpersonal change but seldom mobilize participants to take action in their communities to promote norm and behavior changes. In contrast, the One Man Can program has attempted to avoid accusatory and blaming approaches towards men. It has also developed programs that emphasize the positive role that men can play in bringing about gender equality at the individual, interpersonal, and community levels. Finally, the program sought changes not only at the individual level but at the community level as well.

LIMITATIONS

Given that the sample of men was small and men were recruited from Sonke's partner organizations that were often dedicated to equality and health endeavors, these men may not be representative of the broader population of South African men. While many men attributed numerous changed beliefs and behaviors to the One Man Can program, it is difficult to ascertain the extent to which other programming carried out by Sonke (which saturates radio and TV programs) and by other organizations in these areas also played a role. Given that the study reports on qualitative, cross-sectional data collected up to six months after the close of the OMC program, recall biases may affect the accuracy of responses. These limitations, along with the high likelihood of social desirability biases, suggest that the change reported may be uncharacteristically high. Without the opportunity to triangulate our data with men's partners or wives (who could validate or challenge men' narratives) or collect data longitudinally it is impossible to know whether men's narratives are accurate representations of their beliefs and behaviors or whether the changes described were sustained beyond the six-month follow-up interview. Despite these limitations, however, our results are consistent with studies that show that programs that are "gender transformative"(Gupta and Kambou 2010)—in that they seek to change gender roles and create more gender-equitable relationships—can have a positive impact on attitudes of gender equality in relationships and on health-related behaviors (Barker 2010; Barker, Ricardo, and Nascimento 2007; Dworkin, Treves-Kagan, and Lippman 2013).

CONCLUSIONS

Gender transformative programs have been found to have a positive impact on gender ideologies and health behaviors related to HIV and violence outcomes (Barker et al. 2010; Dworkin, Treves-Kagan, and Lippman 2013). However, most gender transformative programs do not draw on the commonalities between gender oppression and other forms of oppression such as racial inequality to help engage men (Dworkin et al. 2012, 2013). OMC's novel approach can be important because it can reduce resistance to discussions about gender inequalities and women's empowerment by placing these topics in a larger social justice context. Moreover, this approach can press men to understand what is to be gained by redefining masculinities instead of viewing power as a zero sum gain where women gain and men lose.

Ultimately, many men in our sample who participated in OMC embraced emerging conceptions of gender equality and self-reported positive changes in their beliefs and behaviors, especially in the areas of women's rights, beliefs about what it means to be a man, and reduction in alcohol consumption. Researchers and practitioners should not assume that conceptions of masculinity in Africa are unchangeable or that gender relations cannot be improved. The OMC program appears to have made important strides in altering men's attitudes and behaviors, and such programs should be scaled up and emulated elsewhere.

Box 7.1. Summary

Geographic area: South Africa

Global importance of the health condition: HIV and violence are synergistic epidemics, each exacerbating the negative effects of the other, and each is undergirded by relations of gender inequality. The twin epidemics of HIV and violence have led to scientific and NGO efforts to transform gender relations to be more equitable.

Intervention or program: One Man Can is a "gender-transformative" HIV and antiviolence program that is carried out with men across all nine provinces in South Africa. The program content is rights-based and works to reshape norms of masculinity to be less harmful to women and men while pressing men in the direction of more gender equality.

Impact: Men shifted in the direction of more gender equitable beliefs and made health behavior changes including reductions in alcohol, violence, and HIV risk behavior.

Lessons learned: Work with men is a critical facet of transforming gender relations to improve women's empowerment and men's and women's HIV and violence outcomes.

Link between empowerment and health: Gender-transformative interventions that reshape definitions of what it means to be a man are a promising route through which to improve women's empowerment and positively impact women's and men's health.

For a video about Sonke Gender Justice and One Man Can, see https://youtu.be/HWTGTUc3Yho.

Box 7.2. Previous and Contemporary Approaches to Women's Empowerment and Health

PREVIOUS APPROACHES

- Focus on women only and assume that *gender* means "women," so men are left out.

- View men as the source of gender inequality and women's poor health.

- Perceive that men cannot change; masculinity is a fixed state.

- See men as always benefitting (and never suffering) from gender inequality.
- Assume that women-only interventions are sufficient to improve women's health and empowerment.

CONTEMPORARY APPROACHES

- Press beyond women-only approaches and work with men to improve women's empowerment and health.
- Recognize that both women and men are harmed when men adhere to narrow beliefs about what it means to be a man.
- Transform the constraining beliefs and practices of masculinity that shape health.
- Help men to critically reflect on what it means to be a man in their communities, households, and relationships.
- Recognize that masculinities and femininities need to shift to create lasting empowerment and health impacts.
- Highlight commonalities between race, class, and gender oppression to better engage men on gender equality and health issues.

REFERENCES

Barker, G. 2010. Reconceiving the second sex: Men, masculinity and reproduction. *Global Public Health* 5 (6):679–681.

Barker, G., C. Ricardo, and M. Nascimento. 2007. Engaging men and boys in changing gender-based inequity in health: Evidence from programme interventions. Geneva: World Health Organization.

Barker, G., C. Ricardo, M. Nascimento, A. Olukoya, and C. Santos. 2010. Questioning gender norms with men to improve health outcomes: Evidence of impact. *Global Public Health* 5: 539–553.

Colvin, C. 2011. *Executive Summary Report on the Impact of Sonke Gender Justice Network's One Man Can Campaign in Limpopo, Eastern Cape, and Kwa-Zulu Natal, South Africa.* Sonke Gender Justice Network 2009. [accessed Aug 28 2011]. Available from www.sonkegenderjustice.org.

Connell, R. W. 1987. *Gender and Power: Society, the Person and Sexual Politics.* Palo Alto, CA: Stanford University Press.

———. 1995. *Masculinities.* Berkeley: University of California Press.

Dudgeon, M. R., and M. C. Inhorn. 2004. Men's influences on women's reproductive health: Medical anthropological perspectives. *Social Science and Medicine* 59 (7):1379–1395.

Dunkle, K. L., R. K. Jewkes, M. Nduna, J. Levin, N. Jama, N. Khuzwayo, M. P. Koss, and N. Duvvury. 2006. Perpetration of partner violence and HIV risk behaviour among young men in the rural Eastern Cape, South Africa. *AIDS* 20 (16):2107–2114.

Dworkin, S.L. 2015. *Men at Risk: Masculinity, Heterosexuality and HIV Prevention.* New York: NYU Press.

Dworkin, S.L., C. Colvin, A.M. Hatcher, and D. Peacock. 2012. Men's perceptions of women's rights and changing gender relations in South Africa: Lessons for working with men and boys in HIV and antiviolence programs. *Gender and Society* 26 (1):96–120.

———. 2013. Impact of a gender-transformative HIV and anti-violence program on gender ideologies and masculinities in two rural, South African communities. *Men and Masculinities* 16 (2):181–202.

Dworkin, S.L., M.S. Dunbar, S. Krishnan, A.M. Hatcher, and S. Sawires. 2011. Uncovering tensions and capitalizing on synergies in HIV/AIDS and antiviolence programs. *American Journal of Public Health* 101 (6):995–1003.

Dworkin, S.L., R.E. Fullilove, and D. Peacock. 2009. Are HIV/AIDS prevention interventions for heterosexually active men in the United States gender-specific? *American Journal of Public Health* 99 (6):981–984.

Dworkin, S.L., S. Treves-Kagan, and S. Lippman. 2013. Gender transformative interventions to reduce HIV/AIDS and violence with heterosexually-active men: A review of the global evidence. *AIDS and Behavior* 17(9): 2845–2063.

Exner, T., S. Hoffman, S.L. Dworkin, and A.A. Ehrhardt. 2003. Beyond the male condom: The evolution of gender-specific HIV interventions for women. *Annual Review of Sex Research* 14:114–136.

Gupta, G.R., and S.D. Kambou. 2010. Practical and pragmatic: strategically applying gender perspectives to increase the power of global health policies and programs. *Igniting the Power of Community*:265–276.

Higgins, J., S. Hoffman, and S. Dworkin. 2010. Rethinking gender, heterosexual men, and women's vulnerability to HIV/AIDS. *American Journal of Public Health* 100 (3):435–445.

Hirsch, J.S., S. Meneses, B. Thompson, M. Negroni, B. Pelcastre, and C. Del Rio. 2007. The inevitability of infidelity: Sexual reputation, social geographies, and marital HIV risk in rural Mexico. *American Journal of Public Health* 97 (6):986-996.

Hunter, M. 2005. Cultural politics and masculinities: Multiple partners in historical context in Kwa-Zulu-Natal. *Culture, Health, and Sexuality* 7:209–223.

Jakupcak, M., D. Lisak, and L. Roemer 2002. The role of masculine ideology and masculine gender role stress in men's perpetuation of relationship violence. *Psychology of Men and Masculinity* 3: 97–106.

Jewkes, R., K. Dunkle, M.P. Koss, J.B. Levin, M. Nduna, N. Jama, and Y. Sikweyiya. 2006. Rape perpetration by young, rural South African men: Prevalence, patterns and risk factors. *Social Science and Medicine* 63:2949–2961.

Jewkes, R., K. Dunkle, M. Nduna, and N. Shai. 2010. Intimate partner violence, relationship power inequity, and incidence of HIV infection in young women in South Africa: A cohort study. *Lancet* 376 (9734):41–48.

Jewkes, R., M. Nduna, J. Levin, N. Jama, K. Dunkle, N. Khuzwayo, M. Koss, A. Puren, K. Wood, and N. Duvvury. 2006. A cluster randomized-controlled trial to determine the effectiveness of Stepping Stones in preventing HIV infections and promoting safer sexual behaviour amongst youth in the rural Eastern Cape, South Africa: Trial design, methods and baseline findings. *Tropical Medicine and International Health* 11 (1):3–16.

Jewkes, R., Y. Sikweyiya, R. Morrell, and K. Dunkle. 2009. *Understanding Men's Health and Use of Violence: Interface of Rape and HIV in South Africa.* Pretoria, South Africa: Medical Research Council.

———. 2011. The relationship between intimate partner violence, rape, and HIV amongst South African men: A cross-sectional study. *PLoS One* 6(9): 1–6.

Kalichman, S. C., L. C. Simbayi, D. Cain, C. Cherry, N. Henda, and A. Cloete. 2007. Sexual assault, sexual risks and gender attitudes in a community sample of South African men. *AIDS Care* 19 (1):20–27.

Kalichman, S. C., L. C. Simbayi, A. Cloete, M. Clayford, W. Arnolds, M. Mxoli, G. Smith, C. Cherry, T. Shefer, M. Crawford, and M. O. Kalichman. 2009. Integrated gender-based violence and HIV risk reduction intervention for South African men: Results of a quasi-experimental field trial. *Prevention Science* 10 (3):260–269.

Kippax, S., N. Stephenson, R. J. Parker, and P. Aggleton. 2013. Between individual agency and structure in HIV prevention: Understanding the middle ground of social practice. *American Journal of Public Health* 103 (8):1367–1375.

Lippman, S. A., S. Maman, C. MacPhail, R. Twine, D. Peacock, K. Kahn, and A. Pettifor. 2013. Conceptualizing community mobilization for HIV prevention: Implications for HIV prevention programming in the Africa context. *PLoS One* 8(10):e78208. doi:10.1371/journal.pone.0078208.

Lofland, J., and L. Lofland. 1995. *Analyzing Social Settings: A Guide to Qualitative Observation and Analysis.* 3rd edition. Belmont, CA: Wadsworth.

Messner, M. A. 1997. *The Politics of Masculinities: Men in Movements.* Thousand Oaks, CA: Sage.

Peacock, D., and A. Levack. 2004. The men as partners program in South Africa: Reaching men to end gender-based violence and promote sexual and reproductive health. *International Journal of Men's Health* 3 (3):173–188.

Peacock, D., L. Stemple, S. Sawires, and T. Coates. 2009. Men, HIV/AIDS, and human rights. *Journal of Acquired Immune Deficiency Syndromes* 51(S3): S119-S125.

Pronyk, P. M., J. R. Hargreaves, J. C. Kim, L. A. Morison, G. Phetla, C. Watts, J. Busza, and J. D. H. Porter. 2006. Effect of a structural intervention for the prevention of intimate-partner violence and HIV in rural South Africa: A cluster randomised trial. *Lancet* 368 (9551):1973–1983.

Pulerwitz, J., H. Amaro, W. De Jong, S. L. Gortmaker, and R. Rudd. 2002. Relationship power, condom use and HIV risk among women in the USA. *AIDS Care* 14 (6):789–800.

Rehle, T. M., T. B. Hallett, O. Shisana, V. Pillay-van Wyk, K. Zuma, H. Carrara, and S. Jooste. 2010. A decline in new HIV infections in South Africa: Estimating HIV incidence from three national HIV surveys in 2002, 2005 and 2008. *PLoS One* 5 (6):e11094.

Shannon, K., K. Leiter, N. Phaladze, Z. Hianze, A. C. Tsai, M. Heisler, V. Iocopino, and S. Weiser. 2012. Gender inequity norms are associated with increased male perpetrated rape and sexual risks in Botswana and

Swaziland. *PLoS Medicine* 7(1): e28739. doi:10.1371/journal.pone.0028739.
Sonke Gender Justice. n.d. Vision and Mission. http://www.genderjustice.org
.za/about-us/vision-mission/.
UNAIDS Report on the Global AIDS Epidemic. 2012. Geneva: United Nations
Programme on HIV/AIDS. www.unaids.org/sites/default/files/media_asset
/20121120_UNAIDS_Global_Report_2012_with_annexes_en_1.pdf.

Structural (Legal/Policy, Economic) Interventions as Tools of Empowerment

Introduction

SHELLY GRABE, SHERI WEISER, SHARI L. DWORKIN,
JOANNA WEINBERG, AND LARA STEMPLE

Many of the authors included in our book, *Women's Empowerment and Global Health: A Twenty-First-Century Agenda,* share the conceptual understanding that broad structural forces shape empowerment-related processes, which in turn influence women's health (Kabeer 1999). This framework reflects a relatively recent understanding of these interrelationships. As noted in the introduction to the book, much of the early empowerment literature focused instead on individual-level intervention and analysis (Dworkin and Ehrhardt 2007; Perkins and Zimmerman 1995). Such interventions too often assume that individual women have the autonomy to make choices and to act upon them, whereas structural, legal, and policy interventions, in contrast, recognize that individual agency to improve one's health is often constrained by broader social, economic, and political forces (Samman and Santos 2009; Blankenship et al. 2006). Structural interventions that seek to change conditions beyond an individual's sphere of control include efforts to alter policies, laws, institutions, social norms, and economic factors, among other broad influencers (Blankenship, Bray, and Merson 2000; Sumartojo et al. 2000). Although scholarly analyses of structural interventions aiming to improve health and empowerment have increased in recent years (Kerrigan et al. 2006; Pronyk et al. 2006; Raj et al. 2013; Weiser et al. 2015), the potential of these approaches to catalyze change has not been fully realized (Abdul-Quader et al. 2013; Cohen, Scribner, and Farley 2000; Gupta et al., 2008).

In a key article that defined structural interventions for public health, Blankenship et al. (2006) outlined five types of structural programs: (1) community mobilization and community-level interventions (e.g., consciousness-raising among marginalized groups who work together to achieve improved rights and health), (2) the integration of health services at the institutional level (e.g., merging family planning services with HIV services), (3) multisectoral integration (e.g., interventions that combine health and food security objectives), (4) economic and educational interventions (these are examined more in-depth below), and (5) the use of incentives and contingent funding (i.e., receipt of funding is contingent upon the implementation of laws, policies, or behaviors believed to promote public health).

A subset of contingent funding is sometimes referred to as "conditional cash transfers" because the cash given to families or individuals by programs (or governments) is conditioned on one or more health-enhancing behaviors on the part of recipients (such as keeping girls in school). Conditional cash transfers have been found to successfully reduce violence against women, and, in some cases, reduce STI risks for youth (Baird et al. 2012; Heise et al. 2013), although many questions remain about the implementation, evaluation, and ethics associated with such programs, particularly in light of emerging evidence of the effectiveness of unconditional cash transfers for improving health outcomes.

Structural interventions also include intervening through the policy and legal environment. Women's empowerment and health is influenced not only through explicit laws and policies that protect or violate women's human rights but also through broader economic and social policies. As an example of the latter, the implementation of a policy to end school fees may not appear to be a health intervention at first glance, but it contributes to girls' ongoing enrollment and to a reduction in girls' HIV acquisition, even in endemic settings (De Neve et al. 2015; Grown, Gupta, and Kes 2005). Similarly, while some might not initially see women's property rights as a health intervention, scholars have found that strengthening women's access to and control over property has empowering effects that reduce violence against women, minimize their HIV risks, and may influence HIV care and treatment outcomes (Dworkin et al. 2013; Grabe et al. 2012; Hilliard et al. 2016; Lu et al. 2013).

Local, national, and international law also has a tremendous impact on women's health and empowerment. On topics ranging from child marriage to marital rape to female genital mutilation to the criminalization of sex work, laws shape the lived reality of women across the globe.

For example, the rate of abortion for unwanted or mistimed pregnancies varies little from country to country, because women who are desperate to terminate a pregnancy often do so regardless of abortion's legality. But because abortion laws vary widely across nations and even within them, access to safe abortion is inconsistent, leaving the women who must live under restrictive abortion laws at much greater risk of the health complications of unsafe abortion.

The chapters in this section of the book are focused on the linkages between legal, policy, or economic interventions and women's empowerment and health. Among economic interventions, three strategies predominate: microenterprise, property rights, and agricultural and/or food security interventions. The hypothesis driving these strategies is that power inequities between women and men can be reconfigured if women have access to and control over resources. This is particularly important considering that these global statistics have not changed since the 1970s: women perform 66% of the world's work yet earn only 10% of global income and own only 1% of the world's property (UN, 2010). Because poverty and gender subordination intersect in a vicious cycle to worsen women's health, interventions that combine economic empowerment with strategies to directly challenge harmful gender norms are critical tools to interrupt this process.

Economic empowerment has been defined to include the ability to advance economically as well as the power to make and act upon economic decisions (Golla, Malhotra, Nanda, and Mehra 2011). In particular, because many scholars view women's access to and control of resources as crucial to economic empowerment, it can be viewed as both a process of change and a desirable end point (Kabeer 1999). Yet too often, economic empowerment is poorly defined in practice, with interventions trending towards a focus on individual women rather than on the broader societal contexts in which they live. For example, many development programs that aim to empower women through microcredit loans lack other gender-transformative content (Goetz and Gupta 1996; Dworkin 2015). However, evidence suggests that women's receipt of a loan, in and of itself, does little to diversify women's labor, thereby perpetuating traditional occupational structures that failed to challenge male dominance (Ehlers and Main 1988; Kabeer 1994, 2001). One review of microcredit programs conducted in the mid-1990s in Bangladesh found that 63 percent of female loan holders had limited or no control over the loans they had procured (Goetz and Gupta, 1996). In short, it quickly became clear that interventions focusing solely on microcredit lending did not adequately address the other obstacles that constrain women's status and ultimately their health.

Indeed, unequal economic arrangements that favor men both reinforce and are reinforced by social norms. Research has also investigated how the benefits of economic empowerment programs extend beyond strictly financial outcomes. A growing literature suggests promising results, with economic empowerment being linked to improved mental health (World Health Organization 2007), childhood nutrition (Duflo 2003), and reduced HIV risk and intimate-partner violence (Kim, Pronyk, Barnett, and Watts 2008; Vyas and Watts 2009), and broader economic development beyond the economic empowerment of women (Duflo 2012).

In this section of *Women's Empowerment and Global Health: A Twenty-First-Century Agenda,* several scholars present innovative programs that combine a focus on financial or material gain for women (e.g., access to and control over resources, including income or property) with interventions that provide training on gender and women's rights or offer vocational training to women or help mobilize entire communities. Although the interventions presented in this section differ in the strategies they employ, they all emphasize a need to change structural factors in order to influence women's health and well-being.

In chapter 8, Megan Dunbar and Imelda Mudekunye-Mahaka provide an evaluation of SHAZ! (Shaping the Health of Adolescents in Zimbabwe), an intervention designed to mitigate HIV risk among adolescent women and girls in Zimbabwe. SHAZ! is an example of a structural intervention delivered at the individual and small-group levels, pairing reproductive health and HIV services (including screening and treatment for STIs and provision of condoms) with life skills education (including reproductive health education, negotiation skills, and strategies to avoid violence) for both intervention and control participants. The intervention group was also trained in basic financial literacy, and the program sponsored participants to attend their choice of nationally accredited vocational training courses offered through local training institutes. Participants who completed and passed the training were eligible to receive a microgrant valued at US$100 in the form of supplies, additional training, or capital equipment. The previously published SHAZ! randomized control trial reported significant improvements in economic indicators (e.g., food security and income) and HIV risk factors (e.g., transactional sex, lack of condom use, and experience of violence) in the intervention group compared to the control group, and a (nonsignificant) 40 percent reduction in unintended pregnancies. However, there were no significant differences in HIV or herpes simplex virus 2 acquisition in the two groups. The authors of this chapter explore qualitative and process evaluation data to help interpret study findings and to identify what worked, what did not, and why.

This chapter points to the importance of comprehensive gender transformative interventions to impact women's economic empowerment. The authors consider the political and economic context in Zimbabwe at the time of the study to understand why the trial was not successful in reducing HIV and HSV 2 acquisition. This case study underscores the challenges inherent in rigorously evaluating complex and integrated interventions that target vulnerable populations living in resource-poor settings.

In chapter 9, Abigail Hatcher and her colleagues explore how a comprehensive economic intervention—in this case a program combining microfinance, gender equality training, HIV prevention, and community mobilization—may have contributed to women's economic empowerment and reduced levels of violence in rural South Africa. The authors note that many programs' attempts to show the benefits of microfinance have been unsuccessful. Other limitations identified with past microfinance strategies include the strain associated with repayment of loans at high interest rates and the fact that microfinance does not adequately change the gender and class hierarchies that shape women's lives. In contrast, this intervention attempts to influence gender norms in the larger community in addition to increasing women's access to productive resources through microfinance.

The authors analyze data from a six-year ·mixed-methods process evaluation of IMAGE. To do so, they triangulated data from 374 hours of participant observation, thirty-four semistructured interviews, and sixteen focus group discussions with female clients between 18 and 45 who participated in IMAGE. The authors also conducted semistructured interviews with ninety-eight clients, staff, and managers following the trial. They too conclude that gender equality training and community mobilization, coupled with microfinance, may offer more promise than microfinance alone to enhance women's empowerment.

In chapter 10, Carroll Estes examines how the health and economic security of millions of women is impacted at the structural level by U.S. policy and contemporary political trends. She posits that governmental actors and lobbyists are now seeking to dismantle the earned benefits programs of Social Security and Medicare as well as recent health care reforms and the revamped Medicaid program. These changes would disproportionately threaten women's health in view of rising income inequalities and the declining health and economic security among older women as compared to men. This case study outlines three lines of intervention (individual, organizational, and coalitional) undertaken by the author and her colleagues. She identifies herself as a scholar and "organic intellectual" who seeks to combat political and policy hegemony (Gramsci 1971). Estes works in parallel with other scholars and think tanks to challenge the assumptions embedded in current political rhetoric and policy practice. The ultimate goal of these efforts is to subvert the disempowerment of women and all elderly people through fighting for policies that protect these groups. To preserve, protect, and strengthen Social Security and Medicare, Estes and her colleagues are reframing public discourse to destabilize and replace the current ideological hegemony with an alternative model. The alternative is, namely, the continuity and stability of a social contract whereby a government promises specific earned benefits to its people. Her work shows the promise of grassroots social movements, the importance of cross-sectoral alliances, and the role of academicians in carrying out the merger of theory with social action to confront some of the most important political developments in the U.S. domestic sphere today.

Chapter 11, titled "Women's Health and Empowerment after the Decriminalization of Abortion in Mexico City," written by Gustavo Ortiz Millán, documents the impact of the liberalization of Mexico City's abortion law, followed by changes in institutional policies of health centers and hospitals throughout the city. After decades of advocacy by members of the women's movement in Mexico, the legislature reformed Mexico City's abortion laws in 2007 to allow for elective abortion in the first trimester. This was a historic victory for women's reproductive rights in the region. Before the law was reformed, wealthier and more educated women seeking abortion had been able to circumvent the restrictive law, while poorer and/or less educated women had been trapped under the prevailing criminal law, which threatened their health and lives. Thus, intersecting structural inequalities deepened, as the health of poorer women was disproportionately affected by the pre-2007 law. Law reform improved access to safe abortion services for women in Mexico City more evenly across socioeconomic lines, providing them with greater agency over their health and their reproductive lives.

Ortiz Millán's case study also shows that empowerment is as much a process as it is an outcome (Perkins and Zimmerman 1995; Kabeer

1999; Jupp, Ali, Barahona 2010). In addition to recognizing a women's right to have an abortion, law reform in Mexico City reinforced a process of empowerment by reducing abortion-related stigma through enhanced public discussion and awareness about women's reproductive rights. Strategic collaborations between the medical establishment and the women's movement played a key role in ensuring that the new law was implemented properly. After abortion was decriminalized, morbidity and mortality rates attributable to unsafe abortions in Mexico City diminished significantly. Yet because abortion remains criminalized elsewhere in Mexico, women's access to safe abortion remains contingent upon their ability to travel to Mexico City: geographic proximity, financial resources, and other elements of empowerment intersect to inform this access.

Kate Grünke-Horton and Shari L. Dworkin (chapter 12) address the ways in which property rights shape empowerment-related processes, by moving beyond individual- or small-group-level strategies (which remain common in global health interventions) to test a structural, policy-level intervention to improve women's health and empowerment at the community level by working to secure women's property rights. Although property rights violations are an important contributor to women's disempowerment, there is a dearth of literature evaluating the impact of interventions that improve women's property rights. This chapter draws upon data from an academic-community collaboration between the University of California, San Francisco (UCSF), the Kenyan Medical Research Institute (KEMRI), and Grassroots Organization Operating Together in Sisterhood (GROOTS) Kenya. The authors make use of in-depth qualitative interviews with eighty women working with or served by a Community Land and Property Watchdog Model (known as Community Watchdog Group, or CWDG) in Kenya. The Watchdog Model was developed by women who are supported by the network of organizations called GROOTS, which aims to secure women's property rights and reduce the spread and impact of HIV. Investigators interviewed program developers, program implementers, and beneficiaries to explore the effects of a property rights intervention in rural Kenya on women's empowerment and gender equality.

Grünke-Horton and Dworkin's results are focused on the empowerment-related processes that result from rights-based education, community mediation of property disputes, and collaboration with government and local officials to secure women's rights to land and property. In their other published works (Dworkin et al. 2013, 2014; Hilliard et al. 2016;

Lu et al. 2013), these authors linked empowerment processes to health outcomes such as violence and HIV risks, but in this chapter, they emphasize the impact of the program on empowerment-related processes. They found that at both the individual and community level, women perceived that the CWDG model encouraged greater autonomy through increased community involvement, improved rights-based knowledge, and detailed other improvements in agency and social support. The program was also perceived by women to reduce financial dependency on men and challenged harmful gender norms and ideologies.

In the final chapter in the book, "Land Tenure and Women's Empowerment and Health: A Programmatic Evaluation of Structural Change in Nicaragua," Shelly Grabe, Anjali Dutt, and Carlos Arenas describe how changes in land ownership by women, made possible by a recent change in Nicaraguan law, enhanced the social status of women and reduced their exposure to physical and sexual violence. In many parts of the world, women's access to and control over land is determined by marriage. In other contexts, laws protect women's legal right to own land, but a range of entrenched social barriers can prevent women from realizing these rights. Women's inability to enforce their property rights has negative impacts on empowerment, including an increased vulnerability to violence and HIV/AIDS (Dworkin et al. 2013; Grabe 2010; Lu et al. 2013). In most programs, violence against women is addressed through individual level interventions. Here, Programa Productivo, a program run by the Xochilt Acalt Women's Center in rural Nicaragua, employs a different strategy. The program focuses on changing the social structures that put women at *risk* for violence, such as low social status and complete economic dependence on men. Both of these factors are related, in part, to lack of land ownership. The case study highlights land as a key productive asset that can be linked to women's income and empowerment in a sustainable way. It also serves as an important reminder that formal legal rights alone may not be enough to empower women. Sustainable changes in empowerment require intervention on multiple, intersecting components that influence women's lives, all of which can be shaped by both legal and social contexts (Cattaneo and Chapman 2010; Gupta et al. 2008). Xochilt Acalt began as a mobile women's reproductive health-care clinic and has now expanded into a widespread rural network with programs involving agricultural production, education, economic empowerment, and civic participation. Within its agricultural program, Xochilt Acalt mobilized both men and women in the community to support women's land ownership.

Taken together, the six chapters in this section reveal how global advances in women's health are impeded by poverty, limited access to educational and economic opportunities, gender bias and discrimination, unjust laws, and insufficient state accountability. Despite these challenges, each chapter offers hope that structural change—changes in laws, policies, economics, and sociocultural norms—is an effective means of shifting the responsibility for empowerment and health away from individual women exclusively and towards governments, policy makers, and program designers (Blankenship et al. 2006; Grabe 2010). The evidence embodied in these six chapters warrants a much more serious consideration of structural interventions both for women's empowerment and for women's health.

REFERENCES

Abdul-Quader AS, Feelemyer J, Modi S, Stein ES, Briceno A, Semaan S, Horvath T, Kennedy GE, Des Jarlais DC. 2013. Effectiveness of structural-level needle/syringe programs to reduce HCV and HIV infection among people who inject drugs: a systematic review. *AIDS & Behavior* 17(9):2878–2892. http://link.springer.com/article/10.1007%2Fs10461-013-0593-y.

Baird S, Garfein R, McIntosh C, Ozler B. 2012. Effect of a cash transfer programme for schooling on prevalence of HIV and herpes simplex type 2 in Malawi: A cluster randomised trial. *Lancet* 379: 1320–1329.

Blankenship K, Bray SJ, Merson MH. 2000. Structural interventions in public health. *AIDS* 14(S1): S1-S11.

Blankenship K, Friedman S, Dworkin S, Mantell J. 2006. Structural interventions: Challenges and opportunities for interdisciplinary research. *Journal of Urban Health* 83:59–72. www.ncbi.nlm.nih.gov/pmc/articles/PMC1473169/.

Cattaneo LB, Chapman AR. 2010. The process of empowerment: A model for use in research and practice. *American Psychologist* 65:646–659.

Cohen DA, Scribner RA, Farley TA. 2000 A structural model of health behavior: A pragmatic approach to explain and influence health behaviors at the population level. *Preventative Medicine* 30:146–154.

De Neve JW, Fink G, Subramanian SV, Moyo S, Bor J. 2015. Length of secondary schooling and risk of HIV infection in Botswana: Evidence from a natural experiment. *AIDS* 3(8):e470–477. www.thelancet.com/journals/langlo/article/PIIS2214-109X%2815%2900087-X/fulltext.

Duflo E. 2003. Grandmothers and granddaughters: Old age pensions and intra-household allocation in South Africa. Washington DC: World Bank. https://openknowledge.worldbank.org/handle/10986/17173

———. 2012. Women empowerment and economic development. *Journal of Economic Literature* 50: 1051-1079.

Dworkin, SL. (2015). *Men at risk: Masculinity, heterosexuality and HIV/AIDS prevention.* New York: NYU Press.

Dworkin SL, Ehrhardt AA. 2007. Going beyond ABC to include GEM (gender relations, economic contexts, and migration movements): critical reflections on progress in the HIV/AIDS epidemic. *American Journal of Public Health* 97:13–16.

Dworkin SL, Grabe S, Lu T, Kwena Z, Bukusi E, Mwaura-Muiru E. 2013. Property rights violations as a structural driver of women's HIV risks in Nyanza and Western Provinces, Kenya. *Archives of Sexual Behavior* 42:703–715.

Dworkin SL, Lu T, Grabe S, Kwena Z, Mwaura-Muiru E, Bukusi E. 2014. What strategies are needed to secure women's property rights in Western Kenya? Laying the groundwork for a future structural HIV prevention intervention. *AIDS Care* 26:754–757.

Goetz, AM, Gupta, RS. 1996. Who takes the credit? gender, power, and control over loan use in rural credit programs in Bangladesh. *World Development* 24:45–63.

Golla, AM, Malhotra A, Nanda P, Mehra R. 2011. Understanding and measuring women's economic empowerment. International Center for Research on Women: Washington, DC. www.icrw.org/files/publications/Understanding-measuring-womens-economic-empowerment.pdf.

Grabe S. 2010. Promoting gender equality: The role of ideology, power and control in the link between land ownership and violence in Nicaragua. *Analysis of Social Issues and Public Policy* 10:146–170.

———. 2012. An empirical examination of women's empowerment and transformative change in the context of international development. *American Journal of Community Psychology* 49:233–245.

Gramsci A. 1971. *Selections from the prison notebooks* (BQ Hoare and G Nowell-Smith, editor and translator). London, England: Lawrence and Wishart.

Grown C, Gupta GR, Kes A. 2005. Taking action: achieving gender equality and empowering women. UN Millennium Project. London: Earth Scan. www.unmillenniumproject.org/documents/Gender-complete.pdf.

Gupta GR, Parkhurst JO, Ogden JA, Aggleton P, Mahal A. 2008. Structural approaches to HIV prevention. *Lancet* 372:764–775.

Heise L, Lutz B, Ranganathan M, Watts C. 2013. Cash transfers for HIV prevention: Considering their potential. *Journal of the International AIDS Society* 16:1–5. www.ncbi.nlm.nih.gov/pmc/articles/PMC3752431/pdf/JIAS-16-18615.pdf.

Hilliard S, Bukusi E, Grabe S, Lu T, Hatcher A, Kwena Z, Mwaura-Muiru E, Dworkin SL. 2016. How does a community-led property rights program impact violence against women? A qualitative analysis from Western and Nyanza Provinces, Kenya. *Violence Against Women* 21. doi:10.1177/1077801216632613.

Jupp D, Ali SI, Barahona C. 2010. Measuring empowerment? ask them: Qualifying quantitative outcomes from people's own analysis. Studies in Evaluation. Commissioned by Sida, Department for Long-term Program Cooperation, Team for Bangladesh in collaboration with Secretariat for Evaluation. www.oecd.org/countries/bangladesh/46146440.pdf.

Kabeer N. 1994. *Reversed realities: Gender hierarchies in development thought.* London: Verso.

————. 1999. Resources, agency, achievements: Reflections on the measurement of women's empowerment. *Development and Change* 30(3):435–464.

————. 2001. Conflicts over credit: Re-evaluating the empowerment potential of loans to women in rural Bangladesh. *World Development*, 29, 63-84

Kerrigan D, et al. (2006). Environmental-structural interventions to reduce HIV/STI risk among female sex workers in the Dominican Republic. *American Journal of Public Health* 96:120–125.

Kim J, Pronyk P, Barnett T, Watts C. 2008. Exploring the role of economic empowerment in HIV prevention. *AIDS* 22: S57-S71.

Lu T, Kwena Z, Zwicker L, Bukusi E, Maura-Muiru E, Dworkin S. 2013. Securing women's property rights in the era of HIV/AIDS: Barriers and facilitators of implementing a community-led structural intervention in Western Kenya. *AIDS Education and Prevention* 25:151–163.

Oppenheim K. n.d. VII. Contribution of the ICPD Programme of Action to gender equality and the empowerment of women. www.un.org/esa/population /publications/PopAspectsMDG/07_OPPENHEIMMASON.pdf

Perkins DD, Zimmerman MA. 1995. Empowerment theory, research, and application. *American Journal of Community Psychology* 23:569–579.

Pronyk PM, Hargreaves JR, Kim K, Morison LA, Phetla F,Watts C, et al. 2006. Effect of a structural intervention for the prevention of intimate partner violence and HIV in rural South Africa: Results of a cluster randomized trial. *Lancet* 368:1973–1983.

Raj A, Dasgupta A, Goldson I, Lafontant D, Freeman E, Silverman JG. 2013. Pilot evaluation of the Making Employment Needs [MEN] Count intervention: Addressing behavioral and structural HIV risks in heterosexual Black men. *AIDS Care*. Epub 2013/06/19. PubMed PMID: 23767788.

Samman E, Santos ME. 2009. Agency and empowerment: A review of concepts, indicators and empirical evidence. Prepared for the 2009 Human Development Report in Latin America and the Caribbean. Oxford, UK: Oxford Poverty and Human Development Initiative. www.ophi.org.uk/wp-content /uploads/OPHI-RP-10a.pdf.

Sumartojo E, Doll L, Holtgrave D, Gayle H, Merson M. 2000. Enriching the mix: incorporating structural factors into HIV prevention. *AIDS* 14(1):S1–S2.

UNDP. 2010. *Human development report*. New York, NY: Oxford University Press.

Vyas S, Watts C. 2008. How does economic empowerment affect women's risk of intimate partner violence in low and middle income countries? A systematic review of published evidenced. Journal of *International Development* 21: 577-602.

Weiser S, Bukusi E, Steinfeld R, Frongillo EA, Weke E, Dworkin SL, Pusateri K, Shiboski S, Scow K, Butler L, Cohen CR. 2015. Shamba Maisha: Randomized controlled trial of an agricultural intervention to improve HIV health outcomes. *AIDS* 10:1889–1894.

Zimmerman MA. 2000. Empowerment theory: Psychological, organizational, and community levels of analysis. In: Rappaport J, Seidman E, editors. *Handbook of community psychology*. New York: Springer Science. p.43–63.

8

Empowering Adolescent Girls and Women for Improved Sexual Health in Zimbabwe

*Lessons Learned from a Combined
Livelihoods and Life Skills Intervention
(SHAZ!)*

MEGAN S. DUNBAR AND IMELDA MUDEKUNYE-MAHAKA

In Zimbabwe, as in much of sub-Saharan Africa, the prevalence of Human Immunodeficiency Virus (HIV) is high, at 15%, and effective HIV prevention, care, and treatment remains one of its most pressing problems. Among women aged 15–24, HIV prevalence is over two times that of their male counterparts (6% among females compared to 3% among males; ZIMSTAT and ICF International, 2011). Research has shown that much of this disproportionate HIV burden can be attributed to "structural factors"—in particular, gender-based social and economic inequities, which directly or indirectly increase young women's risk for HIV acquisition and transmission (Auerbach, Parkhurst, and Caceres 2011; Sumartojo 2000). In response, a new generation of research and programming has evolved in an effort to address structural factors in HIV prevention (Gibbs et al. 2012; Gupta et al. 2008; Kim et al. 2008; Krishnan et al. 2008; Seeley et al. 2012; Sumartojo et al. 2000).

SHAZ! (Shaping the Health of Adolescents in Zimbabwe) is one such intervention designed to mitigate structural HIV risk among adolescent women and girls in Zimbabwe. SHAZ! is based on a model (figure 8.1) that was developed by integrating the theory of gender and power (Connell 1985; Emerson 1978) with a framework for women's empowerment designed by Kabeer and colleagues (Kabeer 1999; Sen 1999). Drawing upon these writings, SHAZ! conceptualizes empowerment as a process by which adolescent and young women gain the resources, skills, and capacities to drive decision making related to their sexual

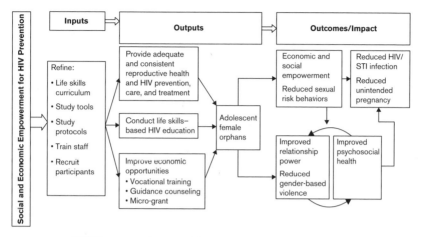

FIGURE 8.1. SHAZ! program logic model.

health and well-being. SHAZ! aims to foster this type of empowerment by (1) increasing participants' access to information and health services; (2) building life skills among participants in communication and relationship negotiation; and (3) promoting economic livelihoods through guidance counseling, vocational skills training, and microgrants. In combination, these interventions are designed to provide participants with greater ability to negotiate safer sex for improved HIV and reproductive health outcomes.

The current iteration of SHAZ! was launched in early 2006 in Chitungwiza, Zimbabwe; a small pilot that had been rolled out in 2004 informed the design of the existing program (Dunbar et al. 2010). A randomized control trial compared the effects of the full SHAZ! intervention (components 1–3 above) to a control condition of life skills education and reproductive health services alone among 315 HIV-uninfected adolescent female orphans, aged 16–19 (n = 158 in the intervention arm, n = 157 in the control arm). The results of this evaluation are described in the following section, "Context and Background," and they have also been presented elsewhere (Dunbar et al. 2009, 2013). The purpose of this case study is to further explore the data—including qualitative and process data—to help interpret these previously reported findings and to identify what worked, what didn't, and why. This case study also highlights how the intervention has been adapted, based on these findings, in an ongoing evaluation of the same model among adolescent and young women living with HIV.

CONTEXT AND BACKGROUND

Zimbabwe has been in the throes of a severe economic and political crisis since the early 2000s, fueled by a government-led land redistribution program that, by 2008, resulted in the collapse of the agricultural sector, skyrocketing inflation, massive unemployment, and widespread civil unrest (Mlambo and Raftoppulous 2010). The Zimbabwean government's response was Operation Murambatsvina (Operation Drive Out Rubbish), a large-scale campaign to forcibly clear slum areas across the country, directly affecting at least 700,000 people through loss of their homes or businesses (Reuters 2008). This overarching context has exacerbated a situation in which adolescent women already faced highly constrained access to educational and economic opportunities and experienced high rates of gender-based violence (Gibbs et al. 2012; Gupta et al. 2008; Kim et al. 2008; Krishnan et al. 2008; Sumartajo 2000; Sumartojo et al. 2000; Seeley et al. 2012), creating an environment of structural HIV risk that cannot be fully addressed through behavioral interventions alone. While economic power and structural interventions to improve economic and educational opportunities have been associated with women's capacity to negotiate safer sex, avoid intimate-partner violence, and generally reduce HIV risk (Baird et al. 2012; Dworkin et al. 2011; Kim et al. 2007; Hallfors et al. 2011; Jewkes et al. 2008; Pronyk et al. 2005, 2006, 2008; Strickland 2004), the dearth of educational and economic opportunities for adolescent women in Zimbabwe drives some to engage in high-risk sex, including early sexual debut, sex with multiple partners, and transactional sex (Dunkle et al. 2004; Gage and Meekers 1994; Haram 1995; Irvin 2000; Komba-Makeka and Liljestrøm 1994; Laga et al. 2001; Nzyuko et al. 1997; Weiss, Whelan, and Gupta 1996). Such risks are even greater for adolescent women who have been orphaned by AIDS or other causes (Gregson et al. 2005; Kang et al. 2007).

SHAZ!, which as described above was designed to address components of this structural risk, was originally developed within the context of a large-scale intervention trial, powered to detect changes in the incidence of HSV 2 (herpes simplex virus 2) as a proxy for HIV infection. However, as the economy in Zimbabwe collapsed in the mid-2000s during the planning process for this large-scale evaluation, the study was scaled back to a phase II randomized control trial (RCT) due to concerns about the feasibility of rolling out a large intervention trial in the midst of the economic crises. This smaller phase II trial was conducted from 2006 to 2008, to assess the potential efficacy of SHAZ! in this challenging economic and political context.

As shown in the description of program components below, all participants received reproductive health and HIV services and a life skills education package, while intervention participants in addition were supported to attend their choice of vocational training courses with access to a microgrant upon successful completion. Control participants were offered access to these components as a standard package because anything less was viewed, in the Zimbabwean context, as unethical. Furthermore, it was considered that this design supported the goal of the evaluation, which was to test the hypothesis that a combined livelihoods and life skills intervention would have greater efficacy, over and above a more standard control condition, on measures of empowerment and sexual behavior and on trends in HIV and HSV 2 incidence and unintended pregnancy. It is important to note that all study participants had either dropped out of or completed their secondary education and were not currently enrolled in school. The research was approved by the Medical Research Council of Zimbabwe, the Committee for the Protection of Human Subjects at the University of California, San Francisco, and the institutional review boards at RTI International and at the Pangaea Global AIDS Foundation. The SHAZ! intervention incorporated three main components:

1. *Reproductive health and HIV services (for both intervention and control participants):* Participants were provided a health screening at every study visit, treated for treatable STIs and minor ailments, and offered condoms and contraceptives. Participants were screened for HIV at entry; those who tested positive were ineligible and were counselled and referred to HIV clinics.

2. *Life skills education (for both intervention and control participants):* The life skills curriculum drew upon Stepping Stones, a previously evaluated training package on HIV/AIDS, gender, and relationships used widely in sub-Saharan Africa. It consisted of fourteen modules delivered to groups of twenty-five women over four to six weeks on HIV/STI and reproductive health education, relationship negotiation skills, strategies to avoid violence, and identification of safe and risky places in the community. Figure 8.2 is an example of a community risk map developed during one of the life skills sessions. The life skills training also included a module conducted by the Red Cross of Zimbabwe on home-based health care.

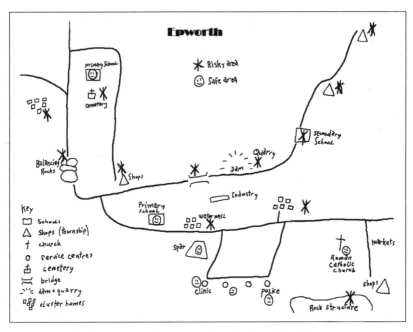

FIGURE 8.2. HIV community risk map developed during a life skills session.

3. *Livelihoods (for intervention participants only):* The livelihoods component provided basic financial literacy, and support for participants to attend their choice of nationally accredited vocational training courses offered through local training institutes. Courses were six months long or less on average, with a practical and a theoretical component. The most popular courses were hairdressing, garment-making, receptionist/secretarial, and nurse's-aide training. Participants who completed and passed their training and developed a business plan received a microgrant valued at US$100 in the form of supplies, additional training, or capital equipment.

To briefly summarize the published findings from the original study (Dunbar et al. 2009, 2010), the results of the evaluation found no statistical difference between study arms (intervention = 158, control = 157) on completion of life skills training (94%) or Red Cross trainings (77%) or in overall retention in data collection visits at 24 months (80%); however, there was a trend towards higher completion among intervention participants. Within the intervention arm, 124 out of 157 participants initiated vocational training, 100 successfully completed training, and 86 received a microgrant—which translates into 54% of the intervention sample overall. The primary reasons for not receiving a start-up grant included not completing vocational training or failing to pass practical exams, not developing a business plan, and relocation. Participation in the full SHAZ! intervention (compared to the control condition) led to significant improvements in all economic indicators (food security, income, and ability to afford medications) and important HIV risk factors (transactional sex, condom use, and experience of violence). Participation also led to a 40% reduction in unintended pregnancy of borderline statistical significance [HR = 0.62, 95% CI (0.38, 1.02)]. While there was no statistically significant difference in the incidence of HIV [HR = 0.94, 95% CI (0.33, 2.69)] or HSV 2 [HR = 1.50, 95% CI (0.70, 3.19)], HSV 2 incidence was higher among intervention participants compared to control participants.

The paper from the original study highlights several potential factors for the mixed results found in this study. On the positive side, the study had several strengths, primarily the rigorous RCT design, the community-based process to design the intervention, and the use of audio computer assisted survey instruments (ACASI) and "young" face-to-face interviewers to improve the reporting of sensitive behaviors. In addition, retention was higher than expected given the political and economic turmoil during the period and the chaotic lives of adolescent orphans who are often shuttled between extended family households. However, the study and the evaluation also faced several challenges. As previously stated, the environment in Zimbabwe at the time of the study made it difficult to test "proof of concept." Only 60% of the participants ultimately received a microgrant due in part to the overarching context and to difficulties in completing vocational training courses and developing business plans. While this was an important finding in itself for ongoing program improvement, such challenges rendered it difficult—if not impossible—to determine the full effect of the livelihoods intervention. Furthermore, the study showed general improvements observed from baseline to endline for several factors (e.g., social support received, relationship power) that were not statistically different across arms. A possible explanation for these findings is that the lack of a true "standard of care" control arm may have diluted intervention effects, given that all participants received life skills training and regular access to health care.

Through a further analysis of data from the original study, including process and qualitative data, the case study description in this chapter aims to improve our understanding and interpretation of the original SHAZ! findings for ongoing program and policy efforts.

METHODS

For the case study described in this chapter, we analyzed retention, attendance, and participation data from the original study, along with qualitative program monitoring data, to explore differences in adherence between study groups by study visit and the reasons behind this attrition. The qualitative program monitoring data consisted of data collected and notes taken during guidance counseling visits with participants conducted throughout the project period. Analysis consisted of reviewing these documents for common themes and issues. In addition, we conducted logistic regression to understand factors related to training completion, defined as having passed practical exams at the end of the training period. Covariates that we evaluated included age, education, socioeconomic status (food security and income), and family demands, such as having children and having to care for sick relatives.

We also compared effects of the intervention on economic and social factors, sexual behavior, and biological outcomes (HIV, HSV 2, and pregnancy) among those who received the microgrant compared to the control participants. This analysis was conducted to better understand the potential effects based on intervention "dose." Ultimately, it is important to understand if participants who completed the livelihoods component of the intervention (the vocational training and microgrant) had better outcomes compared to those in the intervention group who did not complete this component. This will help us understand the relative importance of the economic intervention over and above the life skills education. To help us understand in what ways successful participants (in terms of vocational training and the microgrant) were different from those who did not succeed, we compared baseline demographic characteristics between intervention participants who received the microgrants with those in the intervention arm who did not, as we did in the original analysis between intervention and control participants, and tested whether any differences between them were statistically significant.

TABLE 8.1   RETENTION BY STUDY VISIT AND GROUP

Study visit	Intervention N = 158 (% observed)	Control N = 157 (% observed)
6 months	149 (94)	143 (91)
12 months	142 (90)	137 (87)
18 months	136 (86)	118 (75)
24 months	132 (84)	123 (78)

RESULTS

Study Retention and Intervention Adherence

Table 8.1 presents data on study retention. Among the 315 participants in the study (158 in the intervention group, 157 in the control group), there was no statistical difference in study retention overall. However, an analysis of retention by study arm across all study visits reveals a trend in lower levels of participation among control participants, which was significantly different (statistically speaking) at the 18-months study visit. Similarly, while not statistically significant, fewer control participants completed life skills and Red Cross training compared to intervention participants (table 8.2). These trends in lower participation over time among control participants may have been problematic in terms of understanding the effects of the program if those who dropped out from the control arm were all, for example, younger than those in the intervention arm, or were all more likely to be HIV infected. However, an analysis of intervention versus control participants on demographic factors among those still participating at the end of the study (including age, marital status, and highest level of school completed) showed no statistically significant differences between groups on these factors.

Table 8.2 also shows the proportion of intervention participants who passed vocational training (63%) and who ultimately received a microgrant (54%). In reviewing why these numbers were not closer to the 100% we had expected—given that participants selected their courses based on personal interest and would have welcomed the microgrant—our analysis showed several potential factors at play. First, as highlighted above (and in table 8.1), only 84% of participants were retained for final study visits after two years in the intervention group. While this shows quite a high level of ongoing participation over two years, it does mean that approximately 15% of these participants were not able to

TABLE 8.2   INTERVENTION COMPLETION BY STUDY ARM

Study arm completed	Intervention n = 158 (% observed)	Control n = 157 (% observed)	Total N = 315 (% observed)
Completed life skills training	152 (96)	145 (92)	297 (94)
Passed Red Cross training	129 (82)	115 (73)	244 (77)
Passed vocational training	100 (63)	N/A	N/A
Received microgrant	86 (54)	N/A	N/A

complete the vocational training because they dropped out of the overall program. The main reason for their dropping out was relocation outside of Zimbabwe (45%), a common phenomenon given the economic context at the time, when many were leaving to pursue economic activities in South Africa or other neighboring countries. This reason was followed by returning to formal education (17%) and discontinuation following marriage (2%) or pregnancy (2%).

Among participants who did manage to stay in the program, programmatic monitoring data collected during study visits showed important challenges in successfully completing vocational training and thus being eligible for a microgrant. The most critical of these challenges was the language barrier, given that the nationally accredited vocational training courses we supported participants to attend were conducted in English, not the local Shona language. The project selected these nationally accredited programs to offer the greatest potential benefit to participants for securing employment after training. Our assessment at the time suggested that participants—70% of whom had completed secondary school (which is conducted entirely in English) and 85% of whom had a least two years of secondary education—would be able to successfully navigate training conducted in English. However, this proved to be a greater challenge than anticipated for a large number of participants. Furthermore, the length of the course (six months on average), also posed difficulties for some who experienced family demands—such as household duties, taking care of children or of sick household members, and participating in family businesses. Statistical analysis on factors associated with training completion found that participants who had completed secondary education were nearly three times more likely to complete vocational training and that those reporting that someone in their household was ill were 60% less likely to complete their training. This in turn affected the percentage of participants who received microgrants, given that the provision of grants was conditional on completing vocational training.

Effects by Intervention Dose

Table 8.3 shows the results of an analysis that attempted to understand the effect of the intervention among those who received the microgrant compared to those who didn't receive one. The analysis compares intervention effects on structural and sexual risk factors among all intervention participants (full sample) versus control participants, and intervention participants who received the microgrant (restricted sample) versus control participants. In the analysis among the full sample, intervention participants were less food insecure and more likely to have received an income than control participants. While effect sizes and significance levels among the restricted sample of those who received a microgrant increased for income (e.g., for those receiving their own income, the OR increased from 2.05 to 2.27, and the P value went from $p = 0.02$ to $p = 0.006$) and food security, for other factors, outcome for participants in the full and restricted samples were virtually identical—meaning that there were no measurable differences between the two samples on these factors.

For biological outcomes (e.g., pregnancy, HIV, and HSV 2), participants in the restricted sample (who received microgrants) were less likely to have experienced an unintended pregnancy compared to participants in the full sample [HR = 0.46, 95% CI (0.23, 0.91) vs. HR = 0.62, 95% CI (0.38, 1.02)]. No statistically significant differences were noted between the restricted and full samples for infection with HIV or HSV 2 (table 8.4); however, similar trends were observed: intervention participants in both the full and restricted samples had lower incidence of HIV and higher incidence of HSV 2 infection.

Overall Economic Context

A more detailed analysis of the overarching economic and political context is illustrated by figure 8.3, which shows the gross domestic product (GDP) of Zimbabwe (defined as purchasing power parity or the estimated worth in terms of US dollars) in billions of dollars from the year 2000 to 2008. The study began in February 2006, and it was completed in December 2008. As shown in the graph, GDP fell radically in the final year of the study, just when participants would have experienced the economic benefits of the livelihoods intervention. As described

TABLE 8.3   EFFECT OF THE INTERVENTION COMPARING FULL SAMPLE TO SAMPLE
RECEIVING A MICROGRANT (RESTRICTED SAMPLE)

	Full sample OR (95% CI)	Interaction P value	Restricted sample OR (95% CI)	Interaction P value
Structural factors				
Food insecure				
Intervention (OR, 95% CI)	0.68 (0.60, 0.77)	0.02	0.67 (0.57, 0.80)	0.05
Control (no./total no.[%])	0.83 (0.72, 0.94)		0.83 (0.72, 0.94)	
Received own income				
Intervention (OR, 95% CI)	2.05 (1.79, 2.34)	0.02	2.27 (1.88, 2.73)	0.006
Control (OR, 95% CI)	1.67 (1.48, 1.87)		1.67 (1.48, 1.87)	
Received high social support				
Intervention (OR, 95% CI)	1.19 (1.09, 1.30)	0.94	1.32 (1.18, 1.49)	0.16
Control (OR, 95% CI)	1.19 (1.09, 1.30)		1.19 (1.09, 1.30)	
"High" relationship power score				
Intervention (OR, 95% CI)	1.30 (1.17, 1.44)	0.90	1.38 (1.21, 1.57)	0.44
Control (OR, 95% CI)	1.28 (1.15, 1.43)		1.28 (1.15, 1.43)	
Physical/sexual violence or rape				
Intervention (OR, 95% CI)	0.10 (0.02, 0.67)	0.06	0.42 (0.11, 1.67)	0.60
Control (OR, 95% CI)	0.63 (0.41, 0.96)		0.63 (0.41, 0.96)	
Sexual behavior/risk				
Sexually active in last month				
Intervention (OR, 95% CI)	1.48 (1.32, 1.67)	0.93	1.51 (1.30, 1.75)	0.86
Control (OR, 95% CI)	1.49 (1.33, 1.66)		1.49 (1.33, 1.66)	
Transactional sex in last month				
Intervention (OR, 95% CI)	0.64 (0.50, 0.83)	0.25	0.67 (0.48, 0.94)	0.45
Control (OR, 95% CI)	0.79 (0.62, 1.02)		0.79 (0.62, 1.02)	
Condom use with current partner				
Intervention (OR, 95% CI)	1.79 (1.23, 2.62)	0.25	1.70 (0.98, 2.95)	0.45
Control (OR, 95% CI)	1.29 (0.86, 1.95)		1.29 (0.86, 1.95)	
Contraceptive use current partner				
Intervention (OR, 95% CI)	1.09 (0.74, 1.54)	0.67	1.09 (0.67, 1.78)	0.73
Control (OR, 95% CI)	0.97 (0.67, 1.41)		0.97 (0.67, 1.78)	

Biological outcomes	Full sample HR (95% CI)	P value	Restricted sample HR (95% CI)	P value
HIVM				
Intervention	0.94 (0.33, 2.69)	0.91	0.71 (0.18, 2.73)	0.61
Control	- (Ref)		- (Ref)	
HSV-2				
Intervention	1.50 (0.70, 3.19)	0.30	1.65 (0.72, 3.82)	0.24
Control	- (Ref)		- (Ref)	
Unintended pregnancy				
Intervention	0.62 (0.38, 1.02)	0.06	0.46 (0.23, 0.91)	0.03
Control	- (Ref)		- (Ref)	

NOTE: Ref = reference group.

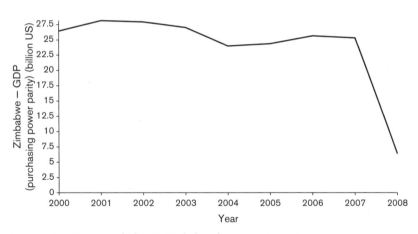

FIGURE 8.3. Economic decline in Zimbabwe from 2007 to 2008

earlier, this rapid decline was the result of a decade-long economic and political crisis, which all but devastated the country.

The overarching political and economic context made it more difficult than it might otherwise have been for the economic intervention to affect the long-term livelihoods of the participants. In addition, many of the SHAZ! participants were displaced through Operation Murambatsvina or had their families' livelihoods destroyed. It is also important to note that qualitative monitoring data suggests that some control participants were translating study reimbursements ($2 a day for transport during two weeks of life skills training and $5 per study visit every six months) into economic opportunities, potentially making it even harder to determine what the effects of the livelihoods intervention would have been if the economic environment had been more stable. Through programmatic data collected during guidance counselling visits, we determined that at least twenty-one participants in the control group used study reimbursements for training and/or to create economic opportunities. As one participant pointed out, "The little money I was getting actually assisted me. . . . It allowed me to attend night school for O-level."

DISCUSSION AND LESSONS LEARNED

As summarized in the previously published manuscript, there were many strengths to the overall evaluation, including the randomized design and the community approach used in designing the intervention over time. However, limitations—including the relative small sample size, the length of the follow-up period, and the fact that only half of the participants received the microgrant—pose challenges to interpreting the mixed outcomes. Through this case study, we attempt to better understand these findings through an assessment of programmatic data and a comparison of outcomes among participants who received the grant compared to control participants.

Findings from this case study point to many lessons learned for ongoing programming not only for SHAZ! but for interventions that are designed to economically empower adolescents in resource-poor settings for improved health. The most important of these lessons is that livelihoods interventions for adolescents should incorporate a wide range of livelihoods options from basic short courses to more advanced training opportunities, including ones in the local language, with flexible hours that allow participants to manage competing demands on their time. These changes would help ensure that a greater proportion of participants could take full advantage of the economic opportunities provided. Furthermore, such interventions must be designed to take into account as much as possible the overarching context, and they must be flexible enough to adapt to changes in this context and to aspects of the intervention that aren't working. While it would have been impossible for us to anticipate the individual effects of the circumstances that befell Zimbabwe during the course of the SHAZ! intervention study, more real-time data collection and analysis during the course of the study would have allowed us to adapt what wasn't working well within these contextual changes. While the main study analysis did show improvements in food security and income generated, which were greater in magnitude among participants in the intervention group than in the control group, the economic crisis no doubt mitigated the potential of the intervention to foster the economic empowerment envisioned in its original design—ultimately hindering the ability of the evaluation to fully test our theory of empowerment.

Unfortunately, the analysis of outcomes among participants who received the microgrants compared to control participants didn't shed much additional light on interpreting study outcomes. In general, findings from the new analysis reinforced the main study findings. In some cases, for example, for the outcome of unintended pregnancy, the magnitude and statistical significance of the effect size increased. However, many unanswered questions remain. For example, why do we see trends towards a reduction in HIV incidence among intervention versus control participants, but at the same time a trend towards an increase in HSV 2 incidence among intervention participants compared to controls? This could simply reflect variation given our small sample size, or a true effect for which we did not have adequate power to prove statistical significance. In any case, it is a perplexing finding given that HIV and HSV 2 incidence should be driven by the same risk factors.

The limitations in interpreting findings from this study point to lessons that could be applied to future studies of similar programs. For example, evaluations of these types of combination interventions need to remain flexible to allow for adaptations along the way, to address programmatic challenges that arise during implementation. Furthermore, proof-of-concept interventions should be implemented in more stable economic and political environments than the one in Zimbabwe during the study period. Such studies should also allow a comparison with a true standard of care control, to more clearly compare the combined effect of the combination intervention to a control condition that is as close to a "do-nothing" group as has been determined to be ethically sound. If shown to be effective in under these conditions, the model could be expanded to more challenging contexts, at which time operational research to tweak and continually improve the project could be incorporated.

The findings from this study have been incorporated into an ongoing evaluation of the next phase of the SHAZ! intervention, entitled SHAZ!-Plus and designed to support adolescent women living with HIV for greater health and well-being. In this evaluation, we have utilized the same components as were implemented in SHAZ! However, we have incorporated a much wider range of livelihoods options, including short, three-day courses conducted in the local language (e.g., soap- and candle-making) and medium-length courses, alongside the nationally accredited vocational training courses that were offered in the original SHAZ! We also provide life skills training courses on weekends and evenings and over shorter periods of time, and we have built into the evaluation regular program reviews of process data and the opportunity to tweak the intervention or its delivery based on these reviews. At the time of publication, we have enrolled 715 participants for a study of 18 months, with over 80% retention. To date, over 82% of the participants exiting the study have completed training and received a microgrant, and we are working towards a target of 85%.

CONCLUSIONS

This SHAZ! case study reflects the challenges inherent in rigorously evaluating combination prevention interventions targeting most-at-risk populations in resource-poor settings, where arguably they are needed most. Such efforts have included interventions to increase gender equity, provide conditional and nonconditional cash transfers, and offer microcredit or other livelihoods opportunities. For instance, IMAGE (Intervention for Microfinance and Gender Equity) merged a curriculum of gender equity and HIV/AIDS education with microfinance for women in South Africa. While no reduction in HIV incidence was observed from its community randomized controlled trial (RCT), results demonstrated effects on related outcomes such as increased assets (Pronyk et al. 2006), a 55% reduction in intimate-partner violence (Pronyk et al. 2006), and increased condom use (Pronyk et al. 2008). In Zimbabwe, an RCT of twenty-five primary schools studied the effects of providing school fees to orphaned girls. HIV was not directly measured, but the study found an 82% reduction in school dropout and marriage rates after two years and more equitable gender attitudes (Hallfors et al. 2011). Recently, an RCT of a cash transfer (CT) program among 1,289 girls attending school in Malawi found lower odds of HIV (OR 0.36, 95% CI [0.14, 0.91]) and HSV 2 (OR 0.24, 95% CI [0.09, 0.65]) among those who received CTs compared to who that did not (Baird et al. 2012). In an effort to identify opportunities to improve the sexual health of young women and girls in sub-Saharan Africa, ongoing work incorporating the lessons learned from this study is of critical importance.

Box 8.1. Summary

Geographical area: Zimbabwe, Southern Africa.

Global importance of the health condition: Zimbabwe is confronting the synergistic plagues of a generalized HIV epidemic and crushing poverty, both of which disproportionately affect adolescent girls and women. Existing behavioral interventions have shown limited impact, in part because they do not address structural factors driving risk.

Intervention or program: SHAZ! was initiated in 2000 and combined access to sexual and reproductive health services and life skills education with support to attend a vocational training course to improve livelihood opportunities. Participants who completed the training were provided with a small start-up grant (equivalent to $100) to support economic activities related to their training.

Impact: Over three hundred adolescent women at risk for HIV were provided with life skills education, economic opportunities through vocational training, and a start-up grant, as well as access to comprehensive HIV and reproductive health care.

Lessons learned: Livelihoods interventions for adolescents aimed at preventing HIV should incorporate a wide range of livelihoods options from basic short courses to more advanced training opportunities, including ones in the local language, with flexible hours that allow participants to manage competing demands on their time. Furthermore, interventions must take into account as much as possible the overarching economic context, and they must be flexible enough to adapt to changes in this context and to aspects of the intervention that aren't working.

Link between empowerment and health: The economic, social, and sexual empowerment of young women and girls can reduce HIV risk even in the context of high HIV risk and poverty.

Box 8.2. Older and Newer Approaches to Livelihoods Development

PREVIOUS APPROACHES

- Assume that a one-size-fits-all approach to livelihoods development for adolescent women will adequately meet their economic needs.

- Assume that all young women are or can be entrepreneurs.

- Perceive that addressing economic empowerment at an individual level addresses gender inequalities and structural barriers to health.

- Think that rigorous intervention evaluations demand static interventions and research design.

NEWER APPROACHES

- Offer a wide variety of livelihoods options that address young women's needs at different levels.

- Utilize interventions that respond to the complexities of the economic and political contexts in which they are situated.

- Using a broader lens on economic empowerment, work to change structural barriers while at the same time working to empower women within existing contexts.

- Allow interventions and evaluations to be flexible so that they respond to dynamic environments.

ACKNOWLEDGMENTS

We would like to acknowledge the participants of the SHAZ! program and all of the wonderful and dedicated SHAZ! staff, without whom the activities described in this chapter would not have been possible.

REFERENCES

Auerbach JD, Parkhurst JO, Caceres CF. 2011. Addressing social drivers of HIV/AIDS for the long-term response: conceptual and methodological considerations. Global Public Health 6 Suppl 3:S293–309. PubMed PMID: 21745027. Epub 2011/07/13. eng.

Baird SJ, Garfein RS, McIntosh CT, Ozler B. 2012. Effect of a cash transfer programme for schooling on prevalence of HIV and herpes simplex type 2 in Malawi: a cluster randomised trial. Lancet 04/07;379(9823):1320–1329.

Connell R. 1985. Theorizing gender. Sociol 19:260–272.

Dunbar, MS, Kang-DuFour, M, Mudekunye I, Lambdin, B, Padian, NS. 2014. SHAZ! phase II intervention results. Plos1. Nov 21;9(11):e113621. doi:10.1371/journal.pone.0113621. eCollection 2014.

Dunbar, MS, Kang-DuFour M, Mudekunye I, Nhamo D, Padian NS. 2009. Economic livelihoods and STI/HIV prevention for orphan girls in Zimbabwe–SHAZ! phase II. 18th International Society for Sexually Transmitted Diseases; London, England. (session organizer and panelists)

Dunbar MS, Maternowska MC, Kang MS, Laver SM, Mudekunye-Mahaka I, Padian NS. 2010. Findings from SHAZ!: a feasibility study of a microcredit and life-skills HIV prevention intervention to reduce risk among adolescent female orphans in Zimbabwe. J Prev Interv Community Apr;38(2):147–161. PubMed PMID: 20391061.

Dunkle KL, Jewkes RK, Brown HC, Gray GE, McIntryre JA, Harlow SD. 2004. Transactional sex among women in Soweto, South Africa: prevalence, risk factors and association with HIV infection. Soc Sci Med 10;59(8):1581–1592.

Dworkin SL, Dunbar MS, Krishnan S, Hatcher AM, Sawires S. 2011. Uncovering tensions and capitalizing on synergies in HIV/AIDS and antiviolence programs. Am J Public Health Jun;101(6):995–1003.

Emerson R, editor. 1978. Sociological theories in progress. Boston: Houghton Mifflin.

Gage AJ, Meekers D. 1994. Sexual activity before marriage in sub-Saharan Africa. Soc Biol 41(1-2):44–60.

Gibbs A, Willan S, Misselhorn A, Mangoma J. 2012. Combined structural interventions for gender equality and livelihood security: a critical review of the evidence from southern and eastern Africa and the implications for young people. J Int AIDS Soc 15 Suppl 1:1–10.

Gregson S, Nyamukapa CA, Garnett GP, Wambe M, Lewis JJ, Mason PR. 2005. HIV infection and reproductive health in teenage women orphaned and made vulnerable by AIDS in Zimbabwe. AIDS Care 17(7):785–794.

Gupta GR, Parkhurst JO, Ogden JA, Aggleton P, Mahal A. 2008. Structural approaches to HIV prevention. Lancet 08/30;372(9640):764–775.

Hallfors D, Cho H, Rusakaniko S, Iritani B, Mapfumo J, Halpern C. 2011. Supporting adolescent orphan girls to stay in school as HIV risk prevention: evidence from a randomized controlled trial in Zimbabwe. Am J Public Health 06;101(6):1082–1088.

Haram L. 1995. Negotiating sexuality in times of economic want: the young and modern Meru women. In: Klepp K-I, Biswalo PM, and Talle A, editors. Young people at risk: fighting AIDS in northern Tanzania. Oslo, Norway: Scandinavian University Press. p. 31–48.

Irvin A. 2000. Taking steps of courage: teaching adolescents about sexuality and gender in Nigeria and Cameroun. New York: International Women's Health Coalition.

Jewkes R, Nduna M, Levin J, Jama N, Dunkle K, Puren A, et al. 2008. Impact of Stepping Stones on incidence of HIV and HSV-2 and sexual behaviour in rural South Africa: cluster randomised controlled trial. BMJ 337:a506. www.bmj.com/content/337/bmj.a506.

Kabeer N. 1999. Resources, agency, achievement: reflections on the measurement of women's empowerment. Dev Change 30(3): 435–464.

Kang M, Dunbar MS, Laver S, Padian NS. 2007. Maternal and paternal orphan status, socio-economic vulnerability, and HIV/STI and pregnancy risk among adolescent girls in Zimbabwe. AIDS Care 20(2):214–217.

Kim J, Pronyk P, Barnett T, Watts C. 2008. Exploring the role of economic empowerment in HIV prevention. AIDS 12;22 Suppl 4:57–71.

Kim JC, Watts CH, Hargreaves JR, Ndhlovu LX, Phetla G, Morison LA, et al. 2007. Understanding the impact of a microfinance-based intervention on women's empowerment and the reduction of intimate partner violence in South Africa. Am J Public Health 10;97(10):1794–1802.

Komba-Malekela B, Liljeström R. Looking for men. 1994. In: Tumbo-Masabo Z, Liljeström R, editors. Chelewa, chelewa: the dilemma of teenage girls. Uppsala, Sweden: Nordiska Africainstitutet. p. 133–149

Krishnan S, Dunbar MS, Minnis AM, Medlin CA, Gerdts CE, Padian NS. 2008. Poverty, gender inequities, and women's risk of human immunodeficiency virus/AIDS. Ann NY Acad Sci 1136:101–110. PubMed PMID: 17954681. Pubmed Central PMCID: 2587136

Laga M, Schwartlander B, Pisani E, Sow PS, Carael M. 2001. To stem HIV in Africa, prevent transmission to young women. AIDS May 4;15(7):931–934. PubMed PMID: 11399966.

Mlambo A, Raftopoulous B. 2010. The regional dimension of Zimbabwe's multi-layered crisis. In: Election processes, liberation movements and democratic change in Africa. Maputo, Mozambique: CMI and IESE.

Nzyuko S, Lurie P, McFarland W, Leyden W, Nyamwaya D, Mandel JS. 1997. Adolescent sexual behavior along the Trans-Africa Highway in Kenya. AIDS. 09;11 Suppl 1:21–26.

Pronyk PM, Hargreaves JR, Kim JC, Morison LA, Phetla G, Watts C, et al. 2006. Effect of a structural intervention for the prevention of intimate-partner violence and HIV in rural South Africa: a cluster randomised trial. Lancet 12/02;368(9551):1973–1983.

Pronyk PM, Kim JC, Abramsky T, Phetla G, Hargreaves JR, Morison LA, et al. 2008. A combined microfinance and training intervention can reduce HIV risk behaviour in young female participants. AIDS. 08/20;22(13):1659-65.

Pronyk PM, Kim JC, Hargreaves JR, Morison L, Makhubele MB, Watts C, Porter JDH. 2005. Integrating microfinance and HIV prevention—perspectives and emerging lessons from rural South Africa. Small Enterprise Dev Sep;16(3): 26–38.

Reuters. 2008 Mar 30. Factbox – Zimbabwe's meltdown. www.reuters.com /article/us-zimbabwe-election-decline-idUSL295874920080330.

Seeley J, Watts CH, Kippax S, Russell S, Heise L, Whiteside A. 2012. Addressing the structural drivers of HIV: a luxury or necessity for programmes? J Int AIDS Soc 15 Suppl 1:1–4.

Sen A. 1999. Development as freedom. Oxford, UK: Oxford University Press.

Strickland RS. 2004. To have and to hold: women's property and inheritance rights in the context of HIV/AIDS in Sub-Saharan Africa. Washington, DC: International Center for Research on Women; June. www.icrw.org/files

/publications/To-Have-and-To-Hold-Womens-Property-and-Inheritance-Rights-in-the-Context-of-HIV-AIDS-in-Sub-Saharan-Africa.pdf.

Sumartojo E. 2000. Structural factors in HIV prevention: concepts, examples, and implications for research. AIDS. Jun;14 Suppl 1:S3-10. PubMed PMID: 10981469.

Sumartojo E, Doll L, Holtgrave D, Gayle H, Merson M. 2000. Enriching the mix: incorporating structural factors into HIV prevention. AIDS 06;14 Suppl 1:1–2.

Weiss E, Whelan D, Gupta GR. 1996. Vulnerability and opportunity: adolescents and HIV/AIDS in the developing world. Washington, DC: International Center for Research on Women.

Wood K, Maforah F, Jewkes R. 1998. "He forced me to love him": putting violence on adolescent sexual health agendas. Soc Sci Med Jul;47(2):233-42. PubMed PMID: 9720642.

Zimbabwe National Statistics Agency (ZIMSTAT) and ICF International. 2012. Zimbabwe demographic and health survey 2010–11. Calverton, MD: ZIMSTAT and ICF International.

9

Is Microfinance Coupled with Gender Training Empowering for Women?

Lessons from the IMAGE Process Evaluation in Rural South Africa

ABIGAIL M. HATCHER, JACQUES DE WET, CHRISTOPHER
BONELL, GODFREY PHETLA, VICKI STRANGE,
PAUL PRONYK, JULIA KIM, LINDA MORISON,
CHARLOTTE WATTS, JOHN PORTER, JAMES R. HARGREAVES

Researchers and practitioners have attempted to intervene on women's empowerment in an effort to improve gender equality, reduce risk of HIV and other sexually transmitted infections, and decrease intimate partner violence (IPV). In such programs, empowerment is often viewed as a multilevel construct that involves critical awareness, participation in groups, and control over decisions (Zimmerman 2000). Empowerment is a process through which individuals, groups, and communities gain mastery over their lives for improved health (Rappaport 1984; Wallerstein and Bernstein 1994), and it can occur at individual, organizational, and societal levels (Zimmerman 2000).

Microfinance, or the extension of small loans to groups of women, has been theorized as an empowering tool for women in poverty, although findings around its effectiveness are mixed. In this case study, we will explore the reasons *why* and *how* one microfinance program may have led to empowerment among women in rural South Africa. Using data from a process evaluation within a randomized controlled trial known as the Intervention with Microfinance for AIDS and Gender Equity (IMAGE), we identified key program elements that contributed to the empowerment of women: encouragement of critical reflection around gender, improved participation in household and community decisions; increased control over financial resources, and collective action among participants to reduce HIV and violence in their communities. In this chapter, we translate findings into practical lessons for both the microfinance and public health fields.

CONTEXT

South Africa is home to the dual epidemics of HIV/AIDS and IPV. Recent estimates place HIV prevalence at 17.8% among individuals aged 15–49, with women of reproductive age disproportionately at risk (*UNAIDS Report* 2010). Moreover, population-based studies estimate that between 24% and 30% of women in South Africa experience IPV in their lifetime (Gass et al. 2011; Jewkes, Levin, and Penn-Kekana 2002).

From a theoretical perspective, gender inequality, HIV/AIDS, and IPV are integrally linked. Violence against women and HIV risk are important consequences of gender inequality (Blankenship et al. 2006; Parker, Easton, and Klein 2000). Conversely, experiencing IPV and living with HIV also serve to reinforce and reproduce gender inequality, both in relationships and in society at large (Jewkes and Morrell 2010). Emerging evidence from South Africa and India shows that IPV is an independent risk factor for HIV acquisition (Jewkes et al. 2010; Decker et al. 2009) and that low sexual relationship power likewise increases HIV risk (Jewkes et al. 2010). For these reasons, women's empowerment may be an important method for improving gender equality alongside reductions in HIV and IPV risk (Campbell 2004; Beeker, Guenther-Grey, and Raj 1998; Sorenson et al. 1998; Kelly 1999).

One potential technique for empowering women is microfinance—a tool for giving poor clients access to financial services, such as savings or small loans. Microfinance has been theorized to be empowering because increased income can become a basis for negotiating clout that improves the household decision-making power of women and strengthens the household economic environment (Johnson and Rogaly 1997; Hadi 2003; Chowdhury and Bhuiya 2001; Pronyk et al. 2006; Littlefield, Hashemi, and Morduch 2003). This may be particularly important for HIV and IPV prevention, since women in poverty tend to experience low sexual relationship power and are often most vulnerable to both HIV acquisition and violence (Rao 1997). Critics note that while microfinance may help entire households to cope with the impact of

HIV, women's status *within* the household may not shift (Garikipati 2008). For example, women may lose control over loan decisions if their partner retains power over financial resources in the household. Moreover, decision making is a complex construct and may be difficult to measure accurately (Mohindra, Haddad, and Narayana 2008).

Early impact studies of microfinance participation showed positive impacts on empowerment for female clients in poverty in developing country contexts (Amin, Becker, and Bayes 1998; Ashraf, Karlan, and Yin 2010; Lakwo 2006; Montgomery and Weiss 2011; Pitt and Khandker 1998; Schuler and Hashemi 1994). In these studies, empowerment was measured using a list of household situations about which women report making a decision alone, making a decision with input from the husband, or deferring to the husband entirely. However, more recent studies of microfinance (with rigorous designs controlling for baseline characteristics and self-selection bias) have not demonstrated comparable results; several trials indicate no measurable improvement in empowerment due to participation in microfinance (Banerjee et al. 2015; Garikipati 2008; Karlan and Zinman 2010; Mohindra, Haddad, and Narayana 2008; Roodman and Morduch 2009; Wakoko 2003; Crépon et al. 2014). In a notable example, scholars reexamined data from an early study of microfinance (Pitt and Khandker 1998) and showed that women who self-selected to microfinance were likely more empowered to begin with, hence nullifying initial claims that microfinance increased empowerment (Roodman and Morduch 2009).

Given the mixed evidence base and inconsistent rigor in study designs, it is difficult to conclude whether microfinance is inherently empowering for women. As a result, some have suggested that empowering clients may require new programs that go beyond simply providing access to financial services (Dunford 2002; Khandker 2005), especially to the extent that poverty also relates to vulnerability, powerless, and dependency (Bhatt 1998). To overcome poverty, impoverished individuals usually require access to a coordinated combination of microfinance and other social services (Khandker 2005; Mosley and Hulme 1998; Bhatt and Tang 2001; Morduch 2000). Indeed, scholars have noted that small increases in income are unlikely to contribute to empowerment unless they are coupled with larger efforts to shift gender norms (Dworkin and Blankenship 2009). Consequently, programs globally have begun to explore an idea called "microfinance plus," which provides clients with a combination of financial and social services, rather than credit alone (Aghion and Morduch 2005).

In the current chapter, we examine the microfinance program Intervention with Microfinance for AIDS and Gender Equity (IMAGE). IMAGE was the first structural intervention in sub-Saharan Africa to measure impact on HIV and violence in a cluster-randomized control trial (Hargreaves et al. 2002). Despite the rigorous design of the IMAGE trial, our team was guided by the notions that trials of complex interventions often fail to answer some critical questions about how outcomes were achieved (Victora, Habicht, and Bryce 2004; Elford et al. 2002) and that it is crucial to combine outcome evaluation with research that is more explanatory in nature (Beeker, Guenther-Grey, and Raj 1998; Wight and Obasi 2003). We therefore conducted a mixed-methods process evaluation during and following the IMAGE trial in order to understand *why* and *how* the intervention achieved its reported outcomes.

PROGRAM DESCRIPTION

Based in a densely populated rural area in Limpopo Province, South Africa, IMAGE combines gender training and HIV prevention with microfinance activities. It is led as a joint effort by the University of the Witswatersrand School of Public Health and London School of Hygiene and Tropical Medicine. IMAGE partners with Small Enterprise Foundation (SEF), a poverty-focused South African microfinance initiative.

Microfinance: To identify eligible households, SEF used a community-driven mapping process through which neighbors ranked the relative wealth of community members (Simanowitz and Nkuna 1998). Next, SEF invited the poorest one-third of women in a neighborhood to participate in its loan program. Groups of five women formed a self-organized "trust group" to apply for loans and share business advice informally. A larger group of forty women met during more formal fortnightly "loan center" meetings to repay loans and decide when to increase funding to fellow women (Hargreaves et al. 2010).

Gender training: Specialized facilitators were recruited from the local area to lead a gender curriculum called Sisters for Life, comprising ten sessions on gender roles, sexual norms, partner communication, HIV prevention, and domestic violence (Kim et al. 2002).

Community mobilization: Following Sisters for Life, loan centers work together to choose several participants to attend a week-long

Natural Leaders Training course on leadership and social mobilization. Upon returning to their loan centers, Natural Leaders assist fellow IMAGE participants in creating Action Plans that tackle community challenges around health and gender-based violence.

SUMMARY OF METHODS AND PUBLISHED QUANTITATIVE FINDINGS

As described in detail elsewhere, IMAGE was evaluated through a cluster-randomized control trial (Pronyk et al. 2006). At the two-year follow-up, women in intervention villages were half as likely to report experiences of intimate partner violence (Kim et al. 2007) and less likely to engage in unprotected sex (Pronyk et al. 2008), and a subgroup reported improved communication with their children around sexuality and health (Phetla et al. 2008). Nine quantitative indicators were developed to measure empowerment: self-confidence, financial confidence, challenging gender norms, autonomy in decision making, perceived contribution to the household, communication within the household, relationship with partner, social group membership, and participation in collective action. Several measures of empowerment were improved among participants in IMAGE, even when adjusting for confounding factors and baseline characteristics (Kim et al. 2007). However, in a follow-up study, empowerment gains through IMAGE (e.g., microfinance plus gender training) were more pronounced than when participants took part in microfinance alone (Kim et al. 2009). This suggests that microfinance alongside gender training may synergistically improve empowerment through both financial and gender norms program content. Nevertheless, previous IMAGE studies have not examined the mechanisms for *why* the program may lead to empowerment or identified program components that provide a plausible argument for *how* these changes may have occurred. Since the *why* and *how* research questions often lie within the realm of process evaluations, in this chapter we analyze process data to craft a richer understanding of previous IMAGE trial results.

METHODS

For the findings presented in this chapter, we conducted a six-year, mixed-method process evaluation, the detailed methods and results of which are reported elsewhere (Hargreaves et al. 2010). In brief, we col-

TABLE 9.1   IMAGE PROCESS EVALUATION DATA COLLECTION METHODS,
2001–2007

Data source	Population	Timeframe/Quantity
		2001–2005
Focus group discussions	Female clients	16 groups
In-depth interviews	Key informants	$n = 15$
	Program drop-outs	$n = 19$
		2005–2007
In-depth interviews	Female clients	$n = 24$
	Staff	$n = 47$
	IMAGE managers	$n = 10$
	Microfinance managers	$n = 12$

NOTE: IMAGE: Intervention with Microfinance for AIDS and Gender Equity.

lected quantitative data in the form of attendance registers, client questionnaires, and financial records. During the IMAGE trial, we conducted 374 hours of participant observation, semistructured interviews ($n = 34$) and focus group discussions ($n = 16$) with female clients, women between 18 and 45 years of age, who participated in IMAGE (table 9.1). Following the IMAGE trial, we collected semistructured interviews with clients, staff, and management ($n = 98$). Interview and focus group discussion guides addressed issues such as the acceptability of the program, experiences with the curriculum, and outcomes of participation in IMAGE.

Focus group discussions and in-depth interviews were transcribed verbatim from digital recordings and, where necessary, translated independently from Sepedi, the local language, into English. Transcripts were analyzed using QSR NVivo (QSR 2002). First, a sample of transcripts were reviewed to establish a thematic code book drawing from the research questions. Intercoder agreement was measured to verifying the coding process. Next, the entire database was broad coded separately by two researchers. This was followed by a second, finer coding to draw out grounded impressions from the data (Miles and Huberman 1994). Analytical reports were written to illustrate all broad codes and fine codes, to illustrate the variation in themes, and to identify areas where research participants converged or diverged in opinion. The quotes cited in this paper are a representative selection from the analytical reports. Ethics approval was granted by the University of Witwatersrand and London School of Hygiene and Tropical Medicine. Participation in research was sought on the basis of informed consent, and anonymity of informants was protected in all research outputs.

FINDINGS

Results are presented using a community psychology lens to examine empowerment, which comprises three interconnected domains: critical awareness, participation, and control over resources. After examining each domain in isolation, we explore the community mobilization aspect of IMAGE, a phase of the program that combined participation, control, and critical awareness.

Empowerment through Critical Awareness

The IMAGE curriculum was facilitated by local women who had vast experience in the culture and day-to-day life of the intervention neighborhoods. To elicit critical reflections on gender subordination as natural versus societally shaped, the IMAGE facilitators asked participants to examine "normal" cultural practices in a new light:

> Often you'll hear people say, "It's natural, it's the way God intended." . . . It's important for people to have the perspective where they can even begin to question those things that seem really natural. (IMAGE manager)

IMAGE activities helped participants to question cultural traditions that had previously seemed natural and unchangeable. One participant explained that IMAGE pushed her to critically assess womens' roles in the tribal court (a local meeting of elders and community leaders), and she shifted from seeing womens' silence in court as "natural" to understanding it as a form of "suppression":

> I was not aware of my culture. For instance, in the tribal court women were not supposed to talk. We would go along with agreement even if we were not happy. We did not know that such things actually suppressed women. We took it as natural. But things are different now; women are doing things for themselves and they are having a say in the court. (female client)

Other women explained that they had internalized subordinated views of women and that IMAGE challenged these. For example, one participant described how she previously condoned IPV given a belief that, under some circumstances, women deserve to be hit by their partners. She described how IMAGE reconfigured her understanding of how oppression is normalized through claims of not only "nature" but also "culture":

> I have realized how easy it is for people to say, "It is our culture that I should beat my wife." I thought it was natural that it happens that way. I thought men were strong and women were weak. After we did a session about culture and roles, I realized that men suppress women and we use culture to justify it. (female client)

The IMAGE approach to empowering women through critical awareness was effective because it drew upon issues that were prominent in the daily lives of clients:

> I got very interested because these were the things that were happening in our homes. I thought, "Wow, we are going to talk about issues that trouble our homes." They do happen and they are everywhere and nobody talks about them. (female client)

A common narrative was that many participants felt compelled to share the knowledge they had acquired through IMAGE. New knowledge had led to a heightened sense of critical awareness.

> Participant 1: I think SEF has given intelligence and knowledge particularly with regard to health issues. Now we are conscious and aware about what is going on around us on health issues. We enjoy them every time.

> Participant 2: I think it is thanks to health facilitators because we finally have come out of the cocoon. (female clients)

Empowerment through Participation

Another technique for empowerment within IMAGE was providing a safe space for discussion, encouraging the voices of participants to emerge. Several participants underscored how safe spaces were fostered through current social institutions in which they were currently embedded, such as the church and the microenterprise loan offices. For example, one woman reported:

> Many of these women never thought that we could talk about violence like this. It was nice because it was in our church but even nicer where everyone had a chance to have a say. (female client)

Successful microfinance seemed to be a prerequisite for active participation, such that stronger loan centers created more active participation by clients:

> Women from good centers tend to be active and participating more than those who come from the average centers, where some of them tend show no interest in everything that happens in the centers. (microfinance manager)

Role-plays and other participatory activities were used as confidence-building tools, giving women an opportunity to share their views in a public setting:

> It was really great. I remember dramas that we did about domestic violence and the end-of-year drama we did for the local community. (female client)

As was anticipated, IMAGE instilled a sense of self-confidence in participants.

Women valued the sense of visibility and confidence that they gained from being involved in IMAGE. Several clients described public speaking as an important skill that they learned through IMAGE:

> I have gained some confidence in terms of public speaking. When there are community meetings, I am now able to stand up and ask questions without being shy. When I came back from the training, I was very enthusiastic and confident. (female client)

Empowerment through Control over Resources

IMAGE clients valued the ability to provide for their families through increased control over financial resources. While the health aspects of IMAGE were valued over time, the most important draw of the program was the improved access to financial resources:

> You have to know that the first thing that will ring in people's mind is money. It is money that will come first because they need it and you must remember these are poor communities. (female client)

Women experienced increased control over resources through their participation in IMAGE. A SEF manager explained that the program improved the quality of microfinance because IMAGE clients were more confident and able to manage their loan centers without relying on loan facilitators:

> IMAGE clients were more empowered than the other clients because they weren't relying much on the MFI staff. IMAGE clients knew their roles, and the training made them aware that "you are an individual; you can do better by yourself." And it built confidence in the clients—when you have confidence you can do anything. (microfinance manager)

Participants explained how improved control over resources led to increased power in intimate relationships:

> MT said that they have learned from the center meetings that domestic violence can be prevented if women stand up against their violent partners. She said we have the power to change the situation. She said that they were told that many women do not work and often depend on their husbands for money and that is when they get beaten because they have no alternative. (female client)

Some participants in our sample also underscored that they had increased power to leave an abusive relationship; this was viewed as a protective effect of the program.

Empowerment through Collective Action

Consistent with Kabeer's definition of power as "power with" (the ability to act with others) and not simply "power to" (e.g., individual-level power), the community mobilization phase of the program was perceived as empowering by women. In particular, women described how, within the community mobilization phase, they could act together to make changes that they identified as important within their community. When a rape prevention committee met with local leaders, it was the first time that women had ever addressed the neighborhood's traditional council. For example, one participant described how collective action gave her confidence to engage with local structures and speak out against injustice:

> We organized a march against women abuse in our area. Many women attended it. It was even published in our local newspaper and many people knew about us. To be a SEF member means to be active and say no to oppression of women. (female client)

Many times, collective action issues were at the intersection of gender equality and health (violence, alcohol, HIV), and other times, these issues were outside of these realms. One participant explained that her loan center brought together local stakeholders in a meeting to address crime:

> SEF women have played an important role in the community. We have organized many meetings. We have organized the all-women meeting, in which we told the chief, civic leader, and the police about the crime in the area. It was the day in which the "women against crime" initiative was formed. (female client)

However, there were some challenges associated with the activities connected to collective action. Some participants felt frustrated about the time burdens associated with collective action or perceived that the issues being tended to should stay at the personal level and should not be taken to the collective level. As described by one female client:

> People do not want to carry our community issues on their shoulders. Rather they prefer to mind their own personal businesses. (female client)

Taking part in collective action was especially challenging at times when clients' priorities were more in line with running a successful small business and repaying their microfinance loan:

> Women do not have time to leave their businesses and concentrate on community activities because SEF does not want to know whether you have spent most of your time helping the community. It wants its money when the repayment time comes. (female client)

To help circumvent the challenges associated with collective action, a majority of participants described ways that they had individually shared information with family, friends, and members of their community. Examples of sharing information included individual conversations with children, talking with groups of adolescents about HIV, talking with friends and relatives about violence in the community, and discussing sexuality more openly. One participant, for example, described sharing information with her children:

> I always talk to my children about the importance of using a condom with their partners [leba lekane ba bona]. (female client)

This sense of sharing lessons with the larger community aligns with IMAGE goals of diffusing the intervention messages. It also serves as a signpost of empowerment—that some women felt compelled to share their understanding of HIV outside the context of the loan center meeting.

DISCUSSION

Structural interventions to bolster gender equity and reduce HIV risks and violence are urgently needed if programs are to sustainably address women's health. This is because programs targeted at individuals may not address the reality of women's lives, in which HIV and violence risk are shaped by broader social and societal norms (Parker, Easton, and Klein 2000; Zierler and Krieger 1997; Kippax et al. 2013). IMAGE is one such structural intervention and is the first randomized trial to merge financial empowerment with gender equality programming. The current study drew on process evaluation findings from IMAGE. Process evaluations can be a critical tool in evaluating how and why interventions influence complex processes such as empowerment on the way to improved health outcomes.

The current study suggests that IMAGE influenced women's empowerment by improving critical awareness, participation, control over resources, and collective action. IMAGE was successful at helping to challenge gender norms and beliefs. Participants viewed their involvement with IMAGE as a challenge to their previous beliefs and social practices, bolstering their critical consciousness and their willingness to act on gender inequality rather than simply learning information. Consistent with quantitative data from the IMAGE study (Pronyk et al. 2006), this process evaluation suggested that participants were more likely to reject traditional gender norms, which suggests that IMAGE helped foster critical awareness, one of the key domains of empowerment mentioned previously.

This qualitative research suggests that participants defined empowerment on the basis of issues that are "close to home," such as improved confidence to speak in public, the ability to share new knowledge with others, and increased power to make decisions affecting the household (Ndlovu 2005). Empowerment through *participation in* the loan center may have been successful because of the solidarity and support women gained from other IMAGE clients (Moniruzzaman 2011). We found that IMAGE clients, like those in other microfinance programs, were able to offer advice to others and earn respect by speaking up at public events (Hays-Mitchell 2000; Holvoet 2005; Kabeer 2001). Our results seem consistent with other scholars who find that microfinance provides the opportunity to strengthen women's networks outside the family—a form of "social capital" that is positive for women and the community at large (Larance 1998). It fosters peer support among participants (Chowa and Sherraden 2012; Pitt and Khandker 1998; Pronyk et al. 2006) and creates group solidarity to solve mutual problems (Hays-Mitchell 1999). Likewise, gaining access to the public sphere of a loan center seemed to offer women more opportunities to have more visibility and influence in the broader community, an outcome that has been noted in other microfinance studies (Holvoet 2005).

In IMAGE, women's *control over resources* may have led to empowerment because access to money was coupled with training on gender norms. Participants in IMAGE reported increased financial decision making, and this has been previously found to impact women's bargaining power in negotiating household roles (Iyengar and Ferrari 2010; Schuler and Hashemi 1994). Some microfinance-only studies have suggested that women's ability to make household decisions improves when income increases (Alam 2012). However, earning more income alone does not necessarily translate into having control over income or choosing how it will be spent (Mayoux 2000; Dworkin and Blankenship 2009). Indeed, recent studies suggest that even when microfinance increases women's income, loans may perpetuate—rather than challenge—traditional gender roles (Haile, Bock, and Folmer 2012; Haase 2012). It seems that, in the case of IMAGE, combining microfinance with intensive training on gender norms was critical for attaining empowerment through the pathway of control over resources.

The *collective action* aspect of IMAGE appeared to be empowering to the women in our study. Similar to other studies, IMAGE seemed to encourage individuals to shift their own behavior and contribute to healthier social norms (Busza and Baker 2004; Gregson et al. 2004) or adopt protective behaviors by learning about HIV in an action-oriented way (Ramirez-Valles 2002). Individual acts of sharing information were widespread among IMAGE clients, and many women reported making measurable changes in their own lives. However, other literature sees community mobilization as a tool for creating broader structural changes in HIV vulnerability (Heise and Elias 1995; Parker, Easton, and Klein 2000; Kippax et al. 2013). In the period between baseline and follow-up, participants in the IMAGE trial were twice as likely to participate in collective action around HIV/AIDS compared to controls (Kim et al. 2006). We found that, although IMAGE sparked distinct examples of collective action, further investment may be required to train and support clients in leading widespread societal change (Beeker, Guenther-Grey, and Raj 1998).

Our findings suggest that IMAGE was empowering for participants, matching other microfinance research showing that social services might offer important gains in self-employment profits (McKernan 2002), client productivity (Noponen and Kantor 2004), and client satisfaction and self-confidence (Dunford 2002). However, other attempts by health researchers to offer microfinance alongside social services have been less successful (Epstein 2006; Gregson et al. 2007). In fact, recent studies have tended to show few measurable effects on empowerment (Banerjee et al. 2015; Garikipati 2008; Karlan and Zinman 2010; Mohindra, Haddad, and Narayana 2008; Roodman and Morduch 2009; Wakoko 2003; Crépon et al. 2014), and media reports have identified suicides and personal trauma associated with forced repayment of loans at high interest (Sharma 2006; Shiva 2004). Some scholars argue that microfinance may be damaging to sustainable development, because it serves as a "poverty trap"—keeping people at low levels of economic activity and a populace in constant debt (Bateman and Chang 2012).

Scholars in recent years have suggested that formal microfinance institutions may be less effective than informal groups, such as women's rotating savings associations (Wakoko 2003). Likewise, microfinance may not adequately change the prevailing gender and class arrangements that shape women's lives (Goetz and Gupta 1996; Jurik 2005). While microfinance may help to change women's level of agency within the household, it is often less successful at redistributing larger resources such as access to health care or participation in political activism around gender equality (Mahmud 2003).

This study is not without important limitations. First, the findings should be interpreted in light of the study setting and context. The region in which IMAGE operated represented an active, fast-growing marketplace, such that financial and empowerment outcomes may have been more pronounced than elsewhere. SEF, as a microfinance lender with a development-oriented approach, may have important differences from other microfinance institutions geared towards maximizing profits. Indeed, when IMAGE initially explored microfinance partnerships, SEF emerged as distinct in terms of its client focus and its relatively benign loan rates (Hargreaves 2013). From a conceptual level, it is possible that income to small groups of women is not purely structural, but rather a social, or group-based, intervention. Scholars argue that perhaps control over harder assets, such as land and property ownership, may provide more structural or enduring protection for women (Dworkin et al. 2013; Weinhardt et al. 2009).

Several methodological challenges are worth noting. Our sampling methodology may have highlighted some voices over others. Program participants may overemphasize positive aspects of an experience due to hopes that researchers have sway over program continuation, although we attempted to address this by purposively sampling program dropouts as well as active clients. Our interpretation of the data may be positively skewed due to personal commitments to the intervention, its implementation, and clients. Lastly, although empowerment was on the causal pathway between IMAGE and both HIV risk behavior and IPV, we did not have sufficient statistical power in the trial to demonstrate that more empowered women had more safer-sex behaviors or fewer experiences with violence. Therefore, this chapter illustrates the potential methods through which IMAGE may have been empowering rather than concluding that it successfully achieved empowerment.

CONCLUSIONS

The Intervention with Microfinance for AIDS and Gender Equity was one of the first structural interventions that merged gender equality with IPV and HIV prevention. Using a process evaluation methodology alongside the randomized control trial of IMAGE allowed us to assess lessons learned, a key step in moving the structural intervention field forward. Despite inherent challenges, our process evaluation suggests that IMAGE was an empowering strategy for delivering microfinance. The intervention seemed to improve women's participation and their control over resources and shaped their skills in critically analyzing gender subordination. We still have much to learn from the resourcefulness of women engaged in empowerment-related programs, but we can conclude that when programs engage in a combination of gender training and community mobilization alongside of microfinance, empowerment is indeed an attainable goal.

Box 9.1. Summary

Geographic area: Rural South Africa.

Global importance of the health condition: HIV and intimate partner violence (IPV) are endemic conditions, disproportionately impacting women of reproductive age in South Africa.

Intervention or program: Microfinance is a structural tool for giving poor clients access to important financial services, such as savings or small loans. Intervention with Microfinance for AIDS and Gender Equity (IMAGE) provided additional gender training for microfinance clients alongside group-based microfinance loans.

Impact: Quantitative indicators from a cluster randomized control trial suggest that IMAGE clients made significant gains in nine domains of empowerment. Our qualitative process evaluation explored *why* and *how* these empowerment gains may have occurred. We learned that IMAGE influenced women's empowerment through several mechanisms: improving women's participation, increasing their control over resources, fostering critical analysis, and encouraging collective action.

Lessons learned: A key lesson for future programs is that microfinance alone is unlikely to foster women's empowerment. Participatory gender training should be paired with microfinance in order to realize gains in women's empowerment.

Link between empowerment and health: Empowerment of IMAGE clients was a key ingredient for the health outcomes of reduced IPV, safer sex, and improved communication with children around sexuality and HIV.

Box 9.2. Mixed Findings on the Effects of Microfinance on Women's Empowerment

Since its inception in the 1970s, microfinance has been theorized to be empowering for women. This is because increased income bolsters the household decision-making power of women. This idea has been harnessed in health fields such as prevention of HIV and intimate partner violence, since poor women tend to experience low sexual relationship power and are often most vulnerable to both HIV acquisition and violence.

Early impact studies of microfinance showed strong links from microfinance to empowerment of poor, female clients. However, more recent studies of microfinance (with rigorous designs controlling for baseline characteristics and self-selection bias) have not demonstrated comparable results. In fact, several recent trials indicate no measurable improvement in empowerment due to participation in microfinance.

Given the mixed evidence base, it is difficult to conclude whether microfinance is inherently empowering for women. Indeed, scholars have noted that small increases in income are unlikely to contribute to empowerment unless they are coupled with larger efforts to shift gender norms. This chapter examines one program that paired participatory gender training with group-based microfinance and examines *how* and *why* it showed an effect on women's empowerment.

ACKNOWLEDGMENTS

We wish to thank those who gave generously to take part in interviews and focus groups. We thank the managing director of SEF, John de Wit, and the many staff who have made this work possible. We also thank John and Joan Gear for support and guidance throughout the study. The IMAGE program has received financial support from Anglo-American Chairman's Fund Educational Trust, AngloPlatinum, Department for International Development (UK), the Ford Foundation, the Henry J. Kaiser Family Foundation, HIVOS, the South African Department of Health and Welfare, and the Swedish International Development Agency.

This chapter is dedicated in loving memory of Lulu Ndlovu, whose spark, talent, and passion made this work possible.

REFERENCES

Aghion, B. A. D., and J. Morduch, eds. 2005. *The Economics of Microfinance.* London: MIT Press.

Alam, S. 2012. The effect of gender-based returns to borrowing on intra-household resource allocation in rural Bangladesh. *World Dev* 40 (6):1164–1180.

Amin, R., S. Becker, and A. Bayes. 1998. NGO-promoted microcredit programs and women's empowerment in rural Bangladesh: Quantitative and qualitative evidence. *J Dev Areas* 32 (2):221–36.

Ashraf, N., D. Karlan, and W. Yin. 2010. Female empowerment: Impact of a commitment savings product in the Philippines. *World Dev* 38 (3):333–344.

Banerjee, A., E. Duflo, R. Glennerster, and C. Kinnan. 2015. The miracle of microfinance? Evidence from a randomized evaluation. *Am Econ J: Appl Econ* 7 (1):22–53.

Bateman, M., and H. J. Chang. 2012. Microfinance and the Illusion of Development: From Hubris to Nemesis in Thirty Years1 *World Econ Rev* 1:33-36.

Beeker, C., C. Guenther-Grey, and A. Raj. 1998. Community empowerment paradigm drift and the primary prevention of HIV/AIDS. *Soc Sci Med* 46 (7):831–842.

Bhatt, E. 1998. Bank of one's own. Consultative Group to Assist the Poorest, Newsletter 5. Washington, DC: World Bank.

Bhatt, N., and S. Y. Tang. 2001. Delivering microfinance in developing countries: Controversies and policy perspectives. *Policy Stud J* 29 (2):319–333.

Blankenship, K. M., S. R. Friedman, S. Dworkin, and J. E. Mantell. 2006. Structural interventions: Concepts, challenges and opportunities for research. *J Urban Health–Bull N Y Acad Med* 83 (1):59–72.

Busza, J., and S. Baker. 2004. Protection and participation: An interactive programme introducing the female condom to migrant sex workers in Cambodia. *AIDS Care* 16 (4):507–518.

Campbell, C. 2004. The role of collective action in the prevention of HIV/AIDS in South Africa. In Hook D., N. Mkhize, P. Kiguwa, and A. Collins, editors. *Critical Psychology in South Africa*. Cape Town, South Africa: Juta/University of Cape Town Press.

Chowa, G., R. Masa, and M. Sherraden. 2012. Wealth effects of an asset-building intervention among rural households in Sub-Saharan Africa. *J Soc Soc Work Res* 3 (4):329-345.

Chowdhury, A., and A. Bhuiya. 2001. Do poverty alleviation programmes reduce inequities in health? The Bangladesh experience. In Leon, D., and G. Walt, editors. *Poverty, Inequality and Health: An International Perspective*. Oxford, UK: Oxford University Press.

Crépon, B., F.Devoto, E. Duflo, and W. Pariente. 2014. *Estimating the Impact of Microcredit on Those Who Take It Up: Evidence from a Randomized Experiment in Morocco*. Cambridge, MA: Massachusetts Institute of Technology.

Decker, M.R., G.R. Seage 3rd, D. Hemenway, A. Raj, N. Saggurti, D. Balaiah, and J.G. Silverman. 2009. Intimate partner violence functions as both a risk marker and risk factor for women's HIV infection: Findings from Indian husband-wife dyads. *J Acquir Immune Defic Syndr* 51 (5):593–600.

Dunford, C. 2002. Building better lives: Sustainable integration of microfinance and education in child survival, reproductive health and HIV/AIDS prevention for the poorest entrepreneurs. In S. Daley-Harris, editor. *Pathways Out of Poverty*. West Hartford, CT: Kumarian Press.

Dworkin, S.L., and K. Blankenship. 2009. Microfinance and HIV/AIDS prevention: Assessing its promise and limitations. *AIDS Behav* 13 (3):462–469.

Dworkin, S.L., S. Grabe, T. Lu, A. Hatcher, Z. Kwena, E. Bukusi, and E. Mwaura-Muiru. 2013. Property rights violations as a structural driver of women's HIV risks: A qualitative study in Nyanza and Western Provinces, Kenya. *Arch Sex Behav* 42 (5):703–713.

Elford, J., L. Sherr, G. Bolding, F. Serle, and M. Maguire. 2002. Peer-led HIV prevention among gay men in London: Process evaluation. *AIDS Care* 14 (3):351–360.

Epstein, H. 2006. The underground economy of AIDS. *Va Q Rev* 82 (1):53–63.

Garikipati, S. 2008. The impact of lending to women on household vulnerability and women's empowerment: Evidence from India. *World Dev* 36 (12):2620–2642.

Gass, J.D., D.J. Stein, DR. Williams, and S. Seedat. 2011. Gender differences in risk for intimate partner violence among South African adults. *J Interpers Violence* Sep; 26(14):2764–2789. www.ncbi.nlm.nih.gov/pmc/articles /PMC3281490/.

Goetz, A.M., and R.S. Gupta. 1996. Who takes the credit? Gender, power, and control over loan use in rural credit programs in Bangladesh. *World Dev* 24 (1):45–64.

Gregson, S., S. Adamson, S. Papaya, J. Mundondo, C.A. Nyamukapa, P.R. Mason, G.P. Garnett, S.K. Chandiwana, G. Foster, and R.M. Anderson. 2007. Impact and process evaluation of integrated community and clinic-based HIV-1 control: A cluster-randomised trial in Eastern Zimbabwe. *PLoS Med* 4 (3):e102.

Gregson, S., N. Terceira, P. Mushati, C. Nyamukapa, and C. Campbell. 2004. Community group participation: Can it help young women to avoid HIV? An exploratory study of social capital and school education in rural Zimbabwe. *Soc Sci Med* 58 (11):2119–2132.

Haase, D. 2012. Revolution, interrupted: Gender and microfinance in Nicaragua. *Crit Sociol* 38 (2):221–240.

Hadi, A. 2003. Promoting health knowledge through micro-credit programmes: Experience of BRAC in Bangladesh. *Health Promot Int* 16 (3):219–227.

Haile, H.B., B. Bock, and H.Folmer. 2012. Microfinance and female empowerment: Do institutions matter? *Womens Stud Int Forum* Jul–Aug; 35 (4):256–265.

Hargreaves, J. 2013, February. Personal communication.

Hargreaves, J., J. Gear, J. Kim, B. Makhubele, K. Mashaba, L. Morison, M. Motsei, C. Peters, J. Porter, P. Pronyk, and C. Watts. 2002. Social interventions for HIV/AIDS: Intervention with Microfinance for AIDS and Gender Equity: IMAGE study, evaluation. Monograph no. 1. Johannesburg, South Africa: Witwatersrand School of Public Health.

Hargreaves, J., A. Hatcher, V. Strange, G. Phetla, J. Busza, J. Kim, C. Watts, L. Morison, J. Porter, P. Pronyk, and C. Bonell. 2010. Process evaluation of the Intervention with Microfinance for AIDS and Gender Equity (IMAGE) in rural South Africa. *Health Educ Res* 25 (1):27–40.

Hays-Mitchell, M. 1999. From survivor to entrepreneur: Gendered dimensions of microenterprise development in Peru. *Environ Plann A* 31: 251–272.

———. 2000. The human rights implications of micro-enterprise development in Peru. In Fenster, T., editor. *Gender, Planning and Human Rights*. London: Routledge. p. 111–124.

Heise, L.L., and C. Elias. 1995. Transforming AIDS prevention to meet women's needs: A focus on developing countries. *Soc Sci Med* 40 (7):931–943.

Holvoet, N. 2005. The impact of microfinance on decision making agency: Evidence from South India. *Dev Change* 36 (1):75–102.

Iyengar, R., and G. Ferrari. 2010. Discussion sessions coupled with microfinancing may enhance the roles of women in household decision-making in Burundi. CEP Discussion Paper no. 1010; Oct. London: Centre for Economic Performance, London School of Economics and Political Science. http://cep.lse.ac.uk/pubs/download/dp1010.pdf.

Jewkes, R.K., K. Dunkle, M. Nduna, and N. Shai. 2010. Intimate partner violence, relationship power inequity, and incidence of HIV infection in young women in South Africa: A cohort study. *Lancet* 376 (9734):41–48.

Jewkes, R., J. Levin, and L. Penn-Kekana. 2002. Risk factors for domestic violence: Findings from a South African cross-sectional study. *Soc Sci Med* 55 (9):1603–1617.

Jewkes, R., and R. Morrell. 2010. Gender and sexuality: Emerging perspectives from the heterosexual epidemic in South Africa and implications for HIV risk and prevention. *J Int AIDS Soc* 13:6.

Johnson, S., and B. Rogaly. 1997. *Microfinance and Poverty Reduction*. London: Oxfam.

Jurik, N.C. 2005. *Bootstrap Dreams: US Microenterprise Development in an Era of Welfare Reform*. Ithaca, NY: Cornell University Press.

Kabeer, N. 2001. Conflicts over credit: Re-evaluating the empowerment potential of loans to women in rural Bangladesh. *World Dev* 29 (1):63–84.

Karlan, D., and J. Zinman. 2010. Expanding credit access: Using randomized supply decisions to estimate the impacts. *Rev Financ Stud* 23 (1):433.

Kelly, J. 1999. Community-level interventions are needed to prevent new HIV infections. *Am J Public Health* 89 (3):299–301.

Khandker, S. 2005. Micro-finance and poverty: Evidence using panel data from Bangladesh. *World Bank Econ Rev* 19:263–286.

Kim, J., G. Ferrari, T. Abramsky, C. Watts, J. Hargreaves, L. Morison, G. Phetla, J. Porter, and P. Pronyk. 2009. Assessing the incremental effects of combining economic and health interventions: The IMAGE study in South Africa. *Bull World Health Organ* 87 (11):824–832.

Kim, J., J. Gear, J. Hargreaves, B. Makhubele, K. Mashaba, L. Morison, M. Motsei, C. Peters, J. Porter, P. Pronyk, and C. Watts. 2002. *Social Interventions for HIV/AIDS Intervention with Microfinance for AIDS and Gender Equity: IMAGE Study*. Monograph no. 2: Intervention. Johannesburg. South Africa: Witwatersrand School of Public Health.

Kim, J., C. Watts, J. Hargreaves, L. Ndlovu, G. Phetla, L. Morison, J. Busza, J. Porter, and P. Pronyk. 2007. Understanding the impact of a microfinance-based intervention on women's empowerment and the reduction of intimate partner violence in South Africa. *Am J Public Health* 97 (10):1794–1802.

Kippax, S., N. Stephenson, R.G. Parker, and P. Aggleton. 2013. Between individual agency and structure in HIV prevention: understanding the middle ground of social practice. *Am J Public Health* 103 (8):1367–75.

Lakwo, A. 2006. *Microfinance, Rural Livelihoods, and Women's Empowerment in Uganda*. Research Report 85. Leiden, Netherlands: African Studies Centre. www.ascleiden.nl/Pdf/rr85lakwo.pdf.

Larance, L.Y. 1998. *Building Social Capital from the Center: A Village Level Investigation of Bangladesh's Grameen Bank*. CSD Working Paper no. 98-4. St. Louis, MO: Center for Social Development, Washington University in St Louis. http://csd.wustl.edu/Publications/Documents/WP98-04_19.Building SocialCapitalFromTheCenter.pdf.

Littlefield, E., S. Hashemi, and J. Morduch. 2003. Is microfinance an effective strategy to reach the millennium development goals? CGAP Focus Note 24. Washington, DC: Consultative Group to Assist the Poor.

Mahmud, S. 2003. Actually how empowering is microcredit? *Dev Change* 34 (4):577–605.

Mayoux, L. 2000. *Micro-finance and the empowerment of women*. Social Finance Programme Working Paper no. 23. Geneva, Switzerland: International Labour Office. www.ilo.org/employment/Whatwedo/Publications /WCMS_117993/lang--en/index.htm.

McKernan, S-M. 2002. The impact of microcredit programs on self-employment profits: Do noncredit program aspects matter? *Rev Econ Stat* 84 (1):93–115.

Miles, M., and A. Huberman. 1994. *Qualitative Data Analysis: An Expanded Sourcebook.* Thousand Oaks, CA: Sage.

Mohindra, K.S., S. Haddad, and D. Narayana. 2008. Can microcredit help improve the health of poor women? Some findings from a cross-sectional study in Kerala, India. *Int J Equity Health* 7:14.

Moniruzzaman, M. 2011. Group management and empowerment lessons from development NGOs in Bangladesh. *J S Asian Dev* 6 (1):67–91.

Montgomery, H., and J. Weiss. 2011. Can commercially-oriented microfinance help meet the millennium development goals? Evidence from Pakistan. *World Dev* 39 (1):87–109.

Morduch, J. 2000. The microfinance schism. *World Dev* 28 (4):617–629.

Mosley, P., and D. Hulme. 1998. Microenterprise finance: Is there a conflict between growth and poverty alleviation? *World Dev* 26 (5):783–790.

Ndlovu, L. 2005. *Empowerment in the eyes of rural women of Makofane, Mabotsa, Ga-Motodi, Alverton, Bothashoek, Riba-Cross, Driekop and Motlolo in Sekhukhuneland, Limpopo Province.* Johannesburg, South Africa: School of Public Health, University of the Witwatersrand.

Noponen, H., and P. Kantor. 2004. Crises, setbacks and chronic problems—The determinants of economic stress events among poor households in India. *J Int Dev* 16 (4):529–545.

Parker, R.G., D. Easton, and C.H. Klein. 2000. Structural barriers and facilitators in HIV prevention: a review of international research. *AIDS* 14 Suppl 1:S22–32.

Phetla, G., J. Busza, J.R. Hargreaves, P.M. Pronyk, J.C. Kim, L.A. Morison, C. Watts, and J.D. Porter. 2008. "They have opened our mouths": Increasing women's skills and motivation for sexual communication with young people in rural South Africa. *AIDS Educ Prev* 20 (6):504–518.

Pitt, M.M., and S.R. Khandker. 1998. The impact of group-based credit programs on poor households in Bangladesh: Does the gender of participants matter? *J Polit Econ* 106 (5):958–996.

Pronyk, P.M., J.R. Hargreaves, J.C. Kim, L.A. Morison, G. Phetla, C. Watts, J. Busza, and J.D.H. Porter. 2006. Effect of a structural intervention for the prevention of intimate-partner violence and HIV in rural South Africa: A cluster randomised trial. *Lancet* 368 (9551):1973–1983.

Pronyk, P.M., J.C. Kim, T. Abramsky, G. Phetla, J.R. Hargreaves, L.A. Morison, C. Watts, J. Busza, and J.D. Porter. 2008. A combined microfinance and training intervention can reduce HIV risk behaviour in young female participants. *AIDS* 22 (13):1659–1665.

QSR NVIVO (Non-numerical Unstructured Data Indexing Searching & Theorizing) qualitative data analysis program Version 6. QSR International Pty, Melbourne, Australia.

Ramirez-Valles, J. 2002. The protective effects of community involvement for HIV risk behavior: A conceptual framework. *Health Educ Res* 17 (4):389–403.

Rao, V. 1997. Wife-beating in rural south India: A qualitative and econometric analysis. *Soc Sci Med* 44 (8):1169–1180.

Rappaport, J. 1984. Studies in empowerment: Introduction to the issue. *Prev Hum Serv* 3 (2 and 3):1–7.

Roodman, D., and J. Morduch. 2009. *The Impact of Microcredit on the Poor in Bangladesh: Revisiting the Evidence*. Working Paper no. 174. Washington, DC: Center for Global Development.

Schuler, S.R., and S.M. Hashemi. 1994. Credit programs, women's empowerment, and contraceptive use in rural Bangladesh. *Stud Fam Plann* 25 (2):65–76.

Sharma, S. 2006. Are micro-finance institutions exploiting the poor? Info-Change News & Features; Aug. http://infochangeindia.org/livelihoods/microfinance/are-micro-finance-institutions-exploiting-the-poor.html.

Shiva, V. 2004. The suicide economy of corporate globalisation. Znet. Countercurrents.org; Apr 5. www.countercurrents.org/glo-shiva050404.htm.

Simanowitz, A., and B. Nkuna. 1998. *Participatory Wealth Ranking Operational Manual*. Tzaneen, South Africa: Small Enterprise Foundation.

Sorenson, G., K. Emmons, M. Hunt, and D. Johnston. 1998. Implications of the results of community intervention trials. *Annu Rev Publ Health* 19:379–416.

UNAIDS Report on the Global AIDS Epidemic 2010. 2010. Geneva, Switzerland: UNAIDS. www.unaids.org/globalreport/Global_report.htm.

Victora, C., J.P. Habicht, and J. Bryce. 2004. Evidence-based public health: Moving beyond randomized trials. *Publ Health Matters* 94 (3):400–405.

Wakoko, F. 2003. *Microfinance and Women's Empowerment in Uganda: A Socioeconomic Approach*. Electronic dissertation. Columbus: Ohio State University. http://rave.ohiolink.edu/etdc/view?acc_num=osu1064325172.

Wallerstein, N., and E. Bernstein. 1994. Introduction to community empowerment, participatory education, and health. *Health Educ Q* 21 (2):141–148.

Weinhardt, L.S., L.W. Galvao, P.E. Stevens, W.H. Masanjala, C. Bryant, and T. Ng'ombe. 2009. Broadening research on microfinance and related strategies for HIV prevention: Commentary on Dworkin and Blankenship (2009). *AIDS Behav* 13 (3):470–473.

Wight, D., and A. Obasi. 2003. Unpacking the "black box": The importance of process data to explain outcomes. In Stephenson, J., J. Imrie, and C. Bonell, editors. *Effective Sexual Health Interventions: Issues in Experimental Evaluation*. Oxford, UK: Oxford University Press.

Zierler, S., and N. Krieger. 1997. Reframing women's risk: Social inequalities and HIV infection. *Annu Rev Publ Health* 18:401–436.

Zimmerman, M. 2000. Empowerment theory: Psychological, organizational, and community levels of analysis. In Rappaport, J., and E. Seidman, editors. *Handbook of Community Psychology*. New York: Kluwer Academic/Plenum.

10

Older U.S. Women's Economic Security, Health, and Empowerment

The Fight against Opponents of Social Security, Medicare, and Medicaid

CARROLL L. ESTES

Research confirms that economic advantages and disadvantages among individuals often persist and accumulate across the life course, leading to significant cumulative health and economic effects (Crystal and Shea 2003; Pescosolido and Kronenfeld 1995; Dannefer 2003; O'Rand 2003, 2006). Virtually all measures of economic disadvantage increase the risk of adverse outcomes, both at the individual and at the population level (Olshansky et al. 2012, Lantz and Pritchard 2010, Scaramella et al. 2008). A preponderance of negative health outcomes are found among low-income women, especially women of color, and those enduring racism, sexism, crime, poor housing, and other stressors (Douthit and Dannefer 2007; Douthit and Marquis 2010). Economic disadvantage (and its opposite, advantage) accumulate via cyclical processes over time and with increasing age (Dannefer 2003; Ferraro, Shippee, and Schafer 2009). The good health and economic security of some older women both emerges from their empowerment and reinforces it. In contrast, the poor health and economic insecurity of disadvantaged older women reinforces their disempowerment and exacerbates it (see also chapter 13 in this volume).

Empowerment operates in both the intrapersonal and interpersonal arenas (Speer 2000) and is influenced by interactions between an individual and the features of his or her social setting (e.g., environmental, economic, and political contexts; Wallerstein and Bernstein 1988; Zimmerman and Warschavsky 1998). Three points are noteworthy when making the link between empowerment and health in older women. First, women are more dependent than men upon the nation-state, and this is true across the life course. Women are acutely vulnerable to the larger political, economic, and global forces that shape state action. Second, women's dependency upon the state increases with age, motherhood, divorce, widowhood, and living alone, while demands for women's unpaid labor in caregiving require many to curtail or quit paid work, leading to further impoverishment (Harrington-Meyer and Herd 2007). The unpaid work caring for children and the financial contributions of middle-aged and older women to parents, in-laws, spouses, adult children, and grandchildren drains them physically and financially (Butler and Zakari 2005; Luo et al. 2012; Musil et al. 2011). Third and finally, U.S. policy produces a "gendered distribution of old age income" (Harrington-Meyer 1996, 551; Estes, Biggs, and Phillipson 2003/2009b; Estes, O'Neill, and Hartmann 2012). Women's smaller incomes at retirement are linked to (1) waged labor, which is itself gendered (23% average lower wage earned than men); (2) nonwaged reproductive labor (largely women's unpaid care work that is not counted towards Social Security benefits but credited as "zero" years outside the labor force); and (3) retirement policies based on a model in which a male breadwinner is assumed to be present if a woman is married and marital status is viewed as a permanent rather than a transient state (Harrington-Meyer 1996). As a consequence of these policies, older women, comprising three-fourths of the elderly poor, receive a smaller dollar amount from every retirement income source than older men (Estes, O'Neill, and Hartmann 2012).

The purpose of this chapter is threefold. First, I detail the ways in which the economic security, health security, and ultimately, the empowerment of women is being undermined by state policy and powerful stakeholders in the United States. Second, I describe three lines of intervention (at the individual, organizational, and coalitional levels) that seek to challenge and subvert attacks on Social Security, Medicare and Medicaid in order to mitigate the resultant negative effects on women's health and economic security. Lastly, I discuss some of the challenges and successes associated with efforts to resist attempts to dismantle Social Security, Medicare, Medicaid, and health care reform.

POLITICAL CONTEXT

The economic and health security of women is under attack by U.S. stakeholders seeking to dismantle the earned benefits programs of Social

Security and Medicare, with some policies under the new health care reform act and the revamped Medicaid program contributing to this erosion of protection. Labeled by some politicians and the media as a "war on women," these attacks threaten women's empowerment and health, particularly in view of rising income inequalities and declining health and economic security in older women as compared to men. Reproductive rights continue to be under assault, with repercussions that reverberate into older age.

The attempted "takedown" of the New Deal and the Great Society is manifested in proposals of conservative politicians and think tanks which incorporates via various congressional budgetary processes (e.g., House Budget Resolution 112 for 2013, known as the "Ryan budget," proposed again in FY 2014, 2015, and 2016, and advanced for 2017 under Ryan's House majority leadership) (1) Social Security cuts, privatization, raising the retirement age, and reductions in cost of living adjustments (COLA); (2) Medicare cuts through federal spending caps, raising the Medicare eligibility age, and privatizing Medicare via vouchers; (3) Medicaid cuts that defund and/or block Medicaid grants (notably, Medicaid is the only public financing of long-term care for elders—primarily women—people with disabilities, and poor children of single mothers); and (4) sixty-one attempts to repeal the 2010 health reforms provided by the Affordable Care Act (ACA)—including the successful 2016 Senate ACA repeal (under the special Omnibus Budget Reconciliation process requiring only fifty-one senators rather than the two-thirds required for federal budgetary enactments; President Obama promised to veto and did so). The repeal of the ACA, if signed into law by the president, would eliminate free preventive health screenings and other health benefits for more than 43 million women. (Significantly, the ACA outlaws discrimination against women by private insurers, for example, by outlawing gender-rating that results in women being charged more for health insurance than men.)

Restricted access to Medicaid affects poor women and children, minorities, the disabled, the aged and the blind. The cost in negative health outcomes as the result of being denied Medicaid coverage is documented, and it is severe (Radley & Schoen 2012). Cuts to Medicaid's long-term nursing-home care and community-based services are particularly harmful for older women. Additionally, long-term care (LTC) in the United States is typically considered women's work, providing little or no pay, no benefits, and with high morbidity and mortality consequences for caregivers (Estes and Zulman 2008). Many women, after a lifetime of caregiving for others, are left in older age without anyone to care for them.

Some argue that these actions are a "denial of basic and civil rights of elders" (International Longevity Center 2006) and are a form of ageism that justifies discrimination in health policies. Ageism, reflected in attitudes, actions, policies, and vocabularies (Macnicol 2012), affects health in a number of ways, including impaired self-esteem, a weakened sense of personal control, memory and immunological deficits, and other risk factors impairing health and empowerment (Herd, Karraker, and Friedman 2012; Levy et al. 2012). For older women, ageism intersects with sex, race, and class discrimination, further curtailing job prospects, economic opportunities, and supportive communities—all risk factors for poor health and higher mortality.

Beginning with Ronald Reagan's presidency (Estes 1991), attacks on the nation's bedrock social insurance programs of Social Security and Medicare multiplied in number and intensity. After the ACA implemented provisions in 2012 to give women access to safe and affordable health and reproductive care, women's reproductive rights became hotly contested. Women in the United States, 98 percent of whom use contraceptives during their childbearing years, now find their rights to health, reproductive care, and even contraception, questioned and denied. More than 120 state initiatives have been proposed or passed that would restrict, defund, or eliminate women's reproductive (and other health) services, while murder and violent threats have shrouded Planned Parenthood clinics. This foreboding treatment of women is further reflected by other state and federal initiatives that have scaled back or repealed provisions to ensure equal pay for women and have decreased funding for programs to prevent violence in families. In addition, significant cuts to Medicaid, children's health, Head Start preschool programs, food stamps, and child care programs have passed in the House in recent years (House Budget Resolutions FY 2012, 2013, 2014, 2015, and 2016). Because most children are raised by mothers (and, increasingly, single women), the negative effects of such cuts on women and families are profound. Moreover, the states that choose not to participate in ACA's Medicaid expansion can effectively deny health care to millions of women, men, and children. Republican governors' resistance and Supreme Court challenges to Medicaid-ACA subsidy provisions have impeded health insurance coverage for millions across the states.

THE FIGHT TO PRESERVE SOCIAL SECURITY, MEDICARE, AND MEDICAID

This case study outlines three lines of intervention undertaken by (1) the author as individual scholar and "organic intellectual" (Gramsci 1971) working in parallel with other scholars and think tanks; (2) the National Committee to Preserve Social Security and Medicare (NCPSSM), a three-million-member national advocacy organization (for which the author was chair of the board of trustees); and (3) cross-movement alliances and coalitions engaging the U.S. public.

Intellectuals and Activists (Individual Level)

As a university sociologist and as a policy scholar, I study efforts to oppose the attacks on Social Security, Medicare, and Medicaid and efforts to mitigate the potential negative effects on women's health and economic security. Four types of sociological practice are relevant in my work (Estes 2008, 2011). As a *professional sociologist*, my objective is to apply sociological knowledge and methodologies in studying (a) ideological constructs (e.g., "Social Security as the problem," the Social Security system as "bankrupt," elders as "greedy geezers") and (b) the agents (the power elites, economic dominants, and structures) behind winning and losing ideas and policies (Estes 1983). As a *policy sociologist*, I study how Social Security, Medicare, and long-term care policy "work" at all levels, including actual and projected outcomes of policy options under debate. As a *critical sociologist*, I seek to demystify the systems of domination that produce injustice and inequality through public (state) policy. Central topics are discourses (public rhetoric and ideological systems that influence policy) and agency (e.g., the work of individuals, groups, and movements aiming to effect social change). I focus on key structural forces of power (the state and the sociocultural realm) and the resources (material, symbolic, organizational, and political) that reinforce and challenge existing power structures. As a *public sociologist*, I work with various communities to bring my and others' work into public dialogue and action.

The ultimate goal of these efforts is to promote alternative frameworks and knowledge to subvert the disempowerment of women and other vulnerable people through state policy. At this level of praxis (social practices in action), I think, write, and work as part of a larger virtual collective of *organic intellectuals*, defined by Gramsci (1971) as those individuals in society who investigate, speak out, and collaborate with (and on behalf of) oppressed communities. The goal is to engage and reframe dominant discourses that shape policy while working on the ground to prevent a takedown of Social Security, Medicare, and Medicaid and, indeed, all programs of the New Deal and the Great Society of the 1960s.

To preserve, protect, and strengthen Social Security and Medicare, our work focuses on reframing elite constructions of reality to destabilize and replace the dominant market ideology with an alternative. The alternative includes the continuity, stability, and security of the social contract between a government and its people and its work towards inclusivity in the interest of social justice.

The National Committee (Organizational Level)

The National Committee to Preserve Social Security and Medicare (NCPSSM) is a nonpartisan, nonprofit organization with three million members and allies who seek to ensure economic and health security for all. Founded in 1982, it has three organizational units: (1) a policy, lobbying, and advocacy arm (C-4 tax status); (2) a political action committee (PAC tax status); and (3) a foundation for education and research (C-3 philanthropic tax status). The NC is 100 percent member-funded and does not endorse or sell any products. National Committee members have been fighting and winning legislative battles around Social Security and Medicare including efforts that (a) stopped President Bush's 2005–2006 campaign to privatize Social Security; (b) thwarted attempts to pass a balanced budget constitutional amendment (H.R.J. Res. 22, 108th Cong. [2004]) and campaigned against the Joint Select Super Committee on Deficit Reduction, both of which sought to cut and privatize Social Security and Medicare; and (3) more positively, made improvements to Medicare via President Obama's health reform policies and helped to secure the passage of ACA in 2010 (www.ncpssm.org).

Due to persistent and accelerated attacks on Social Security, Medicare, and Medicaid under the guise of deficit reduction, the NCPSSM has implemented numerous initiatives, two examples of which are the 2011 Hands Off–No Cuts Campaign and the 2012 Truth Out Campaign to stop Medicare and Social Security privatization and to stop the repeal of "Obamacare," which may again be at risk depending on the outcome of the 2016 election (Massive "no cuts" campaign 2011; "Truth campaign" 2012). Both NCPSSM campaigns involve grassroots volunteers, members, and allies; town hall events with legislators (on the phone and in person); surveys to test messages and poll public opinion; media spots on radio, TV, and Internet; and demonstrations in selected congressional districts. These activities augment the NCPSSM's continuous analysis and work on Capital Hill via lobbying and education campaigns.

Cross-Movement Organizational Action (Coalition Level)

The duration and continuity of the attacks on Social Security since President Reagan's presidency in the early 1980s, as well as overt attacks on Medicare by President George W. Bush, constituted a wake-up call. Bush's sixty-day, sixty-city tour to privatize Social Security and his 2003 Medicare Modernization Act (MMA) that privatized the Part D drug benefit program are tangible evidence of his administration's serious intent to dismantle these landmark programs. The sheer magnitude of money, organization, and power behind the "gut-cut-and-privatize" politics has demanded that individual advocacy organizations band together as a movement. An important example is the establishment of the three-hundred-plus-member Social Security Works (SSW) and its Strengthen Social Security Campaign (SSSC; Altman and Kingson 2015). With funding from a private foundation, many advocacy organizations benefit from the SSW's technical assistance, polling, message development, and campaign staff. Beamish and Lubers (2009) describe the important role of such alliances as "bridging processes" in the development of social movements.

All three levels of action and intervention (individual, organizational, and coalitional) have fomented a "Resistance Movement" (Estes 2008, 128) that is gaining momentum. Voss, 1996 and Einwohner (2002) describe the benefits to social justice organizations of using a series of fortifying strategies to celebrate successes achieved, as organizations and their resistance coalitions expand and evolve. The countermovement of resistance to social security privatization, for example, has achieved some traction.

LESSONS LEARNED

The lessons learned may be understood best through the lens of a two-part theoretical framework. The first part of the framework is a critical political economy of aging (Estes 1979, 1991) within a conflict theory perspective (Weber 1946), which includes three core elements: power, structure, and ideology. The second part of the framework, a constructionist perspective (the idea that society and the meanings that circulate within it are socially constituted and can be modified and changed through social means), is composed of the core elements of discourse, frames, and agency (Estes 1979, 2007, 2011). In this framework, the *dominant ideology* (the idea systems that achieve the most powerful and valued status in a given time) is pivotal in legitimating state policies that profoundly influence the health and economic security of the elderly. Achieving ideological dominance requires the stakeholder capacity to marshal and consolidate economic, political, and cultural resources over a sustained period of time. The winners and losers in ideological battles reflect *dominant social relations* (those who are at the top of power structures and put forward the idea systems that achieve the highest value in society are often the most privileged), and these social relations are shaped by interlocking systems of oppression (Collins 1990)—across gender, race, ethnic status, class, age, (dis)ability, and other axes of inequality. Gramsci's (1971) crucial insight is that beliefs and ideas have the weight of material force, explaining why many people consent to policies that are counter to their own interests, without overt coercion or repression. Thus, Gramsci's concept of *ideological hegemony* (ruling or dominant ideas) help us understand the disparity between people's individual beliefs and their own individual economic situation. Power and agency are crucial to produce and spread the dominant worldview but are also needed to form resistant counterframes. Agency is reflected in the contested processes of framing worldviews. Indeed, according the scholars, "framing itself is an action" (Lakoff and Rockridge Institute 2006, 25; Snow and Benford 1992, 137), while "reframing *is* social change" (Lakoff 2004).

Coinciding with and resurgent subsequent to Ronald Reagan's presidency, the ideology of individualism, with its claims of the superiority of the market, is foundational to attacks on the legitimacy of the public sector in its role in serving the collective public interest. For multiple decades (1980 to present), the ideological hegemony of the market has effectively opened the door to Social Security privatization schemes. This process has occurred through a series of presidentially and congressionally mandated studies and commissions, private foundations and think tanks, and media campaigns operating both nationally and globally (Estes and Phillipson 2003; Estes, Biggs, and Phillipson 2003/2009a; Estes and Wallace 2010).

Early in Reagan's presidency, two conservative think tanks, the Heritage Foundation and the CATO Institute, set out to privatize Social

Security, announcing "a Leninist strategy" to do so (Butler and Germanis 1983). A major lesson learned is about the strength and importance of social constructions of reality in real world politics (e.g., a theorized bankruptcy of Social Security paired with fear campaigns to undermine confidence in the program) and the triple whammy of engaging in a "long war" on economic, political, and symbolic fronts, with the resources to build and sustain it over many decades.

Not surprisingly, "privatization" itself, has achieved ideological hegemony, as evidenced by the ways it is institutionalized and given primacy in public ideology and media, political rhetoric, and organizational forms and practices (Estes 1991; Svihula and Estes 2009). This poses a formidable challenge to the resistance movement to privatization, because the movement of opposition must resist operations and shadow fronts stoked by billions of dollars in financing from U.S.-dominated international organizations (e.g., the World Trade Organization, International Monetary Fund, World Bank) and private funders such as the Koch brothers (CATO Institute founders), Pete Peterson (Peterson Foundation, Concord Coalition), and more. Their institutions and products include think tanks, scholars, reports, testimonies, message machines, press briefings, traveling campaigns, and political operatives promoting "astroturf" movement organizations (e.g., the Tea Party), while co-opting many in the mainstream and digital media. The resurgence of these same interests, which induced Republicans to shut down the government (repeatedly over time), nearly bringing the U.S. economy to a halt unless the ACA was gutted and entitlements were cut, reveals the breadth and influence of these key players, especially in light of the fact that the ACA had already passed.

How did the arguments against the economic and health security of the elderly hold such power? One way to explain this is through what is known as a *crisis motif frame*. Such frames describe current situations in terms of a severe problem that must be acted upon immediately or else catastrophic outcomes will result. Here, the crisis motif frame was the urgent need for privatization campaigns first against Social Security, then Medicare via vouchers and managed care (Estes 2004; Svihula and Estes 2007, 2009), and most recently, new threats to repeal Obamacare. Layered on top are two additional crisis themes: the *deficit crisis* ("apocalyptic deficits," Estes 2011) and the *demographic crisis* of aging ("apocalyptic demography," Robertson 1999). Policy makers and elites in the conservative arm of the U.S. government contend that these crises exist and that they *require* the restructuring of the United States and other Western industrialized welfare states via cuts and belt-tightening (increasing eligibility age).

Given this scenario, a lesson we have learned in our work is the potency of effectively producing and disseminating multiple crisis frames to promote fear and uncertainty en masse, which, in turn, leads the media and the public to acquiesce to and adopt the perspective of the "inevitability" of radical state action (e.g., privatization) to "save" the "unsustainable" Social Security and Medicare systems. The privatization frame is that government is "the problem" and austerity is "the solution," with a shifting of risk and responsibility from the state to individuals and their families (Hacker 2006). An ideology of globalization (Estes 2001) tells us that our economy and way of life (even our democracy) are at stake if we do not cut government "social programs."

Simultaneously, the institution of democracy is being tested via Supreme Court rulings equating money with free speech and corporations with individuals (e.g., the Citizens United ruling). The *inclusionary ethic of citizenship* and the common good are contending with forces advancing a concept of "privatized citizenship," of market morality, where individual responsibility is substituted for social morality (responsibility to community, national, and global commons; Somers 2008, 38). The ideology of individualism obscures understanding of "life course interdependence" where the "quality of life in old age strongly reflects the different costs of life course interdependencies. This includes child rearing, employment, and long-term caregiving in old age, which vary by social class, gender and race" (Twine 1994, 34). It is women's biological and social labor that constitutes that interdependence through the generations. It is women who bear the brunt of these sacrifices. Classical economic models do not attend to this issue, as feminist economist Nancy Folbre (2001) notes.

In spite of formidable odds, the resistance movement is contesting the messages, organizations, and actions that seek to impose the ideological hegemony of individualization, privatization, and globalization because these ideologies undermine democracy, women, communities of color, and social justice. The power of agency is being tested on both sides of the struggle.

Specific to women, the proposed takedown of Social Security, Medicare, Medicaid, and health reform (the ACA) is the historical struggle that confronts women of economic, political, and social disadvantage. Three studies underscore the ultimate consequences of disadvantage. First, Olshansky et al. (2012) find an astounding life expectancy gap of

10 years between white women with 12 or fewer years of education and white women with 16+ years of education; the life-expectancy gap for African American women is 6.5 years, and for Latinas, 2.9 years. Overall, the longevity gap is widening for blacks, Latinos, and the less educated. Second, Arno et al. (2011) report that after Social Security was implemented in 1940, death rates for those 65 and older fell more than for younger persons. This pattern continued through the 1960s and 1970s, when Social Security benefits improved. Third, Schulz and Beach (1999) show how caregiving, for which women are the primary providers, is demonstrated to be a risk factor for mortality. There was a 63-percent higher mortality risk among caregivers who experienced caregiver strain compared to noncaregiver controls. This suggests that being a stressed caregiver is an independent risk factor for mortality among elderly spousal caregivers.

Indeed, societal aging necessitates an "empowerment imperative" in order to ensure economic and health security for all generations (Estes, Casper, and Binney 1993).

CONCLUSION

Research must address the economic and health effects of aging health policy on women across the life course, the changing and contested forms of the nation state, the provision of welfare and threats to democracy. It must pay special attention to the lived situation of women who are racially and/or economically oppressed and to the persistence and deepening of gender, race, ethnicity, class, and age-based inequalities and divisions. Since women are more dependent on the state, they are more vulnerable to uncertainties about policy changes in state action. The risks associated with being female and with growing old as a female are increasing in intensity. This includes the threats of poverty, discrimination, and unceasing demands for women's unpaid caregiving work, which too often compromises their health. Women are hit hard because their work as caregivers is being extended due to policy shifts (e.g., shorter hospitalizations and refusal to adopt policies in the United States that would equalize gender-biased responsibilities). As Glenn (2009) unflinchingly shows, women are "forced to care."

For scholars seeking to support the resistance movement to privatization (or other policy pursuits aimed at women's empowerment), the concept of praxis is pivotal. This chapter offers a small example of how scholars may be called out of ivory towers in the best tradition of engaged social scientists (Hacker et al. 2006), organic intellectuals (Gramsci 1971), public sociologists (Buroway 2005), feminists (Calasanti 2009; Luke and Gore 1992), and race scholars (Omi and Winant 2015; Tippett 2014). It is essential to tap into a shared commitment to critical scholarship and praxis in the cause of active public engagement to ensure that our lives' work is of greatest human consequence. For scholars, this work is formidable and long-term but it is essential to success in the highly contentious struggle to ensure the health and economic security of women, communities of color, the elderly, (dis)abled, and the working class.

Box 10.1. Summary

Geographic area: United States.

Global importance of the health condition: Economic disadvantage accumulates over the life course and impacts women's health and empowerment. Women's economic security and health are continuously threatened by powerful stakeholders who seek to challenge, undermine, and dismantle Social Security, Medicare, Medicaid, and the Affordable Care Act. These programs are critical in light of rising income inequalities and declining health and economic security of impoverished communities. Older women are particularly vulnerable when the budgets of these programs are cut.

Intervention or program: This chapter describes a resistance movement designed to counteract and resist attempts to dismantle Social Security, Medicare, and Medicaid. The resistance movement involves individual scholars working at the micro, meso, and macro levels, a national committee that seeks to secure economic and health security for all, and a cross-movement coalition that is fighting overt attacks to dismantle these landmark programs.

Impact: There is a growing movement of resistance, critique, and protest comprising hundreds of organizations and coalitions spanning race, ethnicity, class, age, gender (sex and sexuality), and disability lines. To date, these efforts have prevented the threats of a "grand bargain" between congressional conservatives and the president that would "reform" Social Security and Medicare by cutting and restructuring these major anti-poverty and health programs.

Lessons learned: Despite impressive progress, social movements such as this one are barely underway and have meager resources in comparison with the billions invested by individuals and organizations representing the top 1 percent to dismantle Social Security, Medicare, and Medicaid.

Link between empowerment and health: Resistance movements challenge the dominant austerity discourses and the policies that flow from them. Resistance movements have emboldened and empowered women and their allies to organize to protect and improve U.S. programs of health and economic security. Their voice and actions have a positive impact on older women's empowerment and health.

Box 10.2. Successes: The Momentum of Social Movements' Resistance to Social Security Attacks, 2005 to 2016

- Victories to celebrate: blocking Social Security privatization and cuts despite strong political and corporate attacks.

 Breaking through grassroots organizations' silos: old and new alliances formed across groups representing the interests of women, people of color, the disabled, youth, the elderly, and the LGBT community.

- Employing new modes of resistance and rapid response: net roots and social media capacity building.

- Developing critical intellectual frameworks: public intellectuals form and engage the media, the public, and the power elites.

- Message development and testing: "The Social Insurance Case."

- Progressive framing of the debate: from deficit and apocalyptic thinking to language of stability, continuity, and benefits as "earned, deserved, and needed."

- Holding congressional and press briefings, broadcasting "Truth Out": refuting myths such as "Social Security is the problem," "the elderly are greedy," and "the system is nearly bankrupt."

- Developing positive alternatives: emancipatory knowledge and action, e-democracy, cross-movement coalitions, and the 99% movement framing the realities of social inequalities by age in terms of women, race, ethnicity, (dis)ability, LGBT, and social class versus the hegemonic ideology of political elites who claim that privatization is the only answer.

REFERENCES

Altman, N.J., and Kingson, E.R. (2015). *Social Security works!* New York: New Press.

Arno, P., House, J.,Viola, D., and Schechter, C.I. (2011, February 17). Social Security and mortality: The role of income support policies and population health in the U.S. *Journal of Public Health Policy,* 1–17. www.palgrave-journals.com/jphp.

Beamish, T.D., and Luebbers, A.J. (2009). Alliance building across social movements: Bridging difference in a peace and justice coalition. *Social Problems,* 56(4), 647-676.

Burawoy, M. (2005). 2004 Presidential address: For public Sociology. *American Sociological Review.* 70(Feb), 4-28.

Butler, F.R., and Zakari, N. (2005). Grandparents parenting grandchildren: Assessing health status, parental stress, and social supports. *Journal of Gerontological Nursing,* 31(3), 43–54.

Butler, S., and Germanis, P. 1983. Achieving a "Leninist" strategy. *Cato Journal,* 3(2), 547-561.

Bytheway, B. (2001). *Ageism.* Philadelphia: Open University Press.

Calasanti, T. (2009). Theorizing feminist gerontology, sexuality, and beyond: An intersectional approach. In V. Bengtson, D. Gans, N.M. Putney, and M. Silverstein (Eds.), *Handbook of theories of aging* (2nd ed., pp.471–485). New York, NY: Springer.

Crystal, S., and Shea, D.G. (2003). Introduction: Cumulative advantage, public policy, and inequality. *Annual Review of Gerontology and Geriatrics,* 22, 1–13.

Cuellar, A., Simmons, A., and Finegold, K. (2012). *The Affordable Care Act and women* (ASPE Research Brief). Washington, DC: Office of the Assistant Secretary for Planning and Evaluation, U.S. Department of Health and Human Services. https://aspe.hhs.gov/report/affordable-care-act-and-women.

Dannefer, D. (2003). Cumulative advantage/disadvantage and the life course: Cross-fertilizing age and social science. *Journal of Gerontology, Series B: Psychological Sciences and Social Sciences,* 58(6), S327–S337.

Dannefer, D., and Phillipson, C. (Eds.). (2010). *SAGE handbook of social gerontology.* London, England: SAGE.

Douthit, K.Z., and Dannefer, D. (2007). Social forces, life course consequences: Cumulative disadvantage and "getting Alzheimer's. In J. Wilmoth and K. Ferraro (Eds.), *Gerontology: Perspectives and issues* (3rd ed., pp. 223–242). New York, NY: Springer.

Douthit, K.Z., and Marquis, A. (2010). Biosocial interactions in the construction of late-life health status. In D. Dannefer and C. Phillipson (Eds.), *SAGE handbook of social gerontology* (pp. 329–342). London, England: SAGE.

Estes, C.L. (1979). *The aging enterprise.* San Francisco: Jossey-Bass.

———. (1991). The Reagan legacy: Privatization, the welfare state, and aging in the 1990s. In J. Myles and J.S. Quadango (Eds.), *States, labor markets, and the future of old age policy* (pp. 59–93). Philadephia: Temply University Press.

———. (2004). Social Security privatization and older women: A feminist political economy perspective. *Journal of Aging Studies*, 18(1): 9–26.

———. (2008). A first generation critic comes of age. *Journal of Aging Studies*, 22 (2): 120–131.

———. (2011). Crises and old age policy. In R. A. Settersten, Jr., and J. L. Angel (Eds.), *Handbook of Sociology of Aging* (pp. 297–320). New York, NY: Springer.

Estes, C. L., and Associates. (2001). *Social policy and aging: A critical perspective*. Thousand Oaks, CA: SAGE.

Estes, C. L., Biggs, S., and Phillipson, C. (2003/2009a). Ageing and globalization. In C. L. Estes, S. Biggs, and C. Phillipson (Eds.), *Social theory, social policy and ageing: A critical introduction* (pp. 102–121). Berkshire, England: Open University Press. (Original work published in 2003).

———. (2003/2009b). *Social theory, social policy and ageing: A critical introduction*. Berkshire, England: Open University Press. (Original work published in 2003)

Estes, C. L., Casper, M. J. and Binney, E. A. (1993). Empowerment imperative. In C. L. Estes and J. H. Swan and Associates. *The long term care crisis* (pp. 241–257). Newbury Park, CA: SAGE.

Estes, C. L. and Goldberg, S. (2003). Healthy Aging Initiative Developmental phase (Unpublished paper for The California Endowment). San Francisco, CA: UCSF, Institute for Health and Aging.

Estes, C. L., Goldberg, S., Williams, E. and Wolin, H. (principal writers). (2009). *AGEnda for action: Building a movement for elder women's advocacy*. San Francisco, CA: Womens Foundation of California.

Estes, C. L., O'Neill, T., and Hartmann, H. (2012). *Breaking the Social Security glass ceiling: A proposal to modernize women's benefits*. Washington, DC: National Committee to Preserve Social Security and Medicare Foundation, National Organization of Women Foundation, and Institute for Women's Policy Research.

Estes, C. L., and Phillipson, C. (2003). The globalization of capital, the welfare state and old age policy. *International Journal of Health Services, 32*(2), 151–164.Estes, C. L., and Wallace, S. P. (2010). Globalization, social policy, and ageing: A North American perspective. In D. Dannefer and C. Phillipson (Eds.), *SAGE handbook of social gerontology* (pp. 513–524). London, England: SAGE.

Estes, C. L., and Zulman, D. (2008). Informalization of long-term caregiving: A gender lens. In C. Harrington and C. L. Estes (Eds.), *Health policy: Crisis and reform in the US health care delivery system.* (pp. 142–151). Boston, MA: Jones and Bartlett.

Ferraro, K. F., Shippee, T. P., and Schafer, M. H. (2009). Cumulative inequality theory for research on aging and the life course. In V. L. Bengtson, D. Gans, N. M. Putney, and M. Silverstein (Eds.), *Handbook of theories of aging* (2nd ed., pp. 413–433). New York, NY: Springer.

Folbre, N. (2001). *The invisible heart: Economics and family values*. New York, NY: Penguin Books.

Folkman, S. (2008.) The case for positive emotions in the stress process. *Anxiety, Stress and Coping*, 21(1), 3–14.

Glenn, E. N. (2012). *Forced to care: Coercion and caregiving in America*. Cambridge, MA: Harvard University Press.

Gramsci, A. (1971). *Selections from the prison notebooks* (B. Q. Hoare and G. Nowell-Smith, Ed. and Trans.). London, England: Lawrence and Wishart.

Hacker, J. S. (2006). *The great risk shift*. New York: Oxford University Press.

Hagestad, G. O., and Dannefer, D. (2001).Concepts and theories of aging: Beyond microfication in social science approaches. In R. H. Binstock and L. K. George (Eds.), *Handbook of aging and the social sciences* (pp. 3–19). New York, NY: Academic Press.

Harrington-Meyer, M. (1996). Making claims as workers or wives: The distribution of Social Security benefits. *American Sociological Review*, 61(3), 449–465.

Harrington-Meyer, M., and Herd, P. (2007). Market friendly or family friendly? The role of the state. In M. Harrington-Meyer and P. Herd (Eds.), *Market friendly or family friendly? The state and gender inequality in old age* (pp. 21–41). New York, NY: Russell Sage Foundation.

Herd, P., Karraker, A., and Friedman, E. (2012). The social patterns of a biological risk factor for disease: Race, gender, socioeconomic position, and C-Reactive Protein. *Journal of Gerontology Series B*, 67B(4), 503–513.

Hildon, Z., et al. (2009). Examining resilience of quality of life (QOL) in the face of health- related psychological adversity at older ages. *The Gerontologist*, 50(1), 36–47.

Hill Collins, P. 1990. *Black feminist thought: Knowledge, consciousness, and the politics of empowerment*. New York: Routledge.

International Longevity Center (ILC)–USA. (2006). *Ageism in America*. New York, NY: Author. www.graypanthersmetrodetroit.org/Ageism_In_America_-_ILC_Book_2006.pdf

Kahn, J. R., and Pearlin, L. I. (2006). Financial strain over the life course and health among older adults. *Journal of Health and Social Behavior*, 47(1), 17–31.

Klein, N. (2000). *No logo: Taking aim at the brand bullies*. London: Flamingo.

Komisar, H., Cubanski, J., Dawson, L., and Neuman, T. (2012, March). *Key issues in understanding the economic and health security of current and future generations of seniors*. Issue Brief Publication #8289. Menlo Park, CA: Henry J. Kaiser Family Foundation. www.kff.org/medicare/upload/8289.pdf

Lakoff, G. 2004. *Don't think of an elephant! Know your values and frame the debate: The essential guide for progressives*. White River Junction, VT: Chelsea Green.

Lakoff, G., and Rockridge Institute. 2006. *Thinking points: Communicating our American values: A progressives handbook*. New York: Farrar, Straus, & Giroux.

Lantz, P. M., and Pritchard, A. (2010). Socioeconomic indicators that really matter for population health. *Preventing Chronic Disease*, 7(4): A74.

Levy, B.R., Zonderman, A.B., Slade, M.D. and Ferrucci, L. (2012). Memory shaped by age stereotypes over time. *Journals of Gerontology Series B: Psychological Sciences and Social Sciences, 67*(4), 432–436.

Luke, C., and Gore, J. (Eds). (1992). *Feminisms and critical pedagogy.* New York: Routledge, Chapman, and Hall.

Luo, Y., LaPierre, T.A., Hughes, M.E., and Waite, L.J. (2012). Grandparents providing care to grandchildren: A population-based study of continuity and change. *Journal of Family Issues, 33*(9), 1143–1167.

Macnicol, J. (2012). Action against age discrimination: US and UK comparisons. *Public Policy and Aging Report, 22*(3), 21–24.

Marmot, M.G. (2004). The status syndrome: How social standing affects our health and longevity. New York, NY: Times Books.

Massive "no cuts" campaign begins. (2011, September 21). *Entitled to Know.* National Committee to Preserve Social Security and Medicare. www.ncpssm .org/EntitledtoKnow/entryid/1851/Massive-No-Cuts-Campaign-Begins.

McEwen, B.S., and Wingfield, J.C. (2003). The concept of allostasis in biology and biomedicine. *Hormones and Behavior, 43*(2), 2–15.

Miller, J. (2011). Social justice work: Purpose driven social science. *Social Problems, 58* (1).

Musil, C.M., Gordon, N.L., Warner, C.B., Zauszniewski, J.A., Standing, T., and Wykle, M. (2011). Grandmothers and caregiving to grandchildren: Continuity, change, and outcomes over 24 months. *The Gerontologist, 51*(1), 86–100.

National Women's Law Center (NWLC). (2012, March). *The health care litigation: What women could lose.* (Fact sheet). Washington, DC: Author. www .nwlc.org/sites/default/files/pdfs/healthlitigationfactsheet.pdf

Nelson, T.D. (2005). Ageism: Prejudice against our feared future self. *Journal of Social Issues 61*(2), 207–221.

Olshansky, S.J., et al. (2012). Differences in life expectancy due to race and educational differences are widening, and many may not catch up. *Health Affairs, 31*: 1803–1813.

Omi, M., and Winant, H. (2015). *Racial formation in the United States* (3rd ed.). New York, NY: Routledge/Taylor & Francis Group.

O'Rand, A.M. (2003). Cumulative advantage theory in aging research. *Annual Review of Gerontology and Geriatrics, 22*(1), 14–30.

———. (2006). Stratification and the life course: Life course capital, life course risks, and social inequality. In R.H. Binstock and L.K. George (Eds.), *Handbook of aging and the social sciences* (6th ed., pp. 145–62). San Diego, CA: Academic Press.

Perry, D. (2012, March-April). Entrenched ageism in health care isolates, ignores and imperils elders. *Aging Today, 33*(2), 1.

Pescosolido, B.A., and Kronenfeld, J. (1995). Health, illness and healing in an uncertain era: Challenges from and for medical sociology [Extra issue]. *Journal of Health and Social Behavior, 35*, 5–33.

Piven, F.F., and Cloward, R.A. (1997). *The breaking of the American social compact.* New York, NY: New Press.

Quadagno, J. (1999). Creating a capital investment welfare state. The new American exceptionalism? *American Sociological Review, 64*(1), 1–11.

———. (2008). *Aging and the life course* (4th ed.). Boston MA: McGraw-Hill.

Radley, D.C., and Schoen, C. (2012). Geographic variation in access to care— The relationship with quality. *New England Journal of Medicine, 367*, 1, 3-6.

Richardson, G.E. (2002). The meta theory of resilience and resiliency. *Journal of Clinical Psychology, 58*(3), 307–321.

Robert, S.A. (1999). Neighborhood socio-economic context and adult health: The mediating role of individual health behavior and psychosocial factors. *Annals of the New York Academy of Sciences, 896*(1), 465–468.

Rogne, L., Estes, C.L., Grossman, B.R., Solway, E., and Hollister, B. (Eds.). (2009). *Social insurance and social justice: Social Security, Medicare and the campaign against entitlements.* New York, NY: Springer.

Sanchez-Jankowski, M. (2008). *Cracks in the pavement: Social change and resilience in poor neighborhoods.* Berkeley, CA: University of California Press.

Scaramella, L.V., Neppl, T.K., Ontai, L.L., and Conger, R.D. (2008 October). Consequences of socioeconomic disadvantage across three generations: Parenting behavior and child externalizing problems. *Journal of Family Psychology, 22*(5), 725–733.

Schulz, R., and Beach, S.R. (1999). Caregiving as a risk factor for mortality: The caregiver health effects study. *Journal of the American Medical Association, 282*(23), 2215–2219.

Singer, B., and Ryff, C.D. (1999). Hierarchies of life histories and associated health risks. *Annals of the New York Academy of Sciences, 896*, 96–115.

Snow D.A., and Benford, D. 1992. Master frames and cycles of protest. In A. Morris and C.M. Mueller (Eds.), *Frontiers in social movement theory* (pp. 133–155). New Haven, CT: Yale University Press.

Sofaer, S., and Able, E. (1990). Older women's health and financial vulnerability: Implications of the Medicare benefit structure. *Women and Health, 16*, 47–67.

Somers, M.R. (2008). *Genealogies of citizenship: Markets, statelessness, and the right to have rights.* New York, NY: Cambridge University Press.

Speer, P.W. (2000). Intrapersonal and interactional empowerment: Implications for theory. *Journal of Community Psychology, 29*(1), 51–61.

Steptoe, A., Feldman, P.J., Kunz, S., Owen, N., Willemsen, G., and Marmot, M. (2002). Stress responsivity and socioeconomic status: A mechanism for increased cardiovascular disease risk? *European Heart Journal, 23*(22), 1757–1763.

Svihula, J., and Estes, C.L. (2007). Social Security politics: Ideology and reform. *Journals of Gerontology: Psychological Sciences and Social Sciences 62B*(2): S79–89.

———. (2009). Social Security privatization: The institutionalization of an ideological movement. In L. Rogne, C.L. Estes, B.R. Grossman, B.A. Hollister, and E. Solway (Eds.), *Social insurance and social justice: Social Security,*

Medicare and and the campaign against entitlements (pp. 217–231). New York, NY: Springer.

Tippett, R., Jones-DeWeever, A., Rockeymoore, M., Hamilton, D., and Darity, W. (2014). *Beyond broke.* Washington, DC: Center for Global Policy Solutions and Duke University Research Network on Racial and Ethnic Inequality. http://globalpolicysolutions.org/wp-content/uploads/2014/04/Beyond_Broke_FINAL.pdf

"Truth campaign" on social security and medicare rolls out this week. (2012, September 12). *Entitled to Know.* National Committee to Preserve Social Security and Medicare. www.ncpssm.org/EntitledtoKnow/entryid/1931/-Truth-Campaign-on-Social-Security-Medicare-Rolls-Out-this-Week.

Twine, F. (1994). *Citizenship and social rights: The interdependence of self and society.* London, England: SAGE.

Voss, K. (1996). The collapse of a social movement: The interplay of mobilizing structures, framing, and political opportunities in the Knights of Labor. In D. McAdam, J. McCarthy, and M. Zaid (Eds.), *Comparative perspectives on social movements: Political opportunities, mobilizing structures, and cultural framings* (pp. 227–258). Cambridge, UK: Cambridge University Press.

Wallerstein, N., and Bernstein, E. (1988). Empowerment education: Friere's ideas adapted to health education. *Health Education and Behavior, 15*(4), 379–394.

Weber, M. (1946). *From Max Weber: Essays in sociology* (H.H. Gerth and C.W. Mills, Ed. and Trans.) New York, NY: Oxford University Press.

Weitz, T., and Estes, C.L. (2001). Adding aging and gender to the women's health agenda. *Journal of Women and Aging, 13*(1), 3–20.

Zimmerman, M.A., and Warschavsky, S. (1998). Empowerment theory for rehabilitation research. *Rehabilitation Psychology, 43*(1), 3–16.

11

Women's Health and Empowerment after the Decriminalization of Abortion in Mexico City

GUSTAVO ORTIZ MILLÁN

On April 24, 2007, Mexico City's Legislative Assembly reformed the city's law on abortion. After public debate on this issue, lawmakers voted 46 to 19 in favor of a bill to decriminalize elective abortion during the first three months of pregnancy. This represented landmark legislation in Latin America and the Caribbean. In the region, most countries have extremely restrictive abortion laws. El Salvador and Nicaragua do not allow abortion in any situation, not even to save the woman's life. Incidence of unsafe abortion in the region is among the highest in the world (Sedgh et al. 2007). Only Cuba, Guyana, and Puerto Rico have laws similar to the one recently passed in Mexico City (UNDESA 2001; Kane 2008).

The decriminalization of abortion in Mexico City was a historic victory for women's movements in Mexico, recognizing women's sexual and reproductive rights and representing a significant step in the empowerment of women through health reform. This reform was a result of a struggle for the decriminalization of abortion in the country for more than thirty years. The abortion reform law also addressed a serious public health issue related to unsafe abortions performed as a result of the previous policy.

Women's movements were not alone in the struggle to pass this legislation; left and center-left political parties introduced the bill in the legislature and, along with Mexico City's Mayor's Office, supported the law when the conservative federal government challenged it before the Supreme

Court. The court upheld the law, but this caused a conservative backlash in seventeen states, leading to modification of local constitutions so that they include an article "protecting the right to life from conception."

Women's rights organizations were active in the political process of getting the law reform in Mexico City passed, and they eventually helped Mexico City's Ministry of Health (MOH) implement the law. Such activism gave women's organizations greater power and more visibility in front of political parties, state congresses, human rights commissions, and other political actors in Mexico. This, in turn, has given such organizations the opportunity to advance some of their goals regarding the promotion of women's reproductive and sexual health. The decriminalization of abortion in Mexico City is an example of how political change influenced women's empowerment in the region, eventually leading to improvements in health outcomes for women.

CONTEXT

Abortion was forbidden in Mexico starting in the mid-nineteenth century (Barraza 2003). However, since Mexico is a federal republic, each state has its own penal code, and abortion laws differ from state to state. Although abortion was still highly restricted by the penal codes of most states, Mexican laws changed gradually during the twentieth century to allow several exceptions for abortion: in all thirty-two states, abortion is permitted when pregnancy results from rape; in twenty-nine, when it threatens a woman's life; in ten states, when pregnancy poses a severe risk to a woman's health; in thirteen, in the case of congenital malformations (GIRE 2012).

Mexico City reformed its overall penal code in 2007, allowing elective abortion during the first trimester. The reform was made possible by a confluence of factors and political movements (Sánchez Fuentes, Paine, and Elliott-Buettner 2008; Shiffman and Smith 2007). A community of policy makers, including the left-wing Partido de la Revolución Democrática (PRD), as well as other center-left political parties, the mayor's office, Mexico City's MOH, and its Human Rights Commission united around the bill decriminalizing abortion. Another important factor was the leadership provided by women coming from the feminist movement in Mexico. A key figure was Marta Lamas, an anthropologist, academic, journalist, and feminist activist, who founded Grupo de Información en Reproducción Elegida (GIRE; Information Group on Reproductive Choice), a non-governmental organization

(NGO) for sexual and reproductive rights. For more than forty years, she fought for abortion rights in Mexico and Latin America. Further leadership came from other women's rights organizations, such as Católicas por el Derecho a Decidir (Catholics for the Right to Decide), Equidad de Género (Gender Equity, founded by the feminist leader Patricia Mercado), International Pregnancy Advisory Services (IPAS) Mexico, and Population Council, Mexico, all of which form, along with GIRE, the Alianza Nacional por el Derecho a Decidir (ANDAR; National Alliance for the Right to Decide, founded in 2002).

These organizations, as well as others, were very successful in mobilizing civil society and in confronting the arguments from the Catholic Church and from prolife organizations that attacked the proposed initiative in the Legislative Assembly. Other members of civil society, including artists, intellectuals, bioethicists, journalists, constitutional experts, physicians, and opinion leaders, also participated in public debates and forums, some organized by the mass media and some by public universities in the city. Many women participated in these forums. The policy community, women's rights NGOs, and many representatives of civil society were united to support this reform in abortion laws. The energy unified around this cause was evident at huge demonstrations throughout Mexico City in 2007, where thousands of women and men showed their support for the reform (Cuenca 2007).

However, a few weeks after the legislation passed, in April 2007, the office of the Attorney General, with the support of the conservative federal government, challenged the law in the Supreme Court, arguing that the legislation was unconstitutional. The NGOs that had formed the alliance ANDAR, as well as others, attempted to change public perception towards abortion through campaigns in newspapers, brochures, and public forums over the ensuing months. The Supreme Court also organized public hearings where activists and health professionals took the opportunity to explain the realities of unsafe abortion across the country. In August 2008, eight out of eleven Supreme Court justices upheld Mexico City's abortion reform law, holding that it did not violate the Constitution and recognizing women's reproductive rights (GIRE 2010). The court's decision was a historic victory for women's movements in Mexico. For the first time in history, the Supreme Court had explicitly recognized the right of women to make decisions about their pregnancies during the first trimester.

However, the reaction in the rest of the country was quite different from the response in Mexico City following the Supreme Court decision.

The court's decision prompted a series of conservative amendments to state constitutions. Seventeen state congresses proposed constitutional amendments guaranteeing a "right to life from conception," even though abortion was already highly restricted in all of those states. The idea was to prevent future state governments from following Mexico City's lead and decriminalize abortion. Two of these state constitutional amendments protecting life from the moment of conception (San Luis Potosí and Baja California) were challenged before the Supreme Court. The court upheld the amendments, and the prolife amendments stand in these states (SCJN 2011) despite the contradiction to the 2007 reform to Mexico City's penal code.

PROGRAM DESCRIPTION

*Activism Education and Training Following
the Adoption of the Law*

Once abortion was decriminalized, Mexico City's government had to guarantee that women would be able to realize their right to have a safe *interrupción legal del embarazo* (ILE; legal interruption of pregnancy). However, at the beginning, it was hard for Mexico City's MOH to implement the ILE program for several reasons: physicians were not trained in the most up-to-date clinical protocols; many physicians declared themselves "conscientious objectors"; and the MOH faced steady opposition from antiabortion groups. During this period the role of women's organizations in implementing these changes was crucial. Some of the organizations that compose ANDAR, as well as some international NGOs with expertise in abortion, played an active role in training health care providers in the public sector on clinical care and counseling issues. IPAS, for example, worked very closely with physicians and nurses in training programs on medical abortion, manual vacuum aspiration (MVA), electric vacuum aspiration (EVA), and dilation and curettage (D & C). IPAS also organized training events and advocacy workshops about sexual and reproductive health at public hospitals and health centers, designed for increasing access to education and safe abortion care.

At the time of the implementation of the law, many obstetrician/gynecologists, nurses, and other health care providers had negative attitudes towards abortion. Many health care providers were hostile and demeaned, stigmatized, and discriminated against abortion seekers. In 1997, an opinion survey revealed that only 15 percent of physicians (obstetrician/gynecologists and internists) in Mexico City agreed to perform elective abortions (Casanueva et al. 1997). In 2007, 85 percent of all obstetricians/gynecologists in public hospitals declared themselves to be conscientious objectors, although some of them performed abortions in their private practices (Malkin and Cattan 2008). According to Contreras et al. (2011), some health care providers took a stand as conscientious objectors to prevent further strain on an already heavy workload. The resulting shortage of trained personnel hindered the implementation of the program.

Over the next several years, women's organizations worked diligently with health care providers on educational programs designed to change attitudes towards performing abortions. For example, IPAS worked with Mexico City's MOH to conduct a "values clarification" program, which was implemented at all of Mexico City's public hospitals and health centers. Through this program, IPAS's trainers offered health care providers background information, materials, instructions, and tips necessary to challenge deeply held assumptions and myths about abortion, moving participants toward acceptance of the sexual and reproductive rights upheld by the new law, including comprehensive abortion care (Schiavon 2012). In part, as a result of programs like this one, attitudes began to change among health care professionals. According to a recent survey, 53 percent of all the obstetrician/gynecologists, nurses, social workers, and other hospital personnel in Mexico City now support the law (Contreras et al. 2011; see also Marván, Álvarez del Río, and Campos 2012). From the outset, Mexico City's government was committed to providing enough physicians trained in abortion care in the public sector, both by hiring nonobjecting obstetrician/gynecologists and providing education to help change the attitudes of already practicing providers.

Mexico City's MOH implemented abortion services in sixteen public hospitals by the time the law entered into force in 2007 and later in three primary health care facilities specializing in abortion services (the most recent one, opened in February 2012, is called Marta Lamas). In these hospitals and health centers, women receive information about the new services. As of December 2011, 112,555 women had received this information (MOH 2011) in the context of seeking care. Women's organizations worked closely with the MOH on the informational materials women receive in these settings. Together, the MOH and various organizations, such as IPAS and GIRE, developed pocket-size cards with all the necessary information about the use of misoprostol and emergency contraception. Women's organizations, such as Equidad de Género, also developed strategies to disseminate information about abortion to the general population, handing out brochures at subway stations and public squares, informing women about where to go and what to do if they needed an abortion (Romero 2012). The MOH also implemented a telephone hotline, called Iletel, where women can get information about the requirements and procedures of the new program; by December 2011, the hotline had received 42,077 calls (MOH 2011).

In Mexico City, women who are considering having an abortion first go through a counseling process where the abortion procedure and its possible risks are explained. During this counseling session, women learn about their options, one of them being carrying the pregnancy to term. At public hospitals and health centers administered by the MOH, service providers have been instructed not to question women about their decision. There are four requirements to accessing abortion services through this program (1) the pregnancy has to be within the first trimester, as confirmed with an ultrasound; (2) after being informed of the procedure and its risks, the woman has to sign an informed consent form; if she is under 18 years old, a parent or legal guardian has to sign it (minors constitute 5.1% of abortion seekers [Mondragón y Kalb et al. 2011]); (3) the woman has to present a valid ID and proof of address; and (4) the woman is also required to come to the visit with a person who can act as a witness and help assume responsibility; this person also has to bring an ID.

The type of abortion procedure women receive is generally based on gestational age. Those at nine weeks gestation or less are offered medical abortion (drug-induced), and those over nine weeks are offered surgical abortion (MVA or EVA). Once these requirements are met, Mexico City residents can obtain an abortion at no cost (there is a sliding scale for out-of-state residents, averaging US$85). For medical abortions, women receive instructions about how to take the misoprostol pills. Medical abortion patients are also required to have a follow-up appointment one or two weeks after the abortion to ensure its completion.

Women's organizations also worked with Mexico City's MOH to improve the quality of abortion services in the years following the 2007 reform—this being an agreement between the organizations and the MOH (Schiavon 2012)—recognizing that if women were to attend abortion clinics, services had to be accessible and acceptable. The Population Council conducted studies of quality of care and patient satisfaction after abortion was decriminalized and found high levels of satisfaction and good quality services overall by 2009, although the study found areas for potential improvement, such as the need for more personalized postabortion contraceptive counseling (Becker et al. 2011; Van Dijk et al. 2011). The public character of MOH-sponsored health centers allows women to hold them accountable and help improve the services provided in the public sector. The public character of these health centers helped abortion seekers understand their right to the services, and it promoted confidence in the quality of the services offered (Amuchástegui et al. 2009).

Equidad de Género and Católicas por el Derecho a Decidir have organized programs that provide support and accompaniment to women seeking abortion care. Women contact these organizations through the Internet or by phone, and representatives of these organizations accompany women through the whole process. The representatives will also accompany women from the surrounding metropolitan area who are seeking an abortion. By 2011, 23.9 percent of all women seeking abortions in Mexico City travel from the neighboring State of Mexico, and 4.1 percent from other states (MOH 2011). Another women's organization, called Balance, created an Internet-accessible fund in 2009 (called María Abortion Fund for Social Justice, or Fondo María) to support women to travel from other states to Mexico City to access these legal abortion services.

Most abortions were initially performed at hospitals, but there has been a shift in abortion care to primary health care facilities and away from hospitals (MOH 2011) over the past several years. When the program was first established, many abortions were performed surgically—using D & C—which entails higher risks for women, but there has been a gradual shift towards higher rates of medical abortions and MVA. Medical abortion and MVA are recommended by the World Health Organization as the safest methods for first trimester abortions (WHO 2003). IPAS and Gynuity, among others, played an active role in facilitating this shift by training providers in the most up-to-date clinical protocols. Gynuity, for example, supported and guided the heads of the ILE program in the MOH in defining and adopting an evidence-based medical abortion protocol now incorporated into the MOH's procedures manual for abortion and post-abortion care. Gynuity also helped to introduce the drugs mifepristone and misoprostol into existing abortion services (Gynuity 2012). The percentage of women undergoing D & C abortions subsequently decreased between 2007 to 2010, from 29% to 2%; while the proportion of women undergoing a misoprostol-only abortion increased from 36% to 64%. Rates of manual vacuum aspiration remains steady: 35% in 2007 and 33% in 2010 (Mondragón y Kalb et al. 2011). Of note, all abortions are performed on an outpatient basis and, for medical abortions, women are provided with the appropriate dose of misoprostol to take home.

From April 2007 to May 2016, 160,170 women underwent an abortion in public hospitals and health centers (GIRE 2016). This number includes both medical and surgical abortions from both public hospitals and primary health care facilities.

Impact of the Legislation Reform on Health Outcomes

Before the implementation of the law, clandestine and unsafe abortions were the third leading cause of maternal mortality in Mexico City—and the fifth leading cause of maternal mortality in the entire country, with sixty maternal deaths per 100,000 live births. Official data from the National Population Council estimated 102,000 induced or spontaneous abortions were taking place in Mexico annually (CONAPO 2000); other studies claim that in 2006 there were 874,747 illegal abortions in Mexico, and 165,455 in Mexico City alone (Juárez et al. 2008). This uncertainty in the data was a result of abortion services being a clandestine phenomenon in most of the country. In 2006, an estimated 149,677 women throughout the country were hospitalized for complications related to induced abortions (Juárez et al. 2008). After abortion was decriminalized, morbidity and mortality rates attributable to unsafe abortions in Mexico City diminished significantly: since 2007, only 2.3% of women undergoing abortions have suffered complications associated with the procedure, all of them mild; there have been no reported cases of major complications (Mondragón y Kalb et al. 2011). The liberalization of abortion laws and the success of Mexico City's new program have changed attitudes towards abortion in a short period of time. At the time the law passed, in 2007, only 38% of Mexico City's population supported the law. The percentage of supporters grew to 63% in 2008 and to 74% in 2009. According to the same opinion survey, 51% of respondents in 2007 thought that the law should be extended to the rest of the country; by 2009, this number had grown to 82.8% (Wilson et al. 2011).

Prior to the law reform, there were inequities in who had access to safe abortion services. Most of the women who had had unsafe abortions were poor, uneducated, married, and already had three or more children; many lived in contexts of domestic violence (Billings et al. 2002; Sousa et al. 2010). In contrast, wealthy women have always had the "right" to have an equally illegal, but safe abortion at a private hospital, with a trained gynecologist, without risking their health. Many wealthy Mexican women also traveled to the United States to have abortions prior to the reform; women who can afford it now travel to Mexico City from other states for the procedure. Thus, restrictive abortion laws in Mexico affected and continue to affect poor women disproportionately, accentuating inequalities in an already unequal society.

DISCUSSION

Decriminalization of abortion in Mexico City in 2007 not only improved health outcomes for women seeking such services throughout the region but also served as a powerful force for women's empowerment in Mexico. Women were empowered through their expanding awareness of their sexual and reproductive rights. Legalization of abortion also played an important role in changing women's views of themselves; as women began receiving high-quality abortion services, provided by the state, they were increasingly assured that their decision to have an abortion was justified. They began to realize that they are entitled to have an abortion if they choose and that they are autonomous when it comes to their own reproductive decisions (Amuchástegui et al. 2009). This shift in attitude was evident to feminists like Marta Lamas, who explained the change in this way:

> In the beginning, when the service started, women still came with shame. But very soon, the attitude with which the service providers received them, telling them that they were entitled to the service and that what they were doing was legal, led to the empowerment of women. Now they come without shame, as if they are saying, "I come to a service I have the right to." Now there's an exercise in citizenship. There are doctors and health care personnel who have long been in the clinics and are amazed at the change in attitude of young women who come to apply for ILE. (Lamas 2012)

Decriminalization not only promoted the empowerment of women, acknowledging their right to have a safe abortion provided by public health centers, but it also empowered women's organizations in Mexico City. First, abortion reforms increased their visibility, since they were active in the public space as they organized demonstrations and public debates, published opinion polls, mobilized intellectuals and civil society, and engaged in other public activities. Second, women's activism during this period, paired with the success of the program, transformed key actors into identifiable political figures, giving them more power to deal with other political actors, such as federal and state congresses, human rights commissions, and Mexico City's MOH, among others.

Organizations such as Equidad de Género are now working closely with national decision makers to apply a gender perspective to emerging public policy movements (Romero 2012). Other organizations, such as the Simone de Beauvoir Leadership Institute (founded by Marta Lamas), Mujeres Trabajadoras Unidas (United Women Workers), Inclusión Ciudadana, and Liderazgo, Gestión y Nueva Política (Leadership, Management, and New Policy, founded by Patricia Mercado), have been working with the government to enhance political participation by women in Mexico. In 2009, they formed a coalition and won, along with the National Women's Institute, a grant from United Nations Women to increase gender equity and women's political participation and economic empowerment in Mexico. As a result of this, more women are holding public offices than ever before (UN Women 2011–2012).

The abortion law reform also promoted the empowerment of women's organizations in the rest of the country. As noted above, the decriminalization of abortion in Mexico City provoked a conservative backlash in the other states, and this motivated women in several states to create women's rights organizations that now fight for the recognition of their sexual and reproductive rights. More than 1,100 women in eleven states have banded together in an organization called Cómplices por la Equidad/Men Engage Mexico, using a legal instrument for the protection of individual rights, called *amparo,* to defend themselves against the states' prolife constitutional amendments, laws that they consider oppose their reproductive rights (Cancino 2010).

For example, in Guanajuato, a state ruled by politicians from the Catholic-conservative Partido Acción Nacional (PAN; National Action Party), a group of women organized an NGO called Las Libres (The Free Ones) in 2000 as a reaction to a proposed revision of the general ban on abortion that threatened to prohibit legal abortions in cases of rape. Las Libres organized public opinion and defeated the revision. After the decriminalization of abortion in Mexico City, Guanajuato's constitution was amended to ban abortion, and enforcement of anti-abortion laws tightened. Las Libres discovered and publicly disseminated information about 130 women who had been incriminated (eleven prosecuted, nine sentenced, and fourteen imprisoned) between 2000 and 2008 as a result of the "crime" of abortion. In 2010, eight women were serving sentences of between twenty-five and twenty-nine years. In the climate of persecution created after the Mexico City law, some states blurred the line between charging a woman with abortion and sentencing her for killing a newborn baby (infanticide). Even some natural miscarriages were considered abortions and women imprisoned as a result. Once these cases were publicized, the information created such a public furor and the activism of women's rights advocates was so strong that the state government was forced to change some women's sentences. For example, some women were released after telling the media that they had been forced to sign confessions after giving birth to babies who were stillborn or premature. Las Libres discovered similar cases in eight other states (Cruz Sánchez 2011; Madrazo 2011; Malkin 2010), leading to increased concern among the public of the impact of tightening abortion laws.

LESSONS LEARNED

After the decriminalization of abortion in Mexico City, Mexican women's organizations reflected on what had happened, concluding that if abortion was to become a political priority in the rest of the country, they had to strengthen their presence in other states. As a result, women's groups started working with a wide range of political actors (e.g., political parties, congresses, governors' and mayors' offices) to create a community of policy makers not only favorable to the decriminalization of abortion countrywide but also to the improvement of existing health care services for women. These organizations also realized that they must build alliances with key members of civil society, such as public health professionals, scientists, bioethicists, lawyers, constitutional experts, intellectuals, academics, opinion leaders, young people, and other social and political actors (Sánchez Fuentes, Paine, and Elliott-Buettner 2008). Indeed, such alliances were being built even before the abortion law reform. In 2004, for example, GIRE helped to found the Colegio de Bioética, an NGO created to promote the study of abortion, assisted reproduction, and other bioethical issues by scientists, lawyers, and philosophers.

Along with the creation of these diverse alliances, women's organizations also learned to work together and divide work strategically. For example, the organizations that compose ANDAR specialize in different aspects of sexual and reproductive rights: GIRE is devoted to the legal aspects; IPAS to the medical and public health aspects; Católicas por el Derecho a Decidir to the ethical and religious aspects; Equidad de Género to the relationship with congresses and local governments, particularly in the more conservative states; and the Population Council is devoted to researching public opinion and to building an evidence base for safe abortion services. These organizations are working together with NGOs in various states to improve health care conditions for women and to create conditions for the decriminalization of abortion beyond the borders of Mexico City.

The decriminalization of elective abortion in Mexico City has made it easier for women's organizations to achieve some of the goals that they have striven towards for more than thirty years. For example, the recent success on decriminalization of abortion has made it easier for groups to work with Mexico City's MOH to improve access to family planning counseling and contraceptive methods. The guidelines of the MOH now state that after an abortion procedure, a woman must be offered a range of contraceptive methods. As a result, there is more information available to abortion seekers about sex education and reproductive health services, and the proportion of women choosing postprocedure contraception has grown. There has been a high acceptance of the intrauterine device (IUD) (41%) and of hormonal methods (19%), suggesting that this service is achieving its goal in attempting to prevent repeat abortions. In 2010, only 1.3% of the women requesting public abortion services had undergone a previous abortion in the MOH program (Mondragón y Kalb et al. 2011).

CONCLUSION

Mexico City's abortion reform legislation was the result of a confluence of factors that made abortion a political priority, but this would not have been possible without the engagement and persistence of women's rights organizations. After the abortion law passed, these organizations worked closely with the MOH to monitor services and to improve the ILE program. The decriminalization of abortion, bolstered by the positive word-of-mouth generated by women who have received the services, are now helping to generate positive attitudes towards sexual and reproductive rights in the greater society (Becker et al. 2011). With respect to women's health, maternal morbidity and mortality due to unsafe abortions has virtually disappeared in Mexico City as result of the reform. Finally, attitudes towards abortion are changing not only in the general population but particularly in women, who are beginning to see access to abortion care as a fundamental human right. Decriminalization and the ILE program are promoting a sense of empowerment in women and are giving women's organizations more visibility and power as political actors than they ever had before throughout Mexico.

Box 11.1. Summary

Geographic area: Mexico City.

Global importance of the health condition: Unsafe abortion is the cause of serious health problems and disability for millions of women around the world each year. It is also a prominent cause of maternal mortality.

Intervention or program: The legalization of elective abortion during the first trimester of pregnancy in Mexico City in 2007 allowed the local Ministry of Health to implement a program called Legal Interruption of Pregnancy (ILE) in publicly funded hospitals and in three primary health care facilities across the city.

Impact: Results of the program show that maternal morbidity and mortality due to unsafe abortion in Mexico City has significantly decreased, if not disappeared.

Lessons learned: The decriminalization of abortion in Mexico City has made it possible for women's organizations to work with Mexico City's political and health communities to improve access to family planning counseling and provision of contraceptive methods.

Link between empowerment and health: The program helped generate in women the idea that their decision to have an abortion is within the realm of human rights, that they are entitled to have access to safe abortion services, and that they have control over decisions influencing their reproductive rights. The decriminalization of abortion in Mexico City also shows how health outcomes among women can be improved through political change that supports women's empowerment.

For a video about Legal Interruption of Pregnancy (ILE), see https://youtu.be/36fcRyGNQjk.

Box 11.2. Factors Behind the Success of the
Decriminalization of Abortion in Mexico City

- The Legal Interruption of Pregnancy (ILE) program was
  established in Mexico City in 2007, the result of a confluence
  of factors that led to successful policy change. A critical
  catalyst was over thirty years of activism by activists in the
  feminist movement across Mexico. These activists helped
  develop legal and political strategies to make abortion a
  political priority, gaining the support of important sectors of
  civil society and of political actors such as local representatives, political parties, Mexico City's Ministry of Health, and
  the Office of the Mayor. Following legal reform, women's
  leaders also aided in upholding the new abortion law when the
  federal government challenged its constitutionality in the
  Supreme Court.

- Women's activists played a key role in helping the Ministry of
  Health assure high quality care in the city's hospitals and
  health centers. They were actively involved in monitoring of
  the quality of services and in helping train physicians and
  nurses in the safest and most up-to-date techniques.

- The program dramatically decreased the number of unsafe
  abortions in Mexico City while improving access to contraceptive methods and counseling services.

- The decriminalization of abortion in Mexico City reinforced
  women's right to have safe abortions in public hospitals and
  health centers. This groundbreaking legal reform altered many
  citizens' attitudes toward abortion, from perceiving it as
  something shameful and illegal to accepting it as a reproductive right. This has helped to develop a stronger sense of
  empowerment in many Mexican women.

ACKNOWLEDGMENTS

Thanks are due to Davida Becker, Gillian Fawcett-García, and Jennifer
Paine, for their very helpful comments and criticism.

REFERENCES

Amuchástegui, A., E. Flores and R. Parrini. 2009. "'Lo bueno es la seguridad':
   la interrupción legal del embarazo como ejercicio de derechos." Letra S 157.
Barraza, E. 2003. Aborto y pena en México. Mexico: Instituto Nacional de
   Ciencias Penales-Grupo de Información en Reproducción Elegida.

Becker, D., C. Díaz-Olavarrieta, C. Juárez, S. G. García, P. Sanhueza, and C. C. Harper. 2011. "Clients' perceptions of the quality of care in Mexico City's public-sector legal abortion program." *International Perspectives on Sexual and Reproductive Health* 37 (4): 191–201.

Billings, D., C. Moreno, C. Ramos, D. González de León, R. Ramírez, L. Villaseñor Martínez, and M. Rivera Díaz. 2002. "Constructing access to legal abortion services in Mexico City." *Reproductive Health Matters* 10 (19): 86–94.

Cancino, F. 2010. "Las reformas antiaborto en 17 estados son impugnadas ante la Corte." CNN Mexico, August 19. http://mexico.cnn.com/nacional/2010/08/19 /las-reformas-antiaborto-en-17-estados-son-impugnadas-ante-la-corte.

Casanueva, E., R. Lisker, A. Carnevale, and E. Alonso. 1997. "Attitudes of Mexican physicians toward induced abortion." *International Journal of Gynecology and Obstetrics* 56 (1): 47–52.

Consejo Nacional de Población (CONAPO). 2000. *Cuadernos de salud reproductiva*. Mexico: CONAPO.

Contreras, X., M. G. van Dijk, T. Sánchez, and P. Sanhueza. 2011. "Experiences and opinions of health-care professionals regarding legal abortion in Mexico City: A qualitative study." *Studies in Family Planning* 42 (3): 183–190.

Cruz Sánchez, V. 2011. "Fin a una década de criminalización por aborto contra mujeres pobres en Guanajuato." *Debate Feminista* 43: 176–191.

Cuenca, A. 2007. "Aprueba ALDF en lo general reforma sobre aborto." *El Universal*. April 24. www.eluniversal.com.mx/notas/420927.html.

Grupo de Información sobre Reproducción Elegida (GIRE). 2010. *Constitutionality of the Abortion Law in Mexico City*. Mexico: GIRE. www.gire.org .mx/publica2/ConstitutionalityAbortionLawMexicoCity_TD8.pdf.

———. 2012. *El aborto en los códigos penales de las entidades federativas 2011*. Mexico: GIRE. www.gire.org.mx/contenido.php?informacion=31.

———. 2016. *Cifras sobre el aborto en el DF*. Mexico: GIRE. www.gire.org .mx/nuestros-temas/aborto/cifras.

Gynuity. 2012. "Gynuity in Mexico." http://gynuity.org/locations/country /mexico/.

Juárez, F., S. Singh, S. García, and C. Díaz Olavarrieta. 2008. "Estimates of induced abortion in Mexico: What's changed between 1990 and 2006?" *International Family Planning Perspectives* 34 (4): 158–168.

Kane, G. 2008. "Abortion law reform in Latin America: Lessons for advocacy." *Gender and Development* 16 (2): 361–375.

Lamas, M. 2001. *Política y reproducción. Aborto: La frontera del derecho a decidir*. México: Plaza y Janés.

———. 2012. "Feminism and legalized abortion in Mexico City." Interview with Gustavo Ortiz Millán. Unpublished.

Madrazo, A. 2011. "Más libres." *Debate Feminista* 43: 192–198.

Malkin, E. 2010. "Many states in Mexico crack down on abortion." *New York Times*, September 22. www.nytimes.com/2010/09/23/world/americas/23mexico .html.

Malkin, E., and N. Cattan. 2008. "Despite new abortion law, Mexico City women face barriers." *New York Times,* August 25. www.nytimes.com/2008 /08/25/world/americas/25iht-mexico.4.15619473.html.

Marván, M.L., A. Álvarez del Río, and Z. Campos. 2012. "On abortion: Exploring psychological meaning and attitudes in a sample of Mexican gynecologists." *Developing World Bioethics*, doi:10.1111/dewb.12005.

Mexico City Ministry of Health (MOH). 2011. *Agenda estadística 2010*. Mexico: MOH. www.salud.df.gob.mx/ssdf/media/Agenda2010/inicio.html.

Mondragón y Kalb, M., A. Ahued, J. Morales Velázquez, C. Díaz Olavarrieta, J. Valencia Rodríguez, D. Becker, and S.G. García. 2011. "Patient characteristics and service trends following abortion legalization in Mexico City: 2007–10." *Studies in Family Planning* 42 (3): 159–166.

Romero, M.E. 2012. "Equidad de Género and legalized abortion in Mexico City." Interview with Gustavo Ortiz Millán. Unpublished.

Sánchez Fuentes, M.L., J. Paine, and B. Elliott-Buettner. 2008. "The decriminalisation of abortion in Mexico City: How did abortion rights become a political priority?" *Gender and Development* 16 (2): 345–360.

Schiavon, R. 2012. "IPAS's experience with legalized abortion in Mexico City." Interview with Gustavo Ortiz Millán. Unpublished.

Sedgh, G., S. Henshaw, S. Singh, E. Åhman, and I.H. Shah. 2007. "Induced abortion: Estimated rates and trends worldwide," *The Lancet* 370 (9595): 1338–1345.

Shiffman, J., and S. Smith. 2007. "Generation of political priority for global health initiatives: a framework and case study of maternal mortality." *Lancet* 370 (9595): 1370–1379.

Sousa, A., R. Lozano, and E. Gakidou. 2010. "Exploring the determinants of unsafe abortion: improving the evidence base in Mexico." *Health Policy and Planning* 25 (4): 300–310.

Suprema Corte de Justicia de la Nación (SCJN). 2011. *Reformas en las constituciones de los estados de Baja California y San Luis Potosí que tutelan el derecho a la vida* (accessed August 27, 2013). Mexico: SCJN. www.scjn.gob.mx/Cronicas/Cronicas%20del%20pleno%20y%20salas/cr-290911-BCyS-LPvida.pdf.

United Nations Department of Economic and Social Affairs (UNDESA). 2001. *Abortion policies: A global review*. New York: UNDESA.

United Nations Women. 2011–2012. *Annual report 2011–2012*. New York: UN Women.

Van Dijk, M., L.J. Arellano Mendoza, A.G. Arangure, A.A. Toriz Prado, A. Krumholz, and E.A. Yam. 2011. "Women's experiences with legal abortion in Mexico City: A qualitative study." *Studies in Family Planning* 42 (3): 167–174.

Wilson, K., S. García, C. Díaz Olavarrieta, A. Villalobos-Hernández, J. Valencia Rodríguez, P. Sanhueza, and Courtney Burks. 2011. "Public opinion on abortion in Mexico City after the landmark reform." *Studies in Family Planning* 42 (3): 175–182.

World Health Organization (WHO). 2003. *Safe abortion: Technical and policy guidance for health systems*. 2nd ed. Geneva: WHO.

12

Impact of a Grassroots Property Rights Program on Women's Empowerment in Rural Kenya

KATE GRÜNKE-HORTON AND SHARI L. DWORKIN

Women's empowerment has become central to the global development agenda since the 1994 United Nations (UN) International Conference on Population and Development (ICPD) in Cairo (McIntosh and Finkle 1995; UN 1994). An increasing focus on bottom-up and grassroots approaches to empowerment emerged from the Fourth World Conference on Women in Beijing in 1995 and is currently championed by women's organizations globally (Goldenberg 2011). This approach is based on an assumption that empowerment comes from within rather than from a third party (Batliwala 2007; Elliott 2008a; Mosedale 2005). Outside entities, such as non-government organizations, can support women in formulating and articulating an empowerment agenda and can also help by providing resources and advocacy. However, women need to define and act upon their goals through negotiation and resistance, both individually and collectively, in order to develop the agency required to achieve empowerment (Kabeer 1999).

Beyond this, there is little consensus on the meaning of empowerment, but many common principles can be seen across the social science, development, and health literature. There is some consensus that empowerment involves the subversion of current power structures (Grabe 2012; Kabeer 2005); having voice and active participation at the community, regional, or national level (Charmes and Wieringa 2003; Narayan-Parker 2002; Zimmerman 2000); and engaging in collective action and solidarity to challenge dominant ideologies that are harmful to gender equality and to women (Kabeer 1999; Romero et al. 2006). A final principle of empowerment is that it is context-specific (Grabe 2012; Nagar and Raju 2003; Romero et al. 2006; Wallerstein 2006; Zimmerman 2000). Thus, numerous scholars argue that empowerment ought to be defined by those whom it affects, rather than by outside entities or institutions. For this chapter, empowerment is defined along the lines of Kabeer's definition above, but we also view it as an iterative process, centered on locally meaningful goals that subvert dominant powers and are defined and evaluated by community members within a specific social context (Cattaneo and Chapman 2010).

In the past decade, women's health and empowerment programs have placed much emphasis on economic empowerment (de Mel, McKenzie, and Woodruff 2012) as a mechanism to improve health outcomes such as HIV risk (Dunbar et al. 2010; Dworkin and Blankenship 2009; Rosenberg et al. 2011), gender-based violence (Jan et al. 2011; Kim et al. 2007), and reproductive health (Dunford 2001). However, income generation initiatives such as microfinance and business training are often limited by their failure to significantly improve women's income and address contextual drivers of gender inequality (Hashemi, Schuler, and Riley 1996; Selinger 2008). Furthermore, skepticism has recently been cast as to whether these programs contribute to a redistribution of gendered power in households or improve women's broader social status (Ali and Hatta 2012; Dupas and Robinson 2009; Holmes et al. 2011).

The limitations of these strategies have led to calls for alternative structural approaches to HIV and violence prevention (Adimora and Auerbach 2010; Coates and Szekeres 2004; Pronyk et al. 2005). One such approach focuses on harder assets such as land and property (Dworkin et al. 2013; Grabe 2010; Lu et al. 2013). In sub-Saharan and Eastern Africa in particular, a woman's land ownership is often tied to her family relations, and a combination of a lack of enforcement of statutory law and honoring customary practices can prevent women from owning property. Furthermore, women who become widowed or separated are frequently stripped of their assets and disinherited, further contributing to economic and social disempowerment (Izumi 2007; Mendenhall et al. 2007; Walsh 2005).

Property rights violations intersect with HIV in complex ways. Women's lack of property ownership has been linked to their likelihood of experiencing both physical and sexual violence (Grabe 2010; Gupta 2006; Izumi 2007; Pandey 2010; Swaminathan, Walker, and Rugadya 2008), which in turn is linked to increased HIV risk (Dunkle et al. 2006;

Jewkes et al. 2010; Jewkes, Levin, and Penn-Kekana 2003; Shi, Kouyou-mdjian, and Dushoff 2013). Asset stripping by in-laws upon the death of a husband (often from HIV/AIDS) frequently results in poverty, home-lessness and migration to slum, market, or beach areas, and the exchange of sex for money, food, shelter, or goods (Aliber and Walker 2006; Dworkin et al. 2013; Henrysson and Joiremen 2009; Walker 2002; Yngstrom 2002). Wife inheritance, whereby widows are passed on to a member of their deceased husband's family, is another common practice that may further contribute to HIV risk (Agot et al. 2010; Dworkin et al. 2013; Izumi 2007). Loss of property and disinheritance leaves many widows unable to pay for medical care, further increasing negative health outcomes (Dworkin et al. 2013; Walsh 2005). Despite the known links between property rights violations, violence, and HIV, there remains a scarcity of research that evaluates the health and empower-ment-related effects of programs focused on women's property rights. The few studies that do exist focus almost exclusively on HIV prevention and violence outcomes, while only one study examines the empower-ment-related effects of property-oriented programs (Grabe 2012).

This chapter draws on qualitative in-depth interview data that was collected as part of an academic/community collaboration between the University of California, San Francisco (UCSF), the Kenyan Medical Research Institute (KEMRI), and Grassroots Organization Operating Together in Sisterhood (GROOTS) Kenya. GROOTS is a network of community-based organizations in Kenya that strive to establish women as catalytic in contributing to and leading their own development. The current analysis is a qualitative exploration into the effects of a grass-roots women's property rights program on empowerment in rural Kenya. By examining women's perceptions of the broader empower-ment-related impacts that resulted from the program, we aim to gain an understanding of the ways in which this collaborative grassroots effort empowers women and contributes to gender equality. The current study focuses on women who sought out GROOTS Kenya to receive assist-ance for a property rights violation, which may have included one or all of the following: land grabbing, asset stripping, disinheritance, or a land boundary dispute. By drawing on in-depth qualitative data from eighty women who were program beneficiaries or who were involved with the development and implementation of the program, we seek to understand the perceived empowerment-related effects of this commu-nity-led model that strives to prevent and mediate women's property rights violations.

In order to explore the dynamics of empowerment within the context of a grassroots property rights watchdog model in rural Kenya, we apply a critical approach to empowerment throughout this chapter, and our theoretical underpinnings draw on feminist standpoint epistemology (Brooks 2007). This approach seeks to build knowledge from women's experiences by placing women at the core of the research process and using women's voices to construct meaning. Consequently, while we draw upon the underlying principles of empowerment already outlined, we also seek to explore participants' own definitions of empowerment. Thus, the aim of this study is to explore how the Community Land and Property Watchdog model (known as the Community Watchdog, or CWDG, model) is perceived to support empowerment at the local level, by those involved in its functioning, and by beneficiaries of the program.

CONTEXT

Kenya is an East African country bordered by Tanzania, Uganda, South Sudan, Ethiopia, Somalia, and the Indian Ocean. It has a population of approximately 44 million, a life expectancy of 63 years, and 1.6 million people (6.3% of the population) living with HIV/AIDS (CIA 2013). Women in Kenya are traditionally viewed as the property of men and have historically had few rights. Approximately 45% of women aged 15–49 report experiencing gender-based violence (KNBS and ICF Macro 2010), which contributes to the disproportionate HIV burden among women: 59.1% of the adult HIV-positive population is female, and in some rural areas HIV prevalence among women is almost double that among men, at 8.0% and 4.3% respectively (KNBS and ICF Macro 2010). Asset stripping and property rights violations, whereby women are disinherited and unlawfully evicted, are common practices, particularly when their husband's death is HIV-related (FIDA 2009; Gupta and Leung 2010). This practice is often enacted through violence (Dworkin et al. 2013; Lu et al. 2013; Walsh 2005), and it perpetuates the continuing disempowerment of women, who are often considered to be second-class citizens in community matters (Orchardson-Mazrui 2006).

The program at the center of this project is the CWDG, which works largely among rural households affected by HIV/AIDS in Kenya to secure women's land and property rights and reduce the spread and impact of HIV (FIDA 2009). The CWDG was developed by GROOTS Kenya, which is part of GROOTS International, a network of community-based organizations formed in response to the Fourth World Conference on Women in Beijing in 1995, as part of the Huairou Commission, a global coalition of grassroots women's initiatives working to enhance women's participation in local, regional, and national development work. The current work focuses on the perceived impact of GROOTS Kenya's flagship property rights program designed in 2005 in response to the enormous number of women's property rights violations in Kenyan communities.

The CWDG is operationalized as local Watch Dog Groups, which are mostly women-led and use a combination of local knowledge and paralegal training for community members to mediate property rights violations, educate communities about women's rights, help women negotiate the formal justice system, and address harmful cultural practices such as wife inheritance (Dworkin et al. 2013; Lu et al. 2013). The CWDG is based in Nairobi and operates in Nairobi County, Homa Bay County, and Kakamega County; it has managed over two hundred cases of women's property rights violations in Kenya (GROOTS Kenya 2008). The CWDG's work is supported by the 2010 Kenyan constitutional reform, which brought significant legal changes in women's right to inherit, access, and own land (Constitution of Kenya 2010). The CWDG works in conjunction with land reform, to ensure that women's property rights are upheld in the cultural contexts of rural Kenya, where customary practices of land inheritance have been at odds with women's legal and constitutional rights (Lu et al. 2013; Walsh 2005).

METHODS

In-depth interviews were conducted by interviewers who were hired through KEMRI Human Resources and who were familiar with the communities in which we worked, but who were external to GROOTS Kenya. Two interviewers attended a two-day training in qualitative research methods and ethical principles of human subjects research led by the Principal Investigator (Shari L. Dworkin). Interview domains focused on what happens to women when their husbands die, what strategies are used to prevent and mediate property rights violations, and the perceived impacts of the program on women in the community. The protocol was approved by the Human Subjects Review Boards at UCSF and KEMRI. Participants were given 500 Kenyan shillings (US$6) for their participation in accordance with Institutional Review Board (IRB) rules in Kenya.

In-depth interviews, conducted in the local language, were carried out at one point in time between January and May of 2011. They were audio recorded and lasted between 1.25 and 2.25 hours. Following completion of the interviews, they were transcribed first into the local language and then into English. We used an open coding process that is typically employed in qualitative methods (Lofland and Lofland 1995). Once the code book was set, we independently coded the remaining interviews and established high concordance between the two reviewers, resolving any discrepancies until consensus was reached. Data analysis was facilitated by Dedoose, a qualitative software program.

In the results that follow, we distinguish between several different types of interviewees. First, women who sought assistance from the CWDG after experiencing a property rights violation will be referred to as "beneficiaries" of the program. Second, women and men who have been trained as paralegals to mediate and resolve property rights violations between beneficiaries and family members will be referred to as "implementers." The third group will be referred to as "developers" as they were involved in the conceptualization and development of the program. While these three terms are used for clarity, it should be acknowledged that those termed "beneficiaries" are also considered to be active agents of change rather than passive beneficiaries, and those termed "developers" and "implementers" are also beneficiaries of the knowledge that is co-constructed by the grassroots model.

FINDINGS

The primary purpose of the CWDG is to enhance and protect women's property and land rights in order to improve economic empowerment and reduce violence and HIV risks at the individual and community level. In line with the study aims, our findings show how the work of the CWDG extends not only to economic and health outcomes but to empowerment-related processes. These findings are presented here as four overarching themes. The first three themes—preventing property rights violations, championing broader rights and knowledge, and providing a support network for rights to be realized—all pertain to the rights-based work of the CWDG and how championing rights leads to empowerment. The fourth overarching theme—challenging gender norms—has four subthemes: (a) enhanced agency, independence, and confidence; (b) increased voice and visibility among women; (c) greater leadership capacity; and (d) increased control among women over their bodies and their health. Each of these results from the challenging of dominant gendered power structures by the CWDG and by the women themselves.

Preventing Property Rights Violations and Securing Property Rights

Women's property rights were a central component of this community-led program. In order to prevent property rights violations and secure land tenure, GROOTS Kenya provided rights-based education to women to ensure that all legal documentation related to inheriting and owning land was in order. The organization emphasized to women the need to secure title deeds and marriage certificates so women could secure their rightful access to and ownership of land, as this implementer explained:

> They have known their rights. Their human rights. And they know what they are supposed to have so that they can be referred to as the legal wife to so and so. . . . Children should be named after that family. You yourself as the wife you must change the ID names and if the husband has left behind any documents, keep them safely. Now women are empowered. (female implementer, age 55, Kakamega County)

If women did not have the necessary paperwork, our interviewees explained that the in-laws could easily claim that the woman was not married to her husband (customary marriages often lack official marriage certificates), facilitating land grabbing and disinheritance. Numerous developers in our sample echoed the importance of legal documentation:

> We taught them [the women] to make sure they had a National Identity Card, we tell them to have a marriage certificate, we taught them to be openly aware of what was owned by their husbands, to not just sit and wait for a miracle to happen to them to do it but to be actively involved. . . . We emphasized micro enterprises, things that women can do together, to come up with a collective ownership of property so that they are able to bail themselves out when the time came. (female developer, age 34, Nairobi County)

With increasing knowledge about how to provide supporting documentation for their property rights, women were more empowered to secure their access to and ownership of land. In addition, if, upon the death of their husband they experienced land grabbing and/or disinheritance, having access to these documents helped them to secure their rightful access to and ownership of land, given that they were the legal next of kin.

Championing Broader Rights and Knowledge

Beyond the direct property-related work of the CWDG, the group also worked to educate the community about women's rights more broadly, situating property rights within the context of women's rights. Through regional changes ongoing throughout Kenya (such as changes in Kenya's 2010 constitution) and GROOTS Kenya's programming, women in the community were informed both about their property rights and about their human rights more broadly. This implementer explained recent changes in community knowledge of property rights:

> People are more aware of their rights. Yes! People are now enlightened. They were ignorant. You know, when a woman was married, she just used to sit in the kitchen. We have told them to get out of the kitchen. You know, the men had been told that women belonged to the kitchen. . . . Right now, we have forced them out of the kitchen and they also know their rights. Yes! (female implementer, age 55, Kakamega County)

In addition to educating community members about women's rights more broadly, the CWDG also taught women what to do and where to go if they experienced violence and discussed the right to access HIV treatment. Participants in our sample made it clear that the presence of the CWDG meant that women knew where to find support for the protection of their rights:

> The CWDG, they have made the community, or even the women in the community, to know their rights, and any violation of the sort, they know rightly where to go. So therefore people are living positively and they know what is happening. (male implementer, age 46, Homa Bay County)

Providing a Support Network for Rights to Be Realized

According to beneficiaries and implementers, prior to the intervention, not only were women unaware of the rights they had, but they were less able to realize them, as there were few support systems within the community. Providing a support network was an important part of encouraging women to realize their rights. The implementation of the CWDG meant women knew where they could receive assistance when they lacked the ability to navigate legal bureaucracies. Several beneficiaries made observations that echoed the following statement when they were explaining the importance of knowing that they were supported:

> I have the power to stop something that is wrong. Before this, women didn't have power, whether something good or bad was happening to them. Our people believed that if something happened to a woman she was to say thank you. If you are beaten you say thank you, if your things are taken away from you say thank you; you have no say. Today I have a say over my things and my thoughts because I know that there is somewhere I can lean on. (female beneficiary, age 39, Homa Bay County)

Beneficiaries frequently reported that they gained knowledge about how to secure their rights and respond to violations of their rights, and when their individual knowledge was insufficient to negotiate their rights, they knew that the CWDG stood in solidarity with them, providing necessary resources. Similarly, a male implementer explained how people in the community were increasingly aware that not only individual women but also numerous community members were sensitized to their rights. He explained the importance of community barazas, open community forum meetings, which were used by the CWDG as a platform for rights-based education in spreading its message to the entire community, including men:

> People in the community are now aware that if they just play around with a widow, there is someone who will fight for them. They just know that there are people who are walking around checking to see if there is anyone oppressing the widow. For me, I see that as a big change because it never used to be like that before. Some men would just play around with a woman and take away everything from her but now when someone hears that he will be taken to court because of taking something that doesn't belong to him, there is some fear. Most of the times the CWDG members stand on the baraza and tell people about women rights and I can say that they are more knowledgeable than before. (male implementer, age 72, Kakamega County)

The CWDG gained a regular speaking platform at community barazas where community leaders and members discussed local issues. In these meetings, the CWDG regularly emphasizes to government stakeholders and community members the multifaceted impacts of property rights violations on the community (Dworkin et al. 2013). In our other work from this project, women reported that because men were aware that women had gained knowledge about their rights, the men felt "watched" by the CWDG. Thus, in that work we reported that beneficiaries perceived that community members were less likely to violate women's rights at the household and community level (Hilliard et al., under review).

Challenging Gender Norms

In addition to educating communities about women's rights (directly in relation to land and property, as well as more broadly) and providing a support network in which rights could be realized, intervening on gender norms was also a key mechanism towards empowering women. Challenges to restrictive gender norms contributed to the subversion of gendered power imbalances. Women in our sample reported that participation in the CWDG helped them challenge notions of subordination, inferiority, silence, and lack of agency. All three groups of participants reported that the CWDG promoted women's independence and confidence, voice and visibility, leadership capacity, and agency over their own bodies and health.

Building Agency, Independence, and Confidence

By teaching women to work actively towards securing income and protecting their own livelihoods, all three categories of participants in our sample (beneficiaries, implementers, developers) perceived that the CWDG has challenged gender norms and moved women towards economic and social self-sufficiency. Financial independence and self-reliance were championed by the CWDG as ways of increasing women's agency. This developer explained how the CWDG encouraged women to become more financially independent:

> We [the CWDG] have taught them to be self-reliant. We should not sit down waiting for a man to bring the flour, to go get the water, to bring everything. . . . We have formed this People of Kenya Enterprise to come and teach them about small businesses, so that they are self-reliant, even if they are told to go to court twice, they can take themselves there. Just don't sit waiting [for] everything to be done for you. So we have taught them to do small businesses, we have also taught them to open their accounts . . . so that one day you can stand on your own and do something for yourself. (female developer, age 42, Kakamega County)

Like many others, this woman explained the importance of financial independence and security. Independence was also encouraged by the CWDG in other forms. This implementer explained that when women were less dependent on men financially, their day-to-day agency was built:

> We usually tell these women, if there is a car in the home learn how to drive it. . . . You must know everything in that home, don't just say that these are men's things. We are all balanced in this world—men, women—are all human beings and if you set yourself to do something, you will. Just don't

wait there. But nowadays most of them have come out and they know: "This I can do. I have to stand up for myself, go buy land, go buy maize, fertilizer and do everything so that I don't go hungry in my home." (female implementer, age 44, Kakamega County)

Additionally, beneficiaries commented that when they perceived themselves to be more equal to men and able to carry out daily tasks related to food and agricultural productivity, they gained a greater degree of autonomy over their homes, families, and livelihoods. They also offered many examples of how women's dependence on men negatively affected their agency and independence and how the CWDG helped them become more self-sufficient:

> This is the area that they [the CWDG group] have brought the biggest change because they have removed us from stigma and brought us to the light. So they have brought a big impact, someone who has removed you from fear and has brought you to the light! You know this has really helped the community because there is no fear in that community. Fear was our biggest problem but now there is no fear because you will find that the Watchdog has taught people how they should take care of themselves. (female beneficiary, age 42, Homa Bay County)

Increasing Women's Voice and Visibility

Participants frequently underscored that prior to the presence of the CWDG, and their use of existing public forums in the form of public barazas, women had very little opportunity to speak in public, and the silencing of women represented a dominant gender norm. The barazas, which had previously been used as a forum to discuss local issues, were now also used by the CWDG not only to educate communities about rights but also to allow women themselves to speak publicly, sharing their personal experiences in solidarity with one another. This implementer explained how women's voices had previously been restricted to the home, but were now being heard at the community level:

> Women were just down, they didn't have a voice, they could not talk during barazas or anywhere, they also didn't know anything. They were just women back benchers; they only knew the kitchen, just cooking food and nothing else, but right now you can even see the Land Tribunal, you just know the Luhya and land issues, it was only the men that were present when it came to land issues, women were not there, so you can see women have been empowered in so many things. (female implementer, age 44, Kakamega County)

Women's increasing community presence and visibility were key to voicing their agenda of defending property and land entitlement and in spreading rights-based messages more broadly. Another beneficiary of the program explained how she gained the confidence to speak publicly since the CWDG has been in her community:

> I used to feel that I have no say, I am just a housewife. My little education, I had discarded it—but at least now I can see we can go far. Sometimes I sit down and I marvel . . . "Am I the one who used to look down upon herself down there in the village and feel that I don't deserve anything? Am I really the one?" So, the CWDG has brought us to a place where we feel that we can now stand before people and talk to them. Even if you are not a good orator, you will talk in your language and they will listen to you. (female implementer, age 37, Kakamega County)

Beneficiaries of the program commonly explained how they were now able to express their points of view publicly:

> I used to be very afraid of standing in front of people and addressing them, even if it were you at that time, I could be asking myself: "What does this girl want by asking me all these questions?" . . . I was not sure of what I am supposed to say, maybe I would say something that is bad. So I feel that they have really given me courage to even stand before people and tell them what I feel. (female beneficiary, age 49, Kakamega County)

It is clear that the very presence of the CWDG was perceived by study participants to build women's public voice, visibility, and solidarity with others in the community.

Encouraging Leadership

Prevailing gender norms in this local community did not previously encourage female leadership. Male domination of positions of authority affected the decision-making power that women had in their communities. GROOTS Kenya emerged out of the Fourth World Conference on Women in Beijing, which emphasized empowerment processes as a means to enable women to contribute to development and leadership in their communities and beyond. In line with these aims, the CWDG encouraged women to become leaders both within the CWDG and in their communities at large.

This developer provided one of many examples of how the CWDG itself had been directly responsible for promoting women's leadership:

> The members of the watchdog groups are really held in high esteem. . . . Some of the members . . . have been elected by their own communities in positions of leadership . . . in the district development committees, district

AIDS committees, social committees, and all that kind of thing. So they are perceived as leaders, they are perceived as champions of human rights, and have been put in positions of leadership to be able to perpetuate even bigger development agendas. (female developer, age 28, Nairobi County)

This also highlights the importance of women's leadership for empowering women beyond preventing, negotiating, and resolving property rights violations. This developer explained how the CWDG builds women's critical leadership skills and how this challenged the assumption that women cannot lead, while simultaneously empowering women:

I think it [the CWDG] really contributed to women's empowerment. [Without the program] I think there would be less empowerment, because generally what I have seen as achievements of the WDG, we have had women who have been elected as village elders just because of being active in the WDG, and this is a position that women never used to take, it was a position that was for the men. . . . It has really enlightened women, for women to understand they need to participate in leadership; it is a vessel to bring women up to leadership. (female developer, age 42, Kakamega County)

This demonstrates how the CWDG provided women with both the support and education for becoming effective leaders, as well as creating an environment that allowed them to practice the skills needed to participate actively in the development of their communities.

Similar to many others in our sample, this developer directly acknowledged the importance of the CWDG in supporting the development of women's rights and leadership skills:

Women are now enlightened, they know their rights, women are even able to contest for some seats. We have an assistant chief now who is a woman. (female developer, age 49, Kakamega County)

The presence of a female assistant chief shows a marked transformation of attitudes towards female leadership, as this is a powerful community leadership position. Beyond becoming leaders within the CWDG and advocating for property rights, being served by the CWDG allowed women to advocate for a wide range of other rights-based issues within the community.

Increasing Agency over Bodies and Health

Women's previous subordinate status in their communities reduced their capacity to control their exposure to health risks, particularly HIV. Several women explained that the existence of CWDG also helped them to protect themselves from HIV risk, challenging ideas that condoms are a sign of infidelity or prostitution, as this beneficiary explains:

> Previously if a woman was found with condoms, they would say, "Now you are a prostitute," but now they will say, "No, my husband, unless you go and find out your HIV status, you have to use this condom, without this, no!" They can even say no to more re-infections, they are now empowered. (female beneficiary, age 43, Kakamega County)

Many women also described how social support networks around the care of their bodies were built because of the assistance offered by the CWDG. Women in our sample specifically perceived this support as breaking their isolation and building their empowerment through stronger social ties and improved health:

> They (the CWDG) embraced me and they told me that "you are not the only one." I just felt as though I had found medicine for my troubles, so I made a habit of going to their meetings and when I could listen to what others were passing through, I felt, "This is normal, [I] am not the only one." I started getting empowered, and that's when I realized that [I] am becoming better, so I started thinking about other women in my community. Coming back, I found that my fellow women had problems and I started talking to them and telling them that "This is the way to go, do this and this." So I became an advisor to my fellow women. (female beneficiary, age 56, Kakamega County)

There was a strong sense of social support and solidarity among women who better understood how to protect themselves from HIV and were empowered to take more control over their own health. As a result, the more-empowered women in the community were able to support and educate other women in the community to protect their health.

DISCUSSION

The findings from this study build on previous research that has shown women's land and property tenure to be deeply interwoven into their ability to gain power and autonomy in their communities (Dworkin et al. 2009). While numerous studies have examined the health-related effects of property rights programming, this work has explored the participants' perceived empowerment-related impacts. Participants, who were both working for and beneficiaries of the CWDG, articulated how this grassroots model played a major role in building the individual- and community-level agency and empowerment of women. They articulated that this was accomplished through championing women's rights, educating women and community members about women's rights, building women's financial independence and day-to-day ability to secure their livelihoods, and challenging gender norms and ideologies that frame women as subservient, inferior, and silent. The CWDG was shown to support women in becoming leaders, both in regards to property rights negotiations and in the broader community arena, recasting women from beneficiaries to agents of change (Asaki and Hayes 2011). In line with previous empowerment research and theory highlighting the need to subvert dominant power structures and challenge dominant ideologies that are harmful to gender equality and women (Grabe 2012; Kabeer 1999; 2005; Romero et al. 2006), these findings show how participants in this sample perceived that the CWDG assisted women in confronting and challenging restrictive gender norms.

Consistent with previous definitions of empowerment as context specific (Grabe 2012; Wallerstein 2006) and with the grassroots approach of the program, we allowed women to define how they and others have been empowered by the CWDG. The qualitative data from this study help fill the gaps in structural empowerment research by providing empirical evidence in support of bottom-up approaches to women's empowerment. The CWDG provides a structural support system that allows and encourages women to empower themselves in ways that are meaningful to them. Due to the rights-based approach of the program, many participants in this study spoke of empowerment in direct relation to rights, such as the right to express one's opinion on matters relevant to the larger community.

Previous work has noted women's internalization of their subordinate status in society and acquiescence to violations of their rights and other gendered inequalities (Kabeer 1999; Shaffer 1998). According to Kabeer (1999), women's increased vocality and visibility in the community allows women to be driven by their own vision and agency; they are able to define their own context-specific empowerment strategies, rather than relying on externally defined agendas. However, while these norms must be challenged in order to press towards gender equality, some skepticism has been expressed about whether voice and visibility translate into real and lasting power (Elliott 2008b).

Additionally, due to the increasing professionalization and globalization of international non-governmental organizations, development agendas may not be fully reflective of women's needs (Nagar and Raju 2003), signifying a need to shift towards more grassroots approaches to empowerment to ensure that women's voices are at the center of their

empowerment. While many structural interventions challenge structural inequalities, they often do so from an external position, potentially reifying a lack of agency among women who are intended beneficiaries of such programs. The grassroots approach of the CWDG allows
women to identify the structures they believe contribute to gendered
power differentials and challenge those structures from within. Our
findings not only supported that these oppressive structures were being
challenged by the model, but the process of challenging them was also
deemed empowering by participants who worked with and sought help
from the CWDG.

Through the use of community baraza meetings, the CWDG not only
spread rights-based education throughout communities but also provided a space for women to challenge attitudes that had previously
silenced them. Additionally, the social support provided by the CWDG
gave women a support network in which they found solidarity. This
was key to encouraging women to continue challenging power imbalances, as they felt safe to do so. The creation of fear among potential
perpetrators, through educating the community about the legal ramifi-
cations of property rights violations, also added to a sense of safety,
creating a context where women trusted the law to provide some protection. The entrenchment of discriminatory practices within Kenyan
culture suggests that constitutional ratification of women's rights is necessary but not sufficient to improve gender equality (FIDA 2009; Welsh,
Duvvury, and Nicoletti 2007). In a context where the formal justice
system provides little support for gender equality (Dworkin et al. 2013;
Izumi 2007; Lu et al. 2013), the CWDG is creating informal practices
that support the realization of women's rights, providing a critical
mechanism for social change at the community level.

There are several limitations to this study. First, the findings are limited to the settings in which the study was conducted (namely, rural
Kenya) and cannot be generalized to other settings in which property
rights violations play a key role in the maintenance of gender inequality.
Second, the participants in this study were either beneficiaries of or
helped to develop and run the CWDG, and therefore they are likely to
express favorable views towards the model. Third, without validated
empowerment measures, we can report on only the perceived impact of
the program, and not on how it affects specific measurable empowerment or health outcomes. Fourth, as a result of the cross-sectional
nature of the data, our results do not explain how empowerment may
evolve over time in relation to the CWDG, nor were we able to examine

the bidirectional and synergistic nature of health and empowerment that is likely operating in this program. While the current findings suggest an increased community-level presence and impact, further longitudinal research is necessary to assess whether the impacts of these changes are long lasting or short lived. Despite these limitations, the findings from this study provide support for the incorporation of grassroots programming into women's development agendas.

CONCLUSIONS

The CWDG is an innovative program that seeks to empower women at the grassroots level. It employs local and legal knowledge to investigate, negotiate, and secure women's property rights, the violation of which had been connected to poor economic livelihoods (Aliber and Walker 2006; Izumi 2007), disruptions to social networks (Welch, Duvvury, and Nicoletti 2007), and health risks such as gender-based violence and HIV (Dworkin et al. 2013; Gupta 2006; Swaminathan, Walker, and Rugadya 2008). Our findings demonstrated that the CWDG model reached beyond property and land tenure rights and empowered women through a number of mechanisms. These included encouraging greater autonomy and community involvement, rights-based education, agency, and social support. It also reduced financial dependency while challenging harmful gender norms and ideologies. Future programs that address structural drivers of gender inequality and negative health outcomes should consider a more holistic approach to women's empowerment by integrating local women's experiences, knowledge, and solutions.

Box 12.1. Summary

Geographic area: Nairobi County, Homa Bay County, and Kakamega County in Central and Western Kenya.

Global importance of the health condition: Women's property rights violations, which are common in this region, have been linked to their likelihood of experiencing both physical and sexual violence and increased HIV risks. While the new Kenyan constitution supports women's right to own property, women's rights are not supported by local customs and practices, and the legal system is expensive and difficult for women in poverty to negotiate. Thus, community-level property rights programming for women is required to address these inequalities and their associated negative health impacts. Few studies examine the health and empowerment-related impacts of programming focused on property rights

Intervention or program: The Community Land and Property Watchdog (CWDG) is a community-led model developed by Grassroots Women Operating Together in Sisterhood (GROOTS) Kenya. The program was developed to prevent HIV and violence against women and is used to secure women's land and property rights as a structural approach to women's empowerment and health.

Impact: Findings show that the CWDG model is perceived in the community to be empowering to women by encouraging greater autonomy through increased community involvement, improving rights-based education, agency, and social support. It is also perceived to reduce financial dependency on men and challenges harmful gender norms and ideologies.

Lessons learned: Structural and economic interventions that are implemented from the bottom up are rarely evaluated in academic/community partnerships. These collaborations are fruitful for exploring the impacts of grassroots empowerment and health interventions.

Link between empowerment and health: Antiviolence and HIV prevention interventions that reshape the structural context in which gendered power operates can positively reshape individual and community-level gender norms and ideologies, which can, in turn, increase women's agency over their bodies and health.

Box 12.2. Previous and Contemporary Debates in Structural Empowerment and Health

PREVIOUS APPROACHES

- Economic empowerment, especially microfinance and training in business skills, has been at the core of structural HIV and antiviolence approaches, seeking to empower women through increasing access to fiscal resources.

- These approaches have resulted in some success in improving women's empowerment and health outcomes.

- Despite these successes, critics of income-oriented empowerment initiatives have emerged, because income gains are minimal and women rarely have control over additional income.

- Failure to truly address the contextual drivers of gender inequalities limits the scope and impact of existing economic empowerment initiatives.

NEW APPROACHES

- Access to and control over harder assets, such as land and property, may provide a more structural basis for empowerment and health.

- A lack of land and property rights has been linked to women's likelihood of experiencing gender-based violence. This impacts HIV risks and can affect HIV treatment outcomes as well.

- Property rights programs seek to challenge gendered power imbalances associated with land and property tenure by supporting women's rights to inherit, access, and own land.

- Property rights programs have shown some success in reshaping violence and HIV outcomes

- More comprehensive approaches to economic empowerment challenge the broad structural drivers of gender inequalities that lead to poor health outcomes for women.

REFERENCES

Adimora, A. A., and Auerbach, J. (2010). Structural interventions for HIV prevention in the United States. *Journal of Acquired Immune Deficiency Syndrome, 55*(S2), S132–S135. doi:10.1097/QAI.ob013e3181fbcb38.

Agot, K. E., Vander Stoep, A., Tracy, M., Obare, B. A., Bukusi, E. A., Ndinya-Achola, J. O., et al. (2010). Widow inheritance and HIV prevalence in Bondo District, Kenya: Baseline results from a prospective cohort study. *PLoS ONE, 5*(11), e14028. doi:10.1371/journal.pone.0014028.s002.

Ali, I., and Hatta, Z. A. (2012). Women's empowerment or disempowerment through microfinance: Evidence from Bangladesh. *Asian Social Work and Policy Review, 6*(2), 111–121. doi:10.1111/j.1753-1411.2012.00066.x.

Aliber, M., and Walker, C. (2006). The impact of HIV/AIDS on land rights: Perspectives from Kenya. *World Development, 34*(4), 704–727. doi:10.1016/j.worlddev.2005.09.010.

Asaki, B., and Hayes, S. (2011). Leaders, not clients: Grassroots women's groups transforming social protection. *Gender and Development, 19*(2), 241–253. doi:10.1080/13552074.2011.592634.

Batliwala, S. (2007). Taking the power out of empowerment—An experiential account. *Development in Practice, 17*(4–5), 557–565. doi:10.1080/09614520701469559.

Brooks, A. (2007). Feminist standpoint epistemology: Building knowledge and empowerment through women's lived experience. In S.N. Hesse-Biber and P.L. Levy (Eds.), *Feminist research practice* (pp. 53–82). Thousand Oaks, California: Sage.

Cattaneo, L.B. and Chapman, A.R. (2010). The process of empowerment: A model for use in research and practice. *American Psychologist, 65*(7), 646–659. doi: 10.1037/a0018854.

Central Intelligence Agency (CIA). (2013). "Kenya." *World Factbook.* Retrieved August 20, 2013 from: www.cia.gov/library/publications/the-world-factbook/geos/ke.html.

Charmes, J., and Wieringa, S. (2003). Measuring women's empowerment: An assessment of the Gender-Related Development Index and the Gender Empowerment Measure. *Journal of Human Development, 4*(3), 419–435. doi:10.1080/1464988032000125773.

Coates, T.J., and Szekeres, G. (2004). A plan for the next generation of HIV prevention research: Seven key policy investigative challenges. *American Psychologist, 59*, 747–757. doi:10.1037/0003–066X.59.8.747.

Constitution of Kenya (2010). National Council for Law Reporting. Nairobi: Kenya.

de Mel, S., McKenzie, D., and Woodruff, C. (2012). *Business training and female enterprise start-up, growth, and dynamics: Experimental evidence from Sri Lanka* (No. 6896). Bonn, Germany: Institute for the Study of Labor (IZA).

Dunbar, M.S., Maternowska, M.C., Kang, M.-S.J., Laver, S.M., Mudekunye-Mahaka, I., and Padian, N.S. (2010). Findings from SHAZ!: A feasibility study of a microcredit and life-skills HIV prevention intervention to reduce risk among adolescent female orphans in Zimbabwe. *Journal of Prevention and Intervention in the Community, 38*(2), 147–161. doi:10.1080/10852351003640849.

Dunford, C. (2001). Building better lives: Sustainable integration of microfinance and education in child survival, reproductive health, and HIV/AIDS prevention for the poorest entrepreneurs. *Journal of Microfinance, 3*(2), 1–25.

Dunkle, K.L., Jewkes, R.K., Nduna, M., Levin, J., Jama, N., Khuzwayo, N., et al. (2006). Perpetration of partner violence and HIV risk behaviour among young men in the rural Eastern Cape, South Africa. *AIDS, 20*, 2107–2114. doi:10.1097/01.aids.0000247582.00826.52.

Dupas, P., and Robinson, J. (2009). *Savings constraints and microenterprise development: Evidence from a field experiment in Kenya* (No. 14693). Cambridge, MA: National Bureau of Economic Research.

Dworkin, S.L., and Blankenship, K. (2009). Microfinance and HIV/AIDS prevention: Assessing its promise and limitations. *AIDS Behavior, 13*(3), 462–469. doi:10.1007/s10461–009–9532–3.

Dworkin, S.L., Grabe, S., Lu, T., Hatcher, A., Kwena, Z., Bukusi, E., and Mwaura-Muiru, E. (2013). Property rights violations as a structural driver of women's HIV risks: A qualitative study in Nyanza and Western provinces, Kenya. *Archives of Sexual Behavior,* Online only. doi:10.1007/s10508–012–0024–6.

Dworkin, S.L., Kambou, S., Sutherland, C., Moalla, K., and Kapoor, A. (2009). Gendered empowerment and HIV prevention: Policy and programmatic pathways to success in the MENA region. *Journal of Acquired Immune Deficiency Virus (51)*, 1–8. doi: 10.1097/QAI.obo13e3181aafd78.

Elliott, C.M. (2008a). *Global empowerment of women: Responses to globalization and politicized religion.* New York, NY: Routledge.

———. (2008b). Introduction: Markets, communities, and empowerment. In C.M. Elliott (Ed.), *Global Empowerment of Women* (pp. 1–21). New York, NY: Routledge.

FIDA. (2009). Women's land and property rights in Kenya—Moving forward into a new era of equality: A human rights report and proposed legislation. *Georgetown Journal of International Law*, 1–126.

Goldenberg, D. (2011). Grassroots women organising for resilient communities around the world. *Institute of Development Studies Bulletin*, 42(5), 74–80. doi:10.1111/j.1759-5436.2011.00255.x.

Grabe, S. (2010). Promoting gender equality: The role of ideology, power, and control in the link between land ownership and violence in Nicaragua. *Analyses of Social Issues and Public Policy*, 10(1), 146–170. doi:10.1111/j.1530-2415.2010.01221.x.

———. (2012). An empirical examination of women's empowerment and transformative change in the context of international development. *American Journal of Community Psychology*, 49, 233–245. doi:10.1007/s10464-011-9453-y.

Grassroots Organization Operating Together in Sisterhood (GROOTS) Kenya. (2008). *Quarterly report*. Nairobi, Kenya: Author.

Gupta, J. (2006). Property ownership of women as protection for domestic violence: The West Bengal experience. In N. Bhatla, S. Chakraborty, and N. Duvvury (Eds.), *Property ownership and inheritance rights of women for social protection: The South Asia experience* (pp. 37–56). Washington, DC: International Center for Research on Women (ICRW).

Gupta, S., and Leung, I.S. (2010). *Turning good practice into institutional mechanisms: investing in grassroots women's leadership.* Geneva: UN Office for Disaster Risk Reduction.

Hashemi, S.M., Schuler, S.R., and Riley, A.P. (1996). Rural credit programs and women's empowerment in Bangladesh. *World Development*, 24(4), 635–653. doi:10.1016/0305-750X(95)00159-A.

Henrysson, E., and Joiremen, S.F. (2009). On the edge of the law: Women's property rights and dispute resolution in Kisii, Kenya. *Law and Society Review*, 43(1), 36–60z. doi:10.1111/j.1540-5893.2009.00366.x.

Hilliard, S., Bukusi, E., Grabe, S., Lu, T., Kwena, Z., and Dworkin, S.L. (2016). Perceived impact of a land and property rights program on violence against women in rural Kenya: A qualitative investigation. *Violence Against Women.* doi:10.1177/1077801216632613.

Holmes, R., Jones, N., Mannan, F., Vargas, R., Tafere, Y., and Woldehanna, T. (2011). Addressing gendered risks and vulnerabilities through social protection: Examples of good practice from Bangladesh, Ethiopia, and Peru. *Gender and Development*, 19(2), 255–270. doi:10.1080/13552074.2011.592637.

Izumi, K. (2007). Gender-based violence and property grabbing in Africa: A denial of women's liberty and security. *Gender and Development, 15*(1), 11–23. doi:10.1080/13552070601178823.

Jan, S., Ferrari, G., Watts, C.H., Hargreaves, J.R., Kim, J.C., Phetla, G., et al. (2011). Economic evaluation of a combined microfinance and gender training intervention for the prevention of intimate partner violence in rural South Africa. *Health Policy and Planning, 26*(5), 366–372. doi:10.1093/heapol /czq071.

Jewkes, R.K., Dunkle, K., Nduna, M., and Shai, N. (2010). Intimate partner violence, relationship power inequity, and incidence of HIV infection in young women in South Africa: A cohort study. *Lancet, 376*(9734), 41–48. doi:10.1016/S0140-6736(10)60548-X.

Jewkes, R.K., Levin, J.B., and Penn-Kekana, L.A. (2003). Gender inequalities, intimate partner violence and HIV preventive practices: Findings of a South African cross-sectional study. *Social Science and Medicine, 56*, 125–134. doi:10.1016/S0277-9536(02)00012-6.

Kabeer, N. (1999). Resources, agency, achievements: Reflections on the measurement of women's empowerment. *Development and Change, 30*(3), 435–464. doi:10.1111/1467-7660.00125.

Kabeer, N. (2005). Is microfinance a 'magic bullet' for women's empowerment? Analysis of findings from South Asia. *Economic and Political Weekly, 40*(44), 4709–4718.

Kenya National Bureau of Statistics (KNBS), ICF Macro. (2010). *Kenya demographic and health survey 2008–2009.* Calverton, Maryland: KNBS and ICF Macro.

Kim, J.C., Watts, C., Hargreaves, J.R., Ndlovu, L.X., Phelta, G., Morison, L., et al. (2007). Understanding the impact of a microfinance-based intervention on women's empowerment and the reduction of intimate partner violence in South Africa. *American Journal of Public Health, 97*(10), 1794–1802. doi:10.2105/AJPH.

Lofland, J., and Lofland, J.H. (1995). *Analyzing social settings: A guide to qualitative observation and analysis.* Detroit, MI: Wadsworth.

Lu, T., Zwicker, L., Kwena, Z., Bukusi, E., Mwaura-Muiru, E., and Dworkin, S.L. (2013). Assessing barriers and facilitators of implementing an integrated HIV prevention and property rights program in Western Kenya. *AIDS Education and Prevention, 25*(2), 151–163. doi:10.1521/ aeap.2013.25.2.151.

McIntosh, A., and Finkle, J.L. (1995). The Cairo Conference on Population and Development: A new paradigm? *Population and Development Review, 21*(2), 223–260. doi:10.2307/2137493.

Mendenhall, E., Muzizi, L., Stephenson, R., Chomba, E., Ahmed, Y., Haworth, A., and Allen, S. (2007). Property grabbing and will writing in Lusaka, Zambia: An examination of wills of HIV-infected cohabiting couples. *AIDS Care, 19*(3), 369–374. doi:10.1080/09540120600774362.

Mosedale, S. (2005). Assessing women's empowerment: Towards a conceptual framework. *Journal of International Development, 17*(2), 243–257. doi:10.1002/jid.1212.

Nagar, R., and Raju, S. (2003). Women, NGOs and the contradictions of empowerment and disempowerment: A conversation. *Antipode, 35*(1), 1–13. doi:10.1111/1467-8330.00298.

Narayan-Parker, D. (2002). *Empowerment and poverty reduction: A sourcebook.* Washington, DC: World Bank.

Orchardson-Mazrui, E. (2006). The impact of cultural perceptions on gender issues. In C. Creighton, F. Yieke, and E. Smith (Eds.), *Gender inequalities in Kenya* (pp. 143–164). Paris, France: United Nations Educational, Scientific, and Cultural Organization (UNESCO).

Pandey, S. (2010). Rising property ownership among women in Kathmandu, Nepal: An exploration of causes and consequences. *International Journal of Social Welfare, 19*(3), 281–292. doi:10.1111/j.1468-2397.2009.00663.x.

Pronyk, P. M., Kim, J. C., Hargreaves, J. R., Makhubele, M. B., Morison, L. A., Watts, C., and Porter, J. D. H. (2005). Microfinance and HIV prevention—Emerging lessons from rural South Africa. *Small Enterprise Development, 16*(3), 26–38.

Romero, L., Wallerstein, N., Lucero, J., Fredine, H. G., Keefe, J., and O'Connell, J. (2006). Woman to woman: Coming together for positive change—using empowerment and popular education to prevent HIV in women. *AIDS Education and Prevention, 18*(5), 390–405. doi:10.1521/aeap.2006.18.5.390.

Rosenberg, M. S., Seavey, B. K., Jules, R., and Kershaw, T. S. (2011). The role of a microfinance program on HIV risk behavior among Haitian women. *AIDS Behavior, 15*(5), 911–918. doi:10.1007/s10461-010-9860-3.

Selinger, E. (2008). Does microcredit "empower"? Reflections on the Grameen Bank debate. *Human Studies, 31*(1), 27–41. doi:10.1007/s10746-007-9076-3.

Shaffer, P. (1998). Poverty and deprivation: Evidence from the Republic of Guinea. *World Development.* 26 (12), 2119–2135.

Shi, C.-F., Kouyoumdjian, F. G., and Dushoff, J. (2013). Intimate partner violence is associated with HIV infection in women in Kenya: A cross-sectional analysis. *BMC Public Health, 13*(512), 1–7.

Strauss, A., and Corbin, J. (1994). Grounded theory methodology. In N. K. Denzin and Y. S. Lincoln (Eds.), *Handbook of qualitative research* (pp. 273–285). Thousand Oaks, CA: Sage.

Swaminathan, H., Walker, C., and Rugadya, M. A. (2008). Women's property rights, HIV and AIDS, and domestic violence: Research findings from two rural districts in South Africa and Uganda. Cape Town, South Africa: HSRC Press.

United Nations. (1994). *Report of the International Conference on Population and Development.* Presented at the International Conference on Population and Development, September; Cairo. www.unfpa.org/sites/default/files/event-pdf/icpd_eng_2.pdf.

Walker, C. (2002). *Land reform in Southern and Eastern Africa: Key issues for strengthening women's access to and rights in land.* Report on a desktop study commissioned by the Food and Agriculture Organization (FAO). http://info.worldbank.org/etools/docs/library/36270/WWalker-Land%20Reform%20and%20Gender.pdf.

290 | Grassroots Property Rights in Kenya

Wallerstein, N. (2006). *What is the evidence on effectiveness of empowerment to improve health?* Copenhagen, Denmark: World Health Organization.

Walsh, J. (2005). Women's property rights violations and HIV/AIDS in Africa. *Peace Review, 17*(2–3), 189–195. doi:10.1080/14631370500332908.

Welch, C. J., Duvvury, N., and Nicoletti, E. (2007). *Women's property rights as an AIDS response: Lessons from community interventions in Africa.* Washington, DC: International Center for Research on Women (ICRW). www .icrw.org/files/publications/Womens-Property-Rights-as- an-AIDS-Response-Lessons-from-Community-Interventions-in-Africa.pdf.

Yngstrom, I. (2002). Women, wives and land rights in Africa: Situating gender beyond the household in the debate over land policy and changing tenure systems. *Oxford Development Studies, 30*(1), 21–40. doi:10.1080 /13600810120011 4886.

Zimmerman, M. A. (2000). Empowerment theory. In J. Rappaport and E. Seidman (Eds.), *Handbook of community psychology* (pp. 43–64). New York, NY: Springer.

13

Land Tenure and Women's Empowerment and Health

A Programmatic Evaluation of Structural Change in Nicaragua

SHELLY GRABE, ANJALI DUTT, AND CARLOS ARENAS

In recent decades the international development field has begun a concerted effort to advocate for women's human rights and empowerment in an effort to address UN Millennium Development Goal 3: "to promote gender equality and empower women." However, it remains unclear what is meant by *empowerment* and what impact a lack of empowerment might have on women's physical and psychological health and well-being.[1] Across the social sciences it is widely agreed that empowerment processes encompass structural inequities and access to material resources, a sense of personal control, and the enhancement of well-being (Cattaneo and Chapman 2010; Zimmerman 1995). Within psychology, *empowerment* has been defined as a sense of personal control and freedom whereby individuals gain agency and mastery over issues of concern to them, enhanced by having access to and control over resources (Rappaport 1987; Zimmerman 1990, 1995). Moreover, although an abundant literature suggests that empowerment is a process whereby multiple components influence each other and may lead to positive outcomes, empirical research does not often identify the components or the links among them (Cattaneo and Chapman 2010; Kabeer 1999; Zimmerman 1995).

In order to examine the role of empowerment in women's health outcomes (i.e., psychological well-being, receipt of violence), this chapter uses an inclusive definition of empowerment that is rooted in psychology but draws on cross-disciplinary perspectives. Early conceptualizations and investigations of empowerment within psychology focused primarily on individual psychological processes such as perceptions of personal control, thereby giving limited attention to context and social structures (Perkins 1995; Riger 1993). However, empowerment theory explicitly links subjective well-being with larger social and political contexts and integrates a critical understanding of the sociopolitical environment with individual outcomes (Perkins and Zimmerman 1995; Zimmerman 1995). Similarly, in the international development literature, although empowerment has largely come to refer to the freedom of choice and action to shape one's life, it is recognized for many marginalized groups that freedom can be severely curtailed by structural inequities (see Mosedale 2005; Narayan 2005, for reviews). Thus, a synthesis of individual and contextual factors is required for the true expansion of opportunities. This chapter presents a case study of a women's organization in Nicaragua that facilitates women's empowerment in part through the ownership of land. The evaluation of this case demonstrates a comprehensive approach to the processes of women's empowerment by measuring and analyzing the multiple components involved—structural, relational, and individual—and the impact they have on women's psychological and physical health.

THE CONTEXT: STRUCTURAL ADJUSTMENTS AND WOMEN'S LANDOWNERSHIP IN NICARAGUA

The global economic policies of the 1980s and 1990s introduced or exacerbated several structural factors that contributed to rising levels of gender inequity throughout the "developing" world[2] (Grabe 2010a; Naples and Desai 2002). Globalization and the structural adjustments that characterized these decades (e.g., withdrawal of subsidized services in the social sector, such as health care) continue to have unique and negative outcomes for women (e.g., feminization of labor and/or poverty; Naples and Desai 2002; Moghadam 2005). A growing body of evidence suggests that institutionalized inequities in the distribution of resources contribute to power imbalances and gender-based norms that can create environments that legitimize and perpetuate women's subordination and negatively impact their health (e.g., Connell 1987; Glick and Fiske, 1999). Although Nicaragua had long been an impoverished country, the shift in presidential power in 1990 brought with it a significant restructuring of social services, resulting in severe cutbacks to public sector commitments to human development goals, including health services.

The Xochilt-Acalt Women's Center in Nicaragua emerged out of this context. The founding members of the center recognized the dire need for health care services for women—particularly women in rural areas. The center started in 1991 as a mobile reproductive and sexual health care clinic serving women in rural communities. Although this type of outreach was important, once the basic health infrastructure was developed, the center evolved over time to comprehensively address the multitude of consequences uniquely confronting women with a lack of institutional power (e.g., food insecurity, high levels of domestic violence; Montenegro, 2004). Thus, in order to address the full range of women's health concerns, new programs were developed in the areas of agricultural production, education, and civic participation that were aimed at connecting women's empowerment with psychological, physical, and sexual health outcomes. Although each program had focused objectives, they had in common gender reflection training that explicitly raised awareness of the role of cultural ideology—that is, social rules, norms, and values that govern gender roles—in human rights violations against women.

The study presented in this chapter reflects an evaluation of one of the center's programs, Programa Productivo. Programa Productivo is an agrarian production program that Xochilt-Acalt developed in 1994 out of a strategic interest in challenging gender norms, thereby providing women with independent economic resources and security. Because landownership throughout Latin America (and most of the world) reflects dominant roles and is a sign of power and control (Deere and Leon 2001; Pena et al. 2008), the program's main initiative was to legally facilitate women's ownership of and titling to land as a means to improve women's status, access to resources, and health and empowerment measures. Women participating in the program received education surrounding their rights as landowners, legal assistance in land titling, and technical training in the area of agricultural production.

Until the last three decades, women's ownership of land in Latin America was restricted because of legal and customary rules that prohibited women from being landowners. Of the Latin American countries that implemented gender-progressive agrarian reform policies in the 1980s, Nicaragua stands out above the rest (Deere 1985). For example, the Agrarian Reform Laws of the 1980s and 1990s that recognized equal rights for both sexes were acknowledged as some of the most forward-looking reforms in Latin America. Moreover, in 1995 a major legislative leap was taken that led to compulsory joint titling for married couples and for those living in stable relationships (FAO 2005).

Nevertheless, data from the rural titling office indicate that between 1979 and 1989, women accounted for only 8–10 percent of beneficiaries under the agrarian reform. These low numbers reflect that land was still being allocated primarily to male "heads of households," whereas titled women were likely widowed or unmarried women living alone (FAO 2005). Thus, despite legislation that positioned Nicaragua as cutting edge in mainstreaming gender in agricultural policy, the relatively low percentage of women landowners reflects the reality that social constructions of gender, combined with cultural practices of restricting women's ownership of land,[3] have historically prohibited women from realizing their legal rights.

In recent years, a small body of literature has emerged examining health and empowerment outcomes of women's landownership. In the first published study in this area, authors found that in Kerala, India, women's receipt of long-term physical violence was inversely related to owning land, a house, or both (Panda and Agarwal 2005). Since that initial publication, investigators have expanded on this research and demonstrated links between landownership and women's negotiating power within the marital relationship, financial decision making, and decreased receipt of physical and sexual violence in West Bengal, Nepal, and Nicaragua, respectively (Grabe 2010b; ICRW 2006; Pandey 2010). Collectively, these studies put forth a framework for investigating landownership as a resource related ultimately to improvements in women's health.

In sum, although property rights may be emerging as one route to addressing women's health and empowerment, deeply entrenched social barriers still prohibit women from taking advantage of opportunities to effectively exercise their rights to own land (Narayan 2005). Because of this, women's organizations have an important role to play in creating the conditions for change in this area (Kabeer 1999). Similarly, there is great need for social scientists in the area of globalization and women's empowerment to evaluate processes involving landownership by defining, measuring, and analyzing the various components of empowerment involved. The following investigation of Programa Productivo was a collaborative project that brought together science and grassroots community advocacy. The expertise of the researcher (Shelly Grabe) ensured theoretically grounded, sound methodology from the lens of social psychology. The expertise of the community collaborator (Carlos Arenas) ensured cultural sensitivity and community relevance to the designed program. The aims of this project support the goals of feminist liberation psychology by focusing on the science of psychology as an instrument for informing social action (Lykes and Moane, 2009). An analysis with the level of complexity presented in the following sections is necessary to lend scientific merit to the understanding of empowerment and increase the acceptability for empowerment approaches among policy makers, especially in regard to impacts on women's health.

METHODS

In order to evaluate the links between landownership and women's empowerment and health, household surveys were administered to two different groups of women in the state of León, Nicaragua. The first group were members of Xochilt-Acalt and were selected by simple random sampling from a list of 380 women involved in Programa Productivo ($N = 124$). The second group of women were randomly selected from neighboring communities in the same municipality that were not actively involved in Xochilt-Acalt ($N = 114$). The total sample size was 238 women. The control group structure allowed for direct comparison of women who were involved in a gender-based social organization aimed at empowerment and women who were not. The study followed field procedures recommended by the World Health Organization (WHO) for conducting violence research in "developing" countries, including hiring and training a local research team to administer the surveys (Ellsberg and Heise 2005). Data were collected in private interviews conducted in Spanish.

Questionnaires included in the survey assessed sociodemographic information, such as age, number of children, and educational history, as well as information about partners, including partner alcohol use. The survey also assessed how regularly women participated in activities with Xochilt-Acalt and whether they owned land. Gender ideology was assessed with a modified version of the Attitudes Towards Women Scale (Spence, Helmreich, and Stapp 1973). Empowerment was assessed with standardized scales indexing power and control within relationships (Sexual Relationship Power Scale: Pulerwitz, Gortmaker, and DeJong 2000; Control: Ellsberg and Heise 2005), financial and household decision making (ICRW 2006), and individual autonomy and mastery (Ryff's Scales of Psychological Well-Being: Ryff 1989). Psychological and physical health outcomes were indexed with standardized scales of self-esteem (Rosenberg Self-Esteem Scale: Baños and Guillén 2000), depression (Center for Epidemiologic Studies—Depression Scale: Grzywacz et al. 2006), and physical, psychological, and sexual violence in the past twelve months (Conflict Tactics Scale: Straus et al. 1996). All questions were translated into Spanish and verified and back-translated to ensure meanings would be conveyed properly in the local context before the survey was piloted. Ethics approval was granted by the University of Wisconsin–Madison.

RESULTS

The average ages of the respondents were in the early to mid forties, and the majority of women had three or more children. Approximately three-quarters of the sample were in relationships that were between six to ten years in duration. Most of the respondents reported being literate, although approximately a quarter of the sample never received formal schooling.

Table 13.1 shows group differences in the proposed process and outcome variables. As can be seen from the table, there are statistically significant differences seen with all the measured variables, with women who were members of Xochilt-Acalt reporting more progressive gender-role ideology conceptions, a greater say in household and financial decision making, more relationship power, less partner control, higher levels of autonomy and mastery, higher levels of self-esteem, lower levels of depression, and less physical and sexual violence in the past twelve months than the control group. Over 40% of women in each group reported experiencing psychological violence in their lifetime, and over 23% reported experiencing physical violence, with estimates of sexual violence being nearly as high. Importantly, women from both groups reported comparable levels of lifetime violence, suggesting that women who participated in Xochilt-Acalt were not a different subset of women who self-selected based on having a priori progressive relationships.

Path models were used to test the proposed processes surrounding women's empowerment and health, namely that participating with Xochilt-Acalt and landownership would lead to greater empowerment and psychological and physical health (Figure 13.1; see Grabe 2010, 2011 for specific details surrounding model building and path analyses). In the first path model, both organization participation and landownership were related to more progressive conceptions in gender-role ideology, which was, in turn, related to higher levels of household but not financial decision-making power, greater relationship power, and less partner control. Neither of the decision-making measures was associated with either indicator of a woman's individual empowerment. In

TABLE 13.1   MEAN DIFFERENCES AMONG XOCHILT-ACALT STUDY VARIABLES

	Xochilt-Acalt members (N = 124) (M, SD)	Control (N = 114) (M, SD)	p	d
Gender ideology	1.84 (.166)	1.62 (.216)	.00	1.16
Household decision making	2.67 (.673)	2.48 (.662)	.02	0.29
Financial decision making	1.94 (.514)	1.81 (.569)	.03	0.24
Relationship power	1.81 (.235)	1.67 (.293)	.00	0.54
Partner control	1.50 (2.45)	2.22 (2.84)	.04	−0.27
Autonomy	1.84 (.150)	1.78 (.165)	.00	0.38
Mastery	1.71 (.137)	1.67 (.140)	.02	0.29
Self-esteem	1.93 (.104)	1.86 (.168)	.00	0.52
Depression	1.69 (.502)	1.83 (.620)	.05	−0.25
12M Physical violence	.067 (.500)	.167 (.651)	.01	−0.17
12M Psychological violence	.372 (.896)	.342 (.910)	.77	0.03
12M Sexual violence	.067 (.309)	.149 (.536)	.00	−0.20
LT Physical violence	.595 (1.122)	.707 (1.444)	.76	−0.09
LT Psychological violence	.959 (1.240)	.911(1.275)	.49	0.04
LT Sexual violence	.438 (.763)	.349(.784)	.35	0.12

NOTES: Mean differences are indicated along with the d = effect size. Effect sizes are calculated as the difference between two means divided by the standardized deviation ($d = [M_1 - M_2/s]$). Effect sizes are computed to assess the magnitude of the difference between groups. According to Cohen (1988) an effect size of 0.2 might be considered "small" (although still a notable difference), whereas values around 0.5 are "medium" effects, and values of 0.8 or higher considered "large" effects. A positive d for gender-role ideology and relationship power indicates that Xochilt-Acalt members scored higher on the study variable. A negative d for partner control indicates that women from Xochilt-Acalt's partners controlled their mobility less.

12M = past twelve months. LT = lifetime.

contrast, relationship power was related to higher levels of autonomy and mastery, and partner control was related to lower levels of women's mastery. Autonomy and mastery were each associated with higher self-esteem and lower depression. Mastery was associated with less psychological violence. The hypothesized model provided a reasonably good fit to the data (i.e., $\chi^2 = 175.82$, $df = 61$, $\chi^2/df = 2.88$, NFI = .81, CFI = .86, RMSEA = .09, AIC = 53.82), but because neither of the decision-making variables served as either significant predictors or outcomes in the hypothesized process, they were dropped from the model and a trimmed model was rerun. Fit statistics from this model indicate a slight improvement ($\chi^2 = 110.34$, $df = 39$, $\chi^2/df = 2.83$, NFI = .87, CFI = .91, RMSEA = .09, AIC = 32.34) over the former.

Next, in order to help explain the mechanisms by which organizational participation and landownership are related to individual empowerment

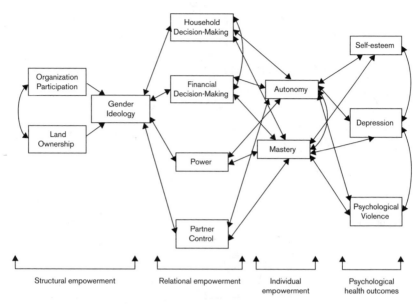

FIGURE 13.1. The hypothesized model. Organizational participation and landownership were hypothesized to predict gender role ideology, which in turn was hypothesized to influence decision making, relationship power, and control, which were expected to predict women's individual empowerment, and, finally, psychological health.

and psychological health, product of coefficients tests were used to test for indirect effects (Sobel 1990). A test of the indirect relation of structural empowerment on relational empowerment suggests that participation in the organization was indirectly related to relationship power ($t = 2.06$, $p = .039$) but not partner control. Landownership was also indirectly related to relationship power ($t = 3.00$, $p = .002$) and partner control ($t = -1.96$, $p = .050$), because it was related to more progressive conceptions of gender-role ideology. Thus, it seems that although participating in the organization and owning land both predict positive outcomes for the participants, actual ownership of land is a more robust predictor of altered gender relations. Nevertheless, since the organization is imperative to facilitating women's ownership over land, participation in the organization was a critical factor in improving women's empowerment outcomes.

Given that the model included multiple components of empowerment, the relations between the empowerment indicators were examined (see Grabe 2011, for more detail). The aim was to evaluate the most commonly used measure of individual empowerment in the development

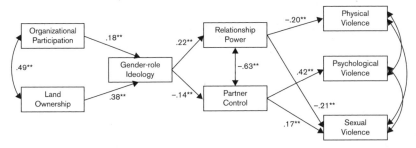

FIGURE 13.2. The relationship between structural power, interpersonal power, and violence. Note: Values are standardized beta weights **p < .01.

literature (i.e., decision making) relative to the additional indicators included in this study. The results suggest that neither measure of decision making was strongly correlated with women's autonomy or mastery nor with women's relationship power or partner control, despite the fact that decision making is often used as a proxy of either agency or relative power within the relationship. In addition, the decision-making scales were not related to any of the psychological health measures. In contrast, relationship power and control, autonomy, and mastery were consistently related to each other and to the health measures.

A second path model was constructed to focus more specifically on the role of power and control in the cycle of domestic violence. As shown in Figure 13.2, women's relationship power predicted fewer episodes of physical and sexual violence, and partner control predicted greater receipt of psychological and sexual violence.

DISCUSSION

Findings from the Xochilt Acalt's Programa Productivo contribute to a growing body of literature that defines and conceptualizes women's empowerment. The evaluation of Xochilt- Acalt's work also supports a theoretical model that suggests that social structures may be associated with health factors that are often linked to subordination and oppression. The results of the study, which show that contexts where power may be unevenly distributed (i.e., women owning land in a situation whereby female landownership defied social roles) may define patterns of personal empowerment, provide support for the suggestion that multiple components of empowerment relate to each other and are critical to understanding the processes surrounding women's empowerment and health.

The study also demonstrates that taking a social psychological approach to the investigation of women's health and empowerment can bridge the theoretical arguments surrounding gender equity with the practical implementation of development interventions. The findings also expose mechanisms surrounding women's subordination and psychological and physical health and provide empirical support that has yet to be demonstrated elsewhere. Moreover, this case study suggests that comprehensive attempts to improve women's health worldwide should involve policies ensuring that appropriate infrastructures exist to support women's abilities to exercise their rights. Although the discourse of human rights is not widely used among psychologists (Kitzinger and Wilkinson 2004), the findings from this evaluation suggest that women's landownership in and of itself, as well as how it relates to other fundamental rights (i.e., violence), may be a requirement of social justice.

In addition, the results support a number of guiding principles and strategies for interventions that can advance the international empowerment agenda and contribute to the aims of social justice articulated in the Beijing Platform for Action (1995). First, the findings suggest that development practitioners should not confuse practical interventions (i.e., those based solely on allocating short-term resources) with strategic interventions (i.e., those with the potential to transform the conditions in which women live). Given the pivotal role of Xochilt-Acalt in administering landownership via Programa Productivo, the findings suggest that it may be most useful to think about resources (i.e., land) as "enabling factors" that catalyze the empowerment process, rather than as ends in themselves (Malhotra and Schuler 2005). Programs may be most effective when policy makers, and those developing interventions, work in collaboration with women's organizations to combine equity in the distribution of resources with a sense of personal power and control to optimally impact health and well-being. In other words, the design of empowerment programs should be based on the potential for women to act on the structures of power that constrain their lives and not on buzzwords that are in favor of a globalized economy.

LESSONS LEARNED

The importance of understanding the process of empowerment is not simply academic. This case study demonstrates that organizational intervention may provide an important and effective means to achieving change. In this case, participating with Xochilt-Acalt was related not only to landownership but also to more progressive gender ideology. Again, although the direction of this relationship cannot be discerned from the model, this link lends support to Freire's (1970) theory of consciousness-raising through group forums as a means to bring about empowerment. Moreover, the results suggest that women's organizational participation was part of the pathway to improving psychological health and reducing violence, although it was not as strong a predictor as owning land. Nevertheless, understanding the benefits associated with participating in the organization suggests that changing laws alone is not enough to bring about significant social change. Organizational intervention can greatly assist in facilitating women's access to land and their related psychological and physical health.

The findings also suggest that while it may be possible that resources serve as catalysts for empowerment, empowering women requires a contextualized understanding of power in different dimensions. For example, the results highlight a relation between structural factors and gender ideology. Although the direction of these effects cannot be discerned from this data, the findings support the notion that resources may provide the material conditions through which inequalities are produced, but cultural ideology plays a critical way in how they are sustained (Glick and Fiske 1999). In particular, women with more progressive gender ideology reported having greater relationship power and were able to withstand partner attempts at control. It is possible that women who are more aware of their sociopolitical environments and who hold beliefs about their rights to exercise their rights are able to exert greater influence in their marital relationships. Perhaps not surprisingly then, higher levels of relationship empowerment were related to women's greater individual empowerment as reflected in measures of autonomy and internal feelings of competence, which, in turn, were related to higher levels of psychological health. Although the empowerment process demonstrated is likely iterative, not linear, the findings suggest that manifestations of power between men and women may not be static but may be malleable under certain conditions. The results also suggest that the most widely relied-upon measure of empowerment in the development literature to date, financial and household decision making, is not a robust or reliable component in the empowerment process.

Finally, the study demonstrates a synergistic relationship between activist-based social organizations and a researcher. Women within the organization were responsible for developing their own strategies for action and the researcher, in the words of Ignacio Martin-Baró (1994), used the discipline of science in the service of social justice by focusing on the oppressive reality of social structures. This study demonstrates that successful collaborations between community-based organizations and social science researchers may be critical in the struggle for social justice.

CONCLUSION

The changes that occurred as a result of the efforts at Xochilt-Acalt are particularly important in the context of the persistently high rates of violence experienced by women globally. However, international calls to improve the well-being of women have led to numerous laws to empower women and improve their health and status. Nevertheless, the barriers to accessing these laws suggest that laws alone are often only one aspect of social change required to effectuate substantial changes (Amnesty International 2005). As such, the success of Xochilt-Acalt, and the potential for generalizing the findings to the issue of property rights as a means to women's empowerment and health, is particularly timely. Not only does the evaluation of Programa Productivo illustrate the mechanisms by which altered structural changes (i.e., fostering women's ownership of land) can bring about significant improvements in women's psychological and physical health, but it provides support for social advocacy and programs aimed at improving women's well-being. Such avenues may be integral to transcending the normative barriers that subordinate women, to enabling greater access to legal, social, and structural support, and ultimately to encouraging women's empowerment.

Although issues of agrarian change and rural development were a major part of the global economic restructuring imposed on "developing" countries in the 1990s, it has been only in very recent years that women's interest in land has emerged as a contested issue (Razavi 2008). Women's property rights have taken on greater importance in light of women's centrality to agricultural livelihoods, an intensification of women's unpaid agricultural labor, increasing levels of poverty, and food scarcity (Razavi, 2008). The findings from Xochilt-Acalt's work suggest, at a minimum, that programs and policies should aim to alter the structural barriers that prohibit women from being landowners. For example, leading organizations that hold empowering women and girls as one of their primary action areas, such as the Clinton Global Initiative (2010), should include facilitating women's access to land as part of their strategic effort to reduce violence against women and girls. Similarly, because women face the risk of land alienation and entitlement failure in the presence of imposed privatization from multilateral lending programs (despite having legal rights), organizational interventions are necessary to ensure that everyone is capable of realizing their rights.

Changing institutional structures shift the responsibility of combating violence from women to policy makers and program implementers, making it possible that women become beneficiaries of legal reform. For example, major foundations, such as the Rural Development Institute (2010), with its Global Center for Women's Land Rights that works to facilitate landownership for women, can use findings from the current study to further their delivery of policy recommendations and programmatic solutions to securing women's land rights. Projects and programs aimed at development in areas involving ownership and control over vital resources can better improve women's rights by altering the complex power structure in which women's subordination is embedded. Finally, perhaps more than most, this area is ripe for interdisciplinary efforts and cooperative collaboration between interventionists, social activists, and researchers working for women's human rights and social justice in an increasingly globalized context. Through collaborative efforts, changes to social policy that effectively grant women human rights and gender-based interventions aimed at transformative relations could lead to the very notions of social justice that are idealized by the international community addressing these issues.

Box 13.1. Summary

Geographic area: Nicaragua.

Global importance of the health condition: Violence against women is the most pervasive human rights violation in the world (UN 2007). Domestic violence, in particular, has become widely recognized internationally as a serious problem with grave implications for women's psychological and physical health (WHO 2005).

Intervention or program: In 1991 the Xochilt-Acalt Women's Center started as a mobile women's reproductive healthcare clinic in León, Nicaragua. Since that time, the center has burgeoned into a widespread rural network with programs aimed at agricultural production, education, economic empowerment, and civic participation. The current case study evaluates a particular aspect of the agricultural production program—landownership—on women's empowerment and health in the region.

Impact: Women landowners involved with Xochilt-Acalt reported more progressive gender ideology, greater say in decision making, more relationship power and control, higher levels of empowerment, greater psychological well-being, and less physical and sexual violence than a control group of women who did not own land.

Lessons learned: Although participation with Xochilt-Acalt played a major role in improving psychological well-being and reducing violence against women, the study also found that owning land played an independent role in promoting women's health.

Link between empowerment and health: Social interventions that alter women's status and shift cultural norms surrounding the capabilities and worth of women increase empowerment, contribute to higher levels of psychological well-being, and reduce women's receipt of violence.

For a video about Xochilt-Acalt Women's Center, see https://youtu.be/Gzxz7jdNhzI.

Box 13.2. Lessons Learned from Rural Nicaragua

In recent decades there has been a focus on women's health and human rights by organizations ranging from the United Nations to grass-roots organizations—all attempting to address UN Millennium Development Goal 3: "to promote gender equality and empower women." In the context of this increased interest, the success of Xochilt-Acalt's efforts to transform women's realities is particularly noteworthy. A major aim of Xochilt-Acalt is to reduce violence against women, an issue frequently addressed with individual-level interventions. However, Xochilt-Acalt recognizes that an individual focus cannot effectively curb violations that are largely social in practice. Instead, its efforts center on altering the social structures that put women at risk for violence, in this case ownership of land when owning land is associated with power and status. By simultaneously addressing issues of violence and women's land rights, the interventions at Xochilt-Acalt reconfigure power relations in a manner that allows women to reach increased levels of health in ways that are socially and experientially just. Furthermore, Xochilt-Acalt centers its change on the desires of women in the local community rather than on interests of foreign partners or donors. A combined focus on social structures and local voices has led to a successful reduction in women's experiences with domestic violence.

NOTES

1. Although an important aim of public health is to address disparate health issues gravely impacting women, many health topics gaining increasing attention in the international arena are violations of women's human rights. While addressing women's health is of critical import, it should be recognized that there are limitations to using "health" versus "human rights" language. Discussions surrounding health may inadvertently obscure the issues of power and inequality that are at the foundation of women's human rights violations.

2. There is no universally recognized definition of a developed country. Former Secretary-General of the United Nations Kofi Annan defined a developed country as "one that allows all of its citizens to enjoy a free and healthy life in a safe environment." Given that many industrialized countries do not meet these criteria, and that the terms *developed*, *under-developed*, and *developing* are often used by so-called First World nations to describe the relatively low economic well-being of another country in a manner that implies inferiority, when used in this chapter these terms will appear in quotation marks to reflect their problematic nature.

3. Despite receiving gender training surrounding joint titling, many titling officers treated the joint titles as "family" titles and recorded fathers and sons on the land titles, rather than husbands and wives.

REFERENCES

Baños, Rosa M., and Verónica Guillén. 2000. Psychometric characteristics in normal and social phobic samples for a Spanish version of the Rosenberg self-esteem scale. *Psychological Reports* 87: 269–274.

Beijing declaration and platform for action. 1995. In *Report of the Fourth World Conference on Women: Beijing, China, 4–15 September 1995*, pp. 1–132. A/CONF.177/20/Rev.1. New York: United Nations (UN). www.un.org/womenwatch/daw/beijing/pdf/Beijing%20full%20report%20E.pdf.

Cattaneo, Lauren B., and Aliya R. Chapman. 2010. The process of empowerment: A model for use in research and practice. *American Psychologist* 65 (7): 646.

Connell, Robert W. 1987. Gender and power: Society, the person, and sexual politics. Stanford, CA: Stanford University Press.

Deere, Carmen D. 1985. Rural women and state policy: The Latin American agrarian reform experience. *World Development* 13 (9): 1037–1053.

———. 2001. *Empowering women: Land and property rights in Latin America*. Pittsburg, PA: University of Pittsburgh Press.

Ellsberg, Mary, and Lori Heise. 2005. *Researching violence against women: A practical guide for researchers and activists*. Washington, DC: World Health Organization, PATH.

Food and Agriculture Organization of the United Nations (FAO). 2004. *A gender perspective on land rights: Equal footing*. Rome, Italy: Gender and Development Service, Sustainable Development Department, FAO. ftp://ftp.fao.org/docrep/fao/007/y3495e/y3495e00.pdf.

————. 2005. Gender and land compendium of country studies: Nicaragua access to land. Rome, Italy: FAO.

Freire, Paulo. 1970. *Pedagogy of the oppressed.* Trans. Myra Bergman Ramos. New York: Continuum.

Glick, Peter, and Susan T. Fiske. 1999. Gender, power dynamics, and social interaction. In *Revisioning Gender,* edited by M.M. Ferree, and J. Lorber, 365–398. Newbury Park, CA: Sage.

Grabe, Shelly. 2010a. Promoting gender equality: The role of ideology, power and control in the link between land ownership and violence in Nicaragua. *Analyses of Social Issues and Public Policy* 10: 146–170.

————. 2010b. Women's human rights and empowerment in a transnational, globalized context: What's psychology got to do with it? In *Feminism and women's rights worldwide,* edited by M.A. Paludi, 17–46. Westport, CT: Praeger/Greenwood Publishing Group.

————. 2011. An empirical examination of women's empowerment and transformative change in the context of international development. *American Journal of Community Psychology* 49, 233–245.

Grzywacz, Joseph G., et al. 2006. Evaluating short-form versions of the CES-D for measuring depressive symptoms among immigrants from Mexico. *Hispanic Journal of Behavioral Sciences* 28 (3): 404–24.

International Center for Research on Women (ICRW). 2006. *Property ownership and inheritance rights of women for social protection: The South Asia experience.* Washington, DC: ICRW.

Lykes, M. Brinton, and Geraldine Moane. 2009. Editors' introduction: Whither feminist liberation psychology? Critical explorations of feminist and liberation psychologies for a globalizing world. *Feminism and Psychology* 19: 283.

Kabeer, Naila. 1999. Resources, agency, achievements: Reflections on the measurement of women's empowerment. *Development and Change* 30 (3): 435–464.

Kitzinger, Celia, and Sue Wilkinson. 2004. Social advocacy for equal marriage: The politics of "rights" and the psychology of "mental health." *Analyses of Social Issues and Public Policy* 4: 173–194.

Malhotra, Anju, and Sidney R. Schuler. 2005. Women's empowerment as a variable in international development. In *Measuring empowerment: Cross-disciplinary perspectives,* edited by Deepa Narayan, 71–88. Washington, DC: World Bank Publications.

Moghadam, Valentine M. 2005. *Globalizing women: Transnational feminist networks.* Baltimore, MD: Johns Hopkins University Press.

Montenegro, Sofía, and Elvira Cuadra. 2004. *The keys to empowerment: Ten years of experiences at the Xochilt-Acalt Women's Center in Malpiasillo, Nicaragua.* Trans. Donna Vukelich. Madison, WI: Wisconsin Coordinating Council on Nicaragua (WCCN).

Mosedale, Sarah. 2005. Assessing women's empowerment: Towards a conceptual framework. *Journal of International Development* 17 (2): 243–257.

Naples, Nancy A., and Manisha Desai, eds. 2002. *Women's activism and globalization: Linking local struggles and transnational politics.* New York: Routledge.

Narayan, Deepa. 2005. Conceptual framework and methodological challenges. In *Measuring empowerment: Cross-disciplinary perspectives,* edited by Deepa Narayan, 3–38. Washington, DC: World Bank Publications.

Panda, Pradeep, and Bina Agarwal. 2005. Marital violence, human development, and women's property status in India. *World Development* 33: 823–850.

Pandey, Shanta. 2010. Rising property ownership among women in Kathmandu, Nepal: An exploration of causes and consequences. *International Journal of Social Welfare:* 281–291.

Peña, Nuaria, et al. 2008. Using rights-based and gender-analysis arguments for land rights for women: Some initial reflections from Nicaragua. *Gender and Development* 16 (1): 55–71.

Perkins, Douglas D., and Marc A. Zimmerman. 1995. Empowerment theory, research, and application. *American Journal of Community Psychology* 23: 569–579.

Perkins, Douglas D. 1995. Speaking truth to power: Empowerment ideology as social intervention and policy. *American Journal of Community Psychology* 23 (5): 765–794.

Pulerwitz, Julie, Steven L. Gortmaker, and William DeJong. 2000. Measuring sexual relationship power in HIV/STD research. *Sex Roles* 42: 637–660.

Rappaport, Julian. 1987. Terms of empowerment/exemplars of prevention: Toward a theory for community psychology. *American Journal of Community Psychology* 15 (2): 121–148.

Razavi, Shahra. 2008. *The gendered impacts of liberalization: Towards "embedded liberalism"?* New York: Routledge.

Riger, Stephanie. 1993. What's wrong with empowerment. *American Journal of Community Psychology* 21 (3): 279–292.

Ryff, Carol D. 1989. Happiness is everything, or is it? Explorations on the meaning of psychological well-being. *Journal of Personality and Social Psychology* 57 (6) (12): 1069–1081.

Spence, Janet T., Robert Helmreich, and Joy Stapp. 1973. A short version of the Attitudes towards Women Scale (AWS). *Bulletin of the Psychonomic Society* 2: 219–220.

Straus, Murray A., Sherry L. Hamby, Sue Boney-McCoy, and David B. Sugarman. 1996. The revised Conflict Tactics Scales (CTS2): Development and preliminary psychometric data. *Journal of Family Issues* 17 (3): 283–316.

United Nations (2007). Ending impunity for violence against women and girls. New York: NY: UN. www.un.org/events/women/iwd/2007/pdf/background .pdf

WHO. (2005). *WHO multi-country study on women's health and domestic violence against women: Summary report of initial results on prevalence, health outcomes and women's responses.* Geneva, Switzerland: World Health Organization.

Zimmerman, Marc A. 1995. Psychological empowerment: Issues and illustrations. *American Journal of Community Psychology* (Special issue: Empowerment theory, research, and application) 23 (5): 581–599.

Conclusions

A Twenty-First-Century Agenda for
Women's Empowerment and Health

SHARI L. DWORKIN AND LARA STEMPLE

In the introduction to this volume, Gita Sen underscored that from the early 1990s on, through the vehicle of major United Nations conferences (the International Conference on Human Rights in Vienna in 1993, the International Conference on Population and Development in Cairo in 1994, and the Fourth World Conference on Women in Beijing in 1995), a human rights-based approach to women's health came into its own. Yet in many ways, empirical analyses of interventions such as those included in this volume have lagged behind these major international achievements. As Sen noted, this is because of the challenges of measuring rights and empowerment for science-based researchers, the politics of studying sex and gender in health fields, and the siloed divides among disciplines, as well as between science and advocacy, academia and community, and theory and practice (Kabeer 1999; Kreiger 2003; Springer, Stellman and Jordan-Young 2012).

The editors and authors of this volume have offered a much-needed correction to bridge these divides. *Women's Empowerment and Global Health: A Twenty-First-Century Agenda* has provided an in-depth examination of numerous women's health and empowerment interventions, policies, and programs that have been implemented recently around the world. Throughout the volume, we took great care to detail *how* interventions work and offered an in-depth exploration of the promises and limitations of designing and implementing interventions on the ground. There are several key takeaways from the body of work in this volume—and these takeaways underscore numerous paths forward in this area of research, practice, and advocacy.

First, as authors and section editors in this volume have argued, and as others in the field have shown, context is not just "background" to global health programming and its implementation. Rather, the centrality of context at the outset of global health programming is indispensable for ensuring that interventions succeed (Gilson et al. 2011; Gupta et al. 2008). That is, it is not adequate to view global health programs through the lens of a one-size-fits-all strategy or a standardized technology, assuming that what works in one location can be easily transported to another. For example, despite the fact that economic empowerment was a strategy used to reduce violence and HIV vulnerability among women in South Africa in the Intervention for Microfinance and Gender Equity (IMAGE; Abigail Hatcher and colleagues, chapter 9), high levels of inflation made it hard for economic programming in Shaping the Health of Adolescents in Zimbabwe (SHAZ!) to succeed (Megan Dunbar and Imelda Mudekunye-Mahaka, chapter 8). Paying close attention to context, then, Dunbar and the team leaned not only on economic empowerment as a strategy, but also on those strategies that supported adolescents in their process of empowerment through a combination of group-based vocational training, life skills education, and livelihood opportunities to reduce their HIV vulnerabilities.

Out of an understanding that context is critical, Victor Robinson, Theresa Hwang, and Elisa Martínez (chapter 5) underscored a second important takeaway reflected throughout the current volume: the need to meaningfully involve local community members so as to ensure that problem definitions and solutions emerge from those who are most affected by a lack of resources, agency, and achievements. Several chapters reinforced this message. For example, Pallavi Gupta, Kirti Iyengar, and Sharad Iyengar in chapter 1 detailed how listening to rural women led programmers to recognize how health systems have failed women who desire to know their pregnancy status. The program they detail instead took reproductive health services to women where they are most needed. Kate Grünke-Horton and Shari Dworkin (chapter 12) underscored how critical it is for local women to define the root causes of their disempowerment and poor health, and in turn these women developed a complex understanding of these drivers. They understood this disempowerment to emerge from a combination of structural inequalities (the lack of land rights, including disinheritance and an inability to afford to adjudicate property disputes), community-level norms (inequitable gender norms among women and men, including the norm that women should not own land), and a lack of rights-based education. The programming took the analysis of root causes and shaped a multi-level program that responded to all of these drivers. In other work, Victor Robinson, Theresa Hwang, and Elisa Martínez (chapter 5), in their examination of a ten-year intervention with sex workers, detailed how it was critical to rely on sex workers' own definitions of empowerment and to synergize programming with sex workers' aspirations and agency, while taking into account that all of these are shaped and constrained by the complex interplay between institutions, communities, the interpersonal level, and cultural norms.

A third critical lesson for future work in this thriving field is understanding the mechanisms and pathways through which empowerment shapes health and vice versa. Paying attention to these pathways allows researchers, practitioners, and advocates to identify the specifics of *how* interventions and policies work, pressing beyond the tendency in global health programming to seek success around a singular quantitative health outcome without a fuller understanding of how outcomes were achieved.

In terms of these mechanisms, Daniel Perlman, Fatima Adamu, Mairo Mandara, Olorukooba Abiola, David Cao, and Malcolm Potts (chapter 3) focused on the role of organizations and girls' groups specifically in building girls' individual agency in areas where gender inequality is particularly exacerbated. These mechanisms were detailed in chapter 4 when Karen Austrian, Judith Bruce, and M. Catherine Maternowska described processes and outcomes of girls' boot camps. Shelly Grabe, Anjali Dutt, and Carlos Arenas (chapter 13) detailed key mechanisms through which empowerment and health were realized, such as gender ideology, gender norms, participation in an advocacy organization, and land ownership. Shari L. Dworkin, Abigail M. Hatcher, Chris Colvin, and Dean Peacock (chapter 7) revealed how individual- and community-level shifts in gender norms (especially concerning what it means to be a man) led to a shift in the direction of more gender equality and increased men's participation in shared decision making in their relationships, leading to less violence against women and reduced HIV vulnerability for both women and men.

Increasingly, interventionists in global health, including rights-based researchers, are attempting to parse out the specific mechanisms (through quantitative mediation/moderation analysis, indicator analysis in rights-based work, and qualitative process evaluations) that shape empowerment and health; this will remain a critical area for future research (Gruskin and Ferguson 2013; Polet et al., 2015; Unnithan 2015).

A fourth major advance that emerges from this volume concerns the need for multisectoral work, whereby sectors that may or may not have previously worked together join forces to make change. Nearly all chapters underscored that advancing empowerment and health outcomes requires intervention and analysis at different levels and requires a number of sectors to join forces to achieve more than any sector can achieve alone. Carroll Estes (chapter 10) reveals how e-democracy, academics who identify as grassroots intellectuals, social justice organizations, and national-level committees worked together to form a cross-movement coalition that fought attempts to dismantle Social Security, Medicare, and Medicaid in the United States. Gustavo Ortiz Millán's work (chapter 11) highlights how the decriminalization of abortion in Mexico City at the legal level made it possible for women's organizations to work with Mexico City's political and health officials to improve access to contraceptive methods. Indeed, Keleher (2010, 179) argues that "programmatic interventions to change gender norms at the level of household and community requires multilevel . . . programs . . . designed to influence the underlying determinants of the problem, and require[s] the protective umbrella of policy and legislative actions that recognize and reinforce the rights of women and girls."

The current collection of case studies illuminates this point. Further, the complexity of this work points to the need for bolstering evaluation methodologies to stretch towards multilevel analysis so as to parse which levels of an intervention impact empowerment and health outcomes. For example, does community-level empowerment shape individual women's empowerment and health? Do structural or policy-level empowerment-related processes shape community and/or individual health, or is it the reverse—or are these mutually reinforcing?

Future work in women's empowerment and health can indubitably be strengthened and pressed even further, particularly thinking across the current works (and sectors) contained in this volume. For example, educational outcomes, such as those chapter 3 focused on, will be compromised if young women do not have economic opportunities in the formal occupational sector following their educational experiences. Economic empowerment, such as that focused on in chapters 8 and 9, may not be achievable without access to and control over land (as shown in chapters 12 and 13), since income is not a "hard asset" and women require harder assets to achieve higher status and clout (Gariki-pati 2008; Prina 2011).

Other pathways forward in the area of women's empowerment and health are illustrated by the limitations of the current volume. First, as one is made acutely aware by the title of the book, the text has largely focused on women, not gender more broadly. Scholars and practition-ers have increasingly pressed the field to examine gender as relational—that is, to take into account the simultaneous nature of masculinity and femininity as points of intervention to improve women's empowerment and the health of both women and men (Connell 1987, 1995; Dworkin et al. 2011, 2015; Messner 1997). This is critical, because scholars have shown that a sole focus on women's empowerment can elicit, at mini-mum, alienation, disconnection, and/or confusion from men, masculin-ist backlash, and at the extreme, violence (Dworkin et al. 2011, 2012, 2015; Kimmel 1996). Moreover, an overwhelming focus on women's *dis*empowerment risks reinforcing the very stereotypes about gendered weakness that feminist scholars and practitioners wish to upend (Stem-ple 2011).

Another reason to eschew an exclusive focus on women is that that work on marginalization across axes of race, sexuality, and age has shown how important it is to work with dominant groups as well in order to meaningfully shift empowerment-related processes; gender relations are no different (Boonzaier and Spiegel 2008; Featherman, Hall, and Krislov 2009; Kimmel 1996; Knight 1997). In fact, the next generation of global health research in this area will likely increasingly test women's empowerment approaches alongside those that are com-bined with masculinities-based work to see if women's health outcomes are improved over and above a control group or if combined mascu-linities and women's empowerment approaches are more effective than women's empowerment approaches alone.

Along these lines, an innovative new randomized trial in South Africa tested just that. Pettifor and her team (2015) tested a women's empower-ment approach alone (a structural intervention: conditional cash trans-fers given to families, conditioned on keeping girls in school) alongside/against a masculinities-and-community-mobilization approach (to shift men in the direction of gender equality) plus the structural women's empowerment approach (a control group was the third arm of the trial). The researchers found that both intervention arms were better than the control arm at reducing violence against women, but it was the com-bined women's empowerment and masculinities/community mobilization arm that led to the best improvements in rates of violence against women (Pettifor et al. 2015). This shows that work with men can synergistically improve what women-focused programming cannot do alone and that it need not be perceived as "diluting" the goals of women's empowerment and health or as taking critical resources away from women (Dworkin et al. 2011; Dworkin 2015).

The next generation of work will also need to press beyond global health approaches with women and men that focus exclusively on gender; it will need to consider the racialized, classed, and sexualized nature of empowerment and health. Intersectionality reveals how it is not just gender relations but also its simultaneity with race, class, sexuality, age, and other key axes of inequality and marginalization that matter for empowerment and health outcomes. For example, lesbian, bisexual, and transgender women have issues that impact them as women and also as sexual minorities; a gender analysis is necessary, but not sufficient, to understand the health implications of these intersecting forces. Global health scholars have been slow to embrace intersectional thinking, which in contrast emerged over twenty-five years ago in law, in the humanities, and in the social sciences (Crenshaw 1991; Hill-Collins 1990, 1999; hooks 1984). It took until 2005–2006 to focus on intersectionality as key to understanding health outcomes (Berger 2005; Dworkin 2005; Schultz and Mullings 2006), and it remains critical to continue to understand this.

Several chapters in the current volume point us in the direction of intersectional analysis to elucidate empowerment and health. For example, chapter 4 examined how it may be important in HIV prevention programming that asks men to change in the direction of more gender equality to link discussions of gender inequality with discussions of racial inequality. Drawing more powerfully on the history of racial or class oppression when discussing with men the need for gender equality and improved health can bolster men's critical awareness of the links between inequalities. Conversations with men could critically engage zero-sum game thinking (that is, when women win, men lose) by including the ways that whites in particular contexts frequently discuss reverse discrimination and disempowerment (or "special rights") when gains for marginalized groups are sought (Boonzaier and Spiegel 2008; Featherman, Hall, and Krislov 2009; Kimmel 1996, 2000; Knight 1994). This kind of engagement—with both women and men—in critical discussion about the ways in which inequalities across social axes are linked to health would press the field even further.

While acknowledging, in conclusion, that the promise of human rights law to ensure women's equality and fulfill the right to health has not yet been realized for many around the world, we also hope to point the way forward. By providing empirical analysis of science-based law and advocacy interventions designed to get us there, by working across disciplines and sectors to uproot harmful gender norms, by trying to understand precisely how empowerment approaches work to improve health, by engaging different contexts and on-the-ground populations in meaningful ways, and by attempting to grapple with tough questions, real limitations, and possibilities for future work—we hope this volume takes us further on the path towards fulfilling the promise of women's health and empowerment.

REFERENCES

Berger, M. (2005). *Workable sisterhood: The political journey of stigmatized women with HIV/AIDS.* Princeton, NJ: Princeton University Press.

Boonzaier, E., and Spiegel, A. D. (2008). Tradition. In N. Shepherd and S. Robins (Eds.), *New South African Keywords* (pp. 195–208). Athens, Ohio: Ohio University Press.

Bowleg, L. (2012). The problem with the phrase "women and minorities": An important theoretical framework for public health. *American Journal of Public Health, 102,* 1267–1273.

Cole, E. (2009). Intersectionality and research in psychology. *American Psychologist, 64,* 170–180.

Connell, R. W. (1987). *Gender and power: Society, the person and sexual politics.* Palo Alto, CA: Stanford University Press.

———. (1995). *Masculinities.* Berkeley: University of California Press.

Crenshaw, K. W. (1991). Mapping the margins: Intersectionality, identity politics, and violence against women of color. *Stanford Law Review, 43,* 1241–1299.

Devault, M. (1999). *Liberating method: Feminism and social research.* Chicago: University of Chicago Press.

Dupas, P., and Robinson, J. (2009). *Savings constraints and microenterprise development: Evidence from a field experiment in Kenya.* Cambridge, MA: National Bureau of Economic Research.

Dworkin, S. L. (2005). Who is epidemiologically fathomable in the HIV/AIDS epidemic? Gender, sexuality, and intersectionality in public health. *Culture, Health, and Sexuality, 7,* 16–23.

———. (2015). *Men at risk: Masculinity, heterosexuality and HIV/AIDS prevention.* New York: NYU Press.

Dworkin, S. L., Colvin, C., Hatcher, A., and Peacock, D. (2012). Men's perceptions of women's rights and changing gender relations in South Africa: Lessons for working with men and boys in HIV and anti-violence programs. *Gender and Society, 26,* 97–120.

Dworkin, S. L., Dunbar, M., Krishnan, S., Hatcher A., and Sawires, S. (2011). Uncovering tensions and capitalizing on synergies in violence and HIV programming. *American Journal of Public Health, 101,* 995–1003.

Dworkin, S. L., Pinto, R. M., Hunter, J., Rapkin, B., and Remien, R. H. (2008). Keeping the spirit of community partnerships alive in the scale up of HIV/AIDS prevention: Critical reflections on the roll out of DEBI (Diffusion of Effective Behavioral Interventions). *American Journal of Community Psychology, 42*(1–2): 51–59. www.ncbi.nlm.nih.gov/pmc/articles/PMC2735211/

Featherman, D., Hall, M., and Krislov, M. (Eds.). (2009). *The next 25 Years: Affirmative action in higher education in the United States and South Africa.* Ann Arbor: University of Michigan Press.

Garikipati, S. (2008). The impact of lending to women on household vulnerability and women's empowerment: Evidence from India. *World Development, 36,* 2620–2642.

Gilson, L. Hanson, K., Sheikh, K., Agyepong, I. A., Ssengooba, F., and Bennett, S. (2011). Building the field of health policy and systems research: Social science matters. *PLoS Medicine, 8,* e10010801. doi:10.1371/journal.pmed.1001079

Gruskin, S., and Ferguson, L. (2013). Using indicators to determine the contribution of human rights efforts to public health efforts. In M. Grodin, D. Tarantola, G. Annan, and S. Gruskin (Eds.), *Health and human rights in a changing world* (pp. 202–210). New York: Routledge.

Gupta, G. R., Parkhurst, J. O., Ogden, J. A., Aggleton, P., and Mahal, A. (2008). Structural approaches to HIV prevention. *Lancet, 372,* 764–775.

Higgins, J., Hoffman, S., and Dworkin, S. L. (2010). Rethinking gender, heterosexual men, and women's vulnerability to HIV. *American Journal of Public Health, 100,* 435–445.

Hill-Collins, P. (1986). Learning from the outsider within: The sociological significance of black feminist thought. *Social Problems, 33,* S14–S32.

———. (1990). *Black feminist thought: Knowledge, consciousness, and the politics of empowerment.* New York: Routledge.

———. (1999). Moving beyond gender: Intersectionality and scientific knowledge. In M. M. Feree, J. Lorber, and B. B. Hess (Eds.), *Revisioning gender* (pp. 261–284). Thousand Oaks, CA: Sage.

———. (2005). *Black sexual politics: African Americans, gender, and the new racism.* New York: Routledge.

hooks, b. (1984). *Feminist theory: From margin to center.* Cambridge, MA: South End Press.

Kabeer, N. (1999). Resources, agency, achievements: Reflection on the measurement of women's empowerment. *Development and Change, 30* (3), 435–464.

Keleher, H. (2010). Gender norms and empowerment: "What works" to increase equity for women and girls. In G. Sen and P. Ostlin (Eds.), *Gender equity in health: The shifting frontiers of evidence and action* (pp. 161–183). New York: Routledge.

Kimmel, M. (1996). *Manhood in America: A cultural history.* New York: Free Press.

———. (2000). Saving the males: The sociological implications of the Virginia Military Institute and the Citadel. *Gender and Society, 14,* 494–516.

Knight, R.H. (1997). How domestic partnerships and gay marriage threaten the family. In R.M. Baird and S.E. Rosenbaum (Eds.), *Same-sex marriage: The moral and legal debate.* Amherst, NY: Prometheus Books.

Kreiger, N. (2003). Gender, sexes, and health: What are the connections—and why does it matter? *International Journal of Epidemiology, 32,* 652–657.

Mazzei, L.A. and Jackson, A.Y. (2009). *Voice in qualitative inequity: Challenging conventional, interpretive, and critical conceptions in qualitative research.* London: Routledge.

Messner, M.A. (1997). *The politics of masculinities: Men in movements.* Thousand Oaks, CA: Sage.

Pettifor, A., et al. (2015). Economic empowerment interventions for the prevention of violence against women and children. Paper presented at the Sexual Violence Research Initiative Forum, Stellenbosch, South Africa.

Polet, F., et al. (2015). Empowerment for the right to health: The use of "most significant change" methodology in monitoring. *Health and Human Rights Journal, 17,* 71–82.

Prina, S. (2011). Do simple savings accounts help the poor to save? Evidence from a field experiment in Nepal. Mimeo, Case Western Reserve University.

Schultz, A.J., and Mullings, L. (2006). *Gender, race, and class: Intersectional approaches.* San Francisco: Jossey-Bass.

Springer, K., Stellman, J.M., and Jordan-Young, R. (2012). Beyond a catalogue of differences: A theoretical frame and good practice guidelines for researching sex/gender in human health. *Social Science and Medicine, 74,* 1817–1824.

Stemple, L. (2011). Human rights, sex, and gender: Limits in theory and practice. *Pace Law Review, 31,* 824.

Thornton Dill, B. (1988). Our mother's grief: Racial ethnic women and the maintenance of families. *Journal of Family History, 13,* 415–431.

Thornton Dill, B., and Baca Zinn, M. (1984). Difference and domination. In B. Thornton Dill and M. Baca Zinn (Eds.), *Women of color in U.S. society* (pp. 3–12). Philadelphia: Temple University Press.

Unnithan, M. (2015). What constitutes evidence in human rights based approaches to health? Learning from lives experiences of maternal and sexual reproductive health. *Health and Human Rights Journal, 17,* 45–56.

Contributors

OLORUKOOBA ABIOLA is a pediatrician who lectures at Ahmadu Bello University, Zaria. She is a fellow of the Population and Reproductive Health Initiative, a collaboration between Ahmadu Bello University and the University of California, Berkeley. Dr. Olorukooba is dedicated to serving vulnerable groups; she works to empower women, facilitate girls' education, and promote health among impoverished youth in northern Nigeria.

FATIMA ADAMU is an Associate Professor in the Department of Sociology, Usmanu Danfodiyo University, Sokoto, and Executive Director of Women for Health, a Department for International Development–funded program aiming to train and support rural girls in Northern Nigeria to begin careers in the health profession. Her research interest is the intersection of gender and power in Muslim societies.

CARLOS ARENAS studied law in Colombia and earned an LLM (Master of Law) at the University of Wisconsin–Madison. He worked for seven years in the Instituto Latinoamericano de Servicios Legales Alternativos, a Latin American human rights NGO based in Bogotá, Colombia, and currently consults on issues related to climate change and displacement.

KAREN AUSTRIAN, PHD, is an Associate in the Population Council's Poverty, Gender, and Youth program and is based in its Nairobi, Kenya, office. Her work focuses on designing and evaluating asset building programs for vulnerable adolescent girls in East and Southern Africa.

CHRISTOPHER BONELL, PHD, MSC, is a Professor of Public Health Sociology at London School of Hygiene and Tropical Medicine. His research is concerned with how social exclusion in the form of poverty or other forms of disadvantage is associated with health risks.

LESLIE R. BRODY, PHD, is a Professor of Psychological and Brain Sciences at Boston University, past Director of the BU Clinical Psychology PhD program (1991–1996), and was the Marion Cabot Putnam Fellow at the Bunting Institute, Radcliffe College (1994–1995). Her research focuses on how gender roles and coping strategies relate to mental and physical health, especially in women with HIV, and since 2008 she has been a co-investigator with the Chicago site of the Women's Interagency HIV study.

JUDITH BRUCE is a Senior Associate and Policy Analyst with the Population Council's Poverty, Gender, and Youth program, based in their New York office. She leads the council's efforts to develop programs that protect the health and well-being and expand the opportunities of the poorest adolescent girls in the poorest communities.

DAVID CAO, MPH, is an Associate Specialist in the School of Public Health at the University of California, Berkeley. His current research is focused on population, reproductive health, and women's empowerment.

MARDGE H. COHEN, MD, is Professor of Medicine at Rush Medical Center and worked as an internist at Cook County Hospital for thirty-one years, where she founded the Cook County Women and Children's HIV Program in 1987 to provide comprehensive medical and psychosocial care to women with HIV and their families. Since 1994, she has led the Chicago consortium of the National Institute of Health's Women's Interagency HIV Study (WIHS), the longest-running cohort study investigating HIV disease progression in women. Since 2004, she has been the Medical Director of Women's Equity in Access to Care and Treatment (WE-ACTx), which supports comprehensive medical and psychosocial care for women and children with HIV and their families in Kigali, Rwanda.

CHRISTOPHER COLVIN, PHD, is an anthropologist, epidemiologist, and Head of the Division of Social and Behavioural Sciences at the School of Public Health and Family Medicine at the University of Cape Town. His research interests include men, masculinity and HIV; health governance and activism; pedagogical approaches in interdisciplinary contexts; and the use of qualitative evidence syntheses (QES) in health policy making.

RUTH C. CRUISE, PHD, is a clinical psychologist at McLean Hospital in the Gunderson Outpatient Program who specializes in cognitive behavioral and dialectical behavioral treatments for at-risk adolescents and adults with suicidality, trauma, and borderline personality disorder. Her research and clinical interests center on the way individuals make meaning of traumatic or difficult experiences and the emotional, cognitive, and behavioral sequelae of the self-narratives they construct.

SANNISHA K. DALE, PHD, EDM, is a Licensed Psychologist and Postdoctoral Fellow in Behavioral Medicine at Massachusetts General Hospital/Harvard Medical School. Her primary research interests include developing effective prevention and intervention strategies to promote resilience and good health outcomes among survivors of trauma and individuals with or at risk for HIV. She is the principal investigator of a K23 award from the National Institute of

Mental Health aimed at developing a behavioral medicine intervention for Black women with HIV and histories of trauma.

JACQUES DE WET, PHD, is a Senior Lecturer in Sociology at the University of Cape Town. His research focuses on social change and identity in postapartheid South Africa, as well as people-centered development.

MEGAN S. DUNBAR is Vice President of Research and Social Policy at Pangaea Global AIDS in Harare, Zimbabwe. Dr. Dunbar engages in research, policy analysis, and advocacy with the aim of ensuring equitable access to prevention, care, and treatment services for those living with and most at risk of acquiring HIV, with a particular focus on adolescent young women and girls.

ANJALI DUTT is a doctoral candidate in Social Psychology at the University of California, Santa Cruz. Her research focuses on understanding individuals' resistance to oppression and efforts to make societies more socially just, particularly in the context of globalization and with a focus on the experiences of women, human rights, and social change.

SHARI L. DWORKIN, PHD, MS, is Professor in the Department of Social and Behavioral Sciences at the University of California, San Francisco (UCSF) and Associate Dean for Academic Affairs in the UCSF School of Nursing. Her research is focused on structural interventions for HIV prevention, treatment, and care and gender-transformative health interventions among heterosexually active men. She is a founding member of the UC Global Health Institute Center of Expertise on Women's Health and Empowerment.

CARROLL L. ESTES, PHD, is Professor of Sociology Emerita, Department of Social and Behavioral Sciences, and Founding Director of the Institute for Health and Aging, University of California, San Francisco. Estes's research is on critical social policy and inequality in economic and health security by race, ethnicity, class, gender, disability, and age.

MONICA GANDHI, MD, is Professor of Medicine and Associate Division Chief (Clinical Operations/Education) of the Division of HIV, Infectious Diseases, and Global Medicine at UCSF/San Francisco General Hospital. Her research focuses on women's health and HIV; her research has shown how antiretroviral adherence can be objectively measured through biomarkers derived from hair samples.

SHELLY GRABE, PHD, is an Associate Professor in Social Psychology at the University of California, Santa Cruz, with affiliations in Feminist Studies and Latin American and Latino Studies. Professor Grabe is engaged in transnational projects in Nicaragua and Tanzania to help demonstrate the role of social movements in promoting social justice aimed at women's justice and empowerment.

KATE GRÜNKE-HORTON, PHD, BN, is a recent graduate from the University of California, San Francisco, in the Department of Social and Behavioral Sciences in the School of Nursing. She specializes in health policy and her interests lie in social movements and women's health. Her dissertation focused on how sex workers influence health policy and social change.

PALLAVI GUPTA worked as the Assistant Research Coordinator at Action Research and Training for Health (ARTH), a nonprofit organization based in Rajasthan, India, at the time of this study. A social scientist by training, her work focuses on public health advocacy, research, and programming, with particular emphasis on reproductive and sexual health rights of young people.

JAMES R. HARGREAVES, PHD, MSC, is Director of the Centre for Evaluation at London School of Hygiene and Tropical Medicine. His research focuses on the socioeconomic epidemiology of HIV/AIDS and tuberculosis and developing interventions to address these public health issues.

ABIGAIL M. HATCHER, MPHIL, is a Senior Researcher at the University of the Witwatersrand and the University of California, San Francisco. A doctoral candidate in public health, she has expertise in the design and testing of interventions for intimate partner violence and HIV engagement in care.

THERESA Y. HWANG, MPA, is the Gender Director at CARE, a leading humanitarian organization fighting global poverty. She provides global leadership on gender equality, child marriage, and capacity building and is an experienced facilitator for gender and diversity trainings.

KIRTI IYENGAR, MD, PHD, is a Senior Coordinator at Action Research and Training for Health (ARTH), and adjunct professor at the Sanford School of Public Policy, Duke University. Her research focuses on health system interventions and task shifting for improving access and quality of reproductive health services with a focus on rights. She designs innovative service delivery approaches in low resource settings and provides programmatic support for implementation of reproductive health programs.

SHARAD IYENGAR, a public health practitioner and researcher, heads Action Research and Training for Health (ARTH), a nonprofit based in Rajasthan, India. His current work focuses on creating opportunities for women to exercise reproductive choice within or despite the health system, tracking home-level maternal-newborn care interventions and assessing referral for emergency obstetric care.

GWENDOLYN A. KELSO, PHD, is a licensed clinical psychologist, serving children, adolescents, and adults at Dana Group Associates in Needham, MA. Her clinical and research interests include identity awareness and development, adult survivors of childhood abuse, working through and healing from loss, and the impact of both social and individual factors on day-to-day functioning.

JULIA KIM, MD, MPH, is a Senior Program Advisor at the Gross National Happiness Centre in Bhutan. Dr. Kim is also a member of the International Expert Working Group for the New Development Paradigm, which was convened by the government of Bhutan. Her background is in public health programs, policy, and research, with a focus on international health and sustainable development.

MAIRO MANDARA, an obstetrician/gynaecologist and an expert in reproductive health and sociocultural issues affecting maternal and child health, is currently serving as the Country Representative of the Bill and Melinda Gates Foundation in Nigeria. Founder of Girl Child Concerns, an NGO based in Kaduna, Nigeria,

Dr. Mandara has promoted girls' education to achieve gender equity and improve maternal and child health for over two decades.

ELISA MARTÍNEZ served for a decade as CARE USA's inaugural gender equity advisor and led CARE International's Strategic Impact Inquiry on Women's Empowerment. She is now a doctoral student in Sociology at the University of Massachusetts, studying the politics of impact measurement in struggles for development and social change.

M. CATHERINE MATERNOWSKA, PHD, MPH, formerly of the Bixby Center for Global Reproductive Health, currently works at the UNICEF Office of Research–Innocenti, in Florence, Italy. For well over two decades, Maternowska has led research and managed donor-financed programming on child protection and sexual and reproductive health, with expertise in gender-based violence policy, prevention, care, and treatment.

HABIBA MOHAMED is the Founder and Director of Women and Development Against Distress in Africa (WADADIA). She has been a consultant Outreach Manager for the Fistula Foundation since 2014 and Field Coordinator for One By One since 2011.

LINDA MORISON is a Senior Lecturer working on the Clinical Psychology Programme at the University of Surrey. Her research focuses on cost-effective and feasible ways of preventing and relieving psychological distress within different populations.

IMELDA MUDEKUNYE-MAHAKA is the Country Director of Pangaea Zimbabwe. She oversees the implementation of Pangaea programs and is the director of the SHAZ! Project, which serves the health and livelihood needs of adolescent girls and young women in Zimbabwe. Formerly with the University of Zimbabwe-UCSF Collaborative Research Programme in Women's Health, she has over a decade of experience working with adolescent girls and young women in HIV and reproductive health and in behavioral research.

GUSTAVO ORTIZ MILLÁN, PHD, is Research Professor at the Institute for Philosophical Research, National Autonomous University of Mexico. He is the author of *La Moralidad del Aborto* (The Morality of Abortion; 2009, Siglo Press XXI: Mexico City) and *Aborto, Democracia y Empoderamiento* (Abortion, Democracy, and Empowerment; 2014, Fontamara Press: Mexico City).

PAIGE PASSANO, MPH, is the Director of the Sahel Leadership Program for the OASIS Initiative, a project of the College of Natural Resources, and the Bixby Center for Population, Health and Sustainability at the University of California, Berkeley. Her primary interests are how culture and social norms can restrict access to health and education—and how local communities can take action to break multigenerational patterns of deprivation.

DEAN PEACOCK, MSW, is founding director of Sonke Gender Justice, a South African non-governmental organization (NGO) working across Africa to address HIV and AIDS, prevent GBV, and promote gender equality, human rights and social justice. He is an Honorary Senior Lecturer at the University of Cape Town's School of Public Health and an Ashoka Fellow.

DANIEL PERLMAN, PHD, is a medical anthropologist with more than thirty years' experience planning, implementing, and evaluating community health and education programs in Asia, Africa, and Latin America. He is currently the Director of the Centre for Girls Education—a partnership between Ahmadu Bello University and the School of Public Health, University of California, Berkeley.

GODFREY PHETLA is a Director at the Department of Trade and Industry in South Africa. He leads research and policy analysis on entrepreneurship and small business promotion.

LINDSEY POLLACZEK, MPH, led the evaluation of Let's End Fistula Programme for her Master's project at the UCLA Fielding School of Public Health in 2012. She is the Program Director for Fistula Foundation and has been working in Kenya for the Action on Fistula initiative since 2014.

JOHN PORTER, PHD, is Professor of International Health at London School of Hygiene and Tropical Medicine. His research focuses on the ethics and practice of infectious disease policy, public health and human rights.

MALCOLM POTTS, PHD, is Professor of Maternal and Child Health at University of California, Berkeley, and co-founder of the OASIS Initiative, which focuses on the interlinkages between population, food security, and health in the Sahel region of Africa. He is dedicated to improving food security, educational attainment, and access to family planning.

PAUL PRONYK, MD, PHD, is the Chief of Child Survival and Development at UNICEF Indonesia. His research spans the fields of maternal child health and nutrition, structural interventions for gender and HIV, and the health and social impacts of economic development programs.

VICTOR ROBINSON is an independent consultant based in the United States and India. His work focuses on social dynamics of power, culture, and gender in development contexts.

GITA SEN, PHD, is Director of the Ramalingaswami Centre on Equity and Social Determinants of Health at the Public Health Foundation of India and Adjunct Professor of Global Health and Population at the Harvard School of Public Health. She is a pioneer in the area of gender, women's empowerment, development, and health. Her recent work includes research and policy advocacy on the gender dimensions of population policies and the equity dimensions of health.

LARA STEMPLE, JD, is the Director of Graduate Studies and the Director of the Health and Human Rights Law Project at University of California, Los Angeles, School of Law. She teaches and writes in the areas of human rights, global health, gender, sexuality, HIV/AIDS, and incarceration.

VICKI STRANGE is a senior research officer at the Social Science Research Unit of the Institute of Education, London. Her research has focused on understanding complex interventions for improving the health of women and young people.

LYNISSA R. STOKES, PHD, is a clinical psychologist currently teaching at the College of Public Health and Human Sciences at Oregon State University. Her primary research interests include the prevention of HIV and STDs/STIs among at-risk minority women, men, and couples and the influence of partner, relationship, and contextual factors on sexual risk and protective behaviors. She is the first author of a recently published article on individual, interpersonal, and structural power influences on condom use patterns among rural Latino young adult men and women.

DALLAS SWENDEMAN, PHD, MPH, is Co-Director of the Center of Expertise in Women's Health, Gender and Empowerment of the University of California Global Health Initiative. He is also faculty in the Department of Psychiatry and Biobehavioral Sciences in the David Geffen School of Medicine at UCLA and in the Department of Epidemiology at the UCLA Fielding School of Public Health. His empowerment-related research focuses on the conceptualization, measurement, and impacts of empowerment-oriented interventions through a fifteen-year mixed-methods research partnership with the Sonagachi Project/Durbar program in Kolkata and West Bengal, India, working with sex workers and their families.

PAULA TAVROW, PHD, is an Adjunct Associate Professor at University of California, Los Angeles, Fielding School of Public Health and has been conducting research in Western Kenya since 1997. She is a founding member of the UC Global Health Institute Center of Expertise on Women's Health and Empowerment and served as its first Co-Director.

CHARLOTTE WATTS, PHD, is Chief Scientific Adviser at the United Kingdom Department for International Development. Dr. Watts is also head of the Social and Mathematical Epidemiology Group at London School of Hygiene and Tropical Medicine and founder of the Gender, Violence and Health Centre. Her research aims to provide evidence on how to reduce women's vulnerability to HIV and violence and to address the structural forces that help shape their vulnerability.

KATHLEEN M. WEBER, RN, BS, BSN, is the Project Director and a Co-Investigator on the Chicago Women's Interagency HIV Study (WIHS) Consortium. Her research affiliation is with the Hektoen Institute of Medicine and the CORE Center at Cook County Health and Hospitals System.

JOANNA WEINBERG, JD, LLM, is Senior Lecturer in Law at Hastings College of the Law and Associate Adjunct Professor of Law, Policy, and Ethics at the Institute for Health and Aging, University of California, San Francisco. Her primary research and writing involve bioethics, aging, and end-of-life care; human subjects protection; and health policy and public health.

SHERI WEISER, MD, is Adjunct Associate Professor of Medicine in the University of California, San Francisco, School of Medicine. Dr. Weiser's research examines the relationships between poverty, HIV-related health behaviors, and health outcomes in underserved populations in resource-rich and resource-poor settings. She is particularly interested in the role of targeted food assistance and sustainable food production strategies in improving models of HIV care delivery to underserved populations in the United States and globally.

Index

abortion: contraception availability in
India, 33–35; counseling process for, in
Mexico City, 256; incrimination from,
260–61; Indian services for, 33–35;
lack of, 6; legality of, 181; maternal
mortality from, 258; MTP Act for, 34;
percentage of safe in India, 45 fig.;
pregnancy tests and, 34–35; in rape
cases, 260; stigmas of, 185; types of,
256–58
abortion decriminalization in Mexico City,
185, 263, 311; Católicas por el Derecho
a Decidir for, 257, 262; challenges to,
253; conservative reaction to, 253–54;
context of, 252–54; education and
training after, 254–58; as empowerment,
259–61; Equidad de Género for, 256,
257, 260, 262; feminist movements for,
252–53; healthcare provider opposition
to, 254–55; health impacts of, 258–59;
ILE program from, 254, 262–63; Lamas
on, 259; MOH abortion service after,
255–56; outcomes of, 261–63; overview
of, 251–52; poverty and, 184, 258–59;
primary healthcare facilities in, 257–58;
prolife opposition to, 260–61; rights
improvements from, 262; service quality
after, 256–67; success factors of, 264;
Supreme Court on, 253; values
clarification program on, 255; women's
organizations for, 256–57, 259–62, 264

ACA. *See* Affordable Care Act
ACASI. *See* audio computer assisted survey
instruments
Accredited Social Health Activists (ASHAs),
35–36; performance of, 48–49. *See also*
Indian fertility control intervention
Acquired Immune Deficiency Syndrome
(AIDS), 8. *See also* Human Immunodeficiency Virus
Action Research & Training for Health
(ARTH), 30–32, 34–35; CHW training
by, 36 fig.; educational materials
distributed by, 37 fig.; number of
pregnancy tests done by, 39 fig.;
pregnancy test conductors, 39 fig.;
wall painting from, 37. *See also* Indian
fertility control intervention
Adolescent Data Guides: of girls in
Kenya, 100 fig.; from Population
Council, 98
adolescent girls: disadvantagement of,
93; Haiti and Kenya vulnerabilities
of, 95–96; Haiti context for, 97–98;
Kenya context for, 96–97; Safe and
Smart Savings Program for Vulnerable
Adolescent Girls, 102; SHAZ! for,
with HIV risk, 190–91; Sierra Leone
Adolescent Girls Network, 104;
Zimbabwe structural risks of, 192. *See
also* Shaping the Health of Adolescents
in Zimbabwe

microfinance plus, 212
microgrants, 196, 198–99, 202–3;
intervention with, 200 *table*
Ministry of Health (MOH), Mexico, 252,
254, 262; abortion service implementation from, 255–56; women's organizations influence on, 264
miscarriages, 261
MMA. *See* Medicare Modernization Act
MMR. *See* maternal mortality ratio
MOH. *See* Ministry of Health
MOS-HIV. *See* Medical Outcome Study
MTA. *See* Medical Termination of
Pregnancy
multisectoral work, 311

Nari Mukti Sangha (NMS): with sex
workers in Bangladesh, 119, 121, 124,
129–30, 136n26; structure and power
changes from, 129–30
National Committee to Preserve Social
Security and Medicare, U.S. (NCPSSM),
236, 237–38
National Institutes of Health (NIH), U.S.,
25, 73, 141
National Population Council, Mexico, 258
National Rural Health Mission (NRHM),
India, 33–34
NCPSSM. *See* National Committee to
Preserve Social Security and Medicare,
U.S.
negotiation skills, 80
NGO. *See* non-governmental organization
NHIF. *See* Kenyan National Hospital
Insurance Fund
Nicaragua,: land ownership in, 186; lessons
from rural, 304. *See also* land ownership
in Nicaragua study; Xochilt Acalt
Women's Center
Nigeria, northern: early marriage in, 73–75,
84–85; Hausa people in, 73–75; public
education in, 75–76, 84–86. *See also*
Centre for Girls Education program
Nigerian Universal Basic Education Act of
2004, 76
NIH. *See* National Institutes of Health
NMS. *See* Nari Mukti Sangha
non-governmental organization (NGO), 26,
262; to grassroots approaches, 281–82;
on masculinity, 160; support roles of,
267
NRHM. *See* National Rural Health Mission

Obama, Barack, 237

obstetric fistula, 21–22; afflictions from,
57–58; care for, 58–59; in Kenya,
58–59; overview of, 57. *See also* Let's
End Fistula Program
older women: ageism toward, 235;
empowerment and health of, 232–33;
empowerment barriers for, 139–40; in
gender roles and coping study on
HIV, 147; income of, 233; research
on, 242. *See also* gender roles and
coping study on HIV; Social Security,
Medicare, and Medicaid preservation
case study
OMC. *See* One Man Can
One By One, 60
One Man Can (OMC) program, 160, 171;
CATs in, 163; context of, study, 161–63;
discussion of, study, 168–69; as gender
transformative, 170; health behavior
changes from, 167–68; interviews of,
164; masculinity defined by, 162; men's
view of women's empowerment from,
165; relationship power shifts from,
166; on South Africa racial inequality,
162–63; study limitations on, 169–70;
study methods of, 163–64; study results
of, 164
Operation Murambatsvina, 192, 202
oppression, 170
Ortiz Millán, Gustavo, 184–85, 311

Partido Acción Nacional (PAN), Mexico,
260
Partido de la Revolución Democrática
(PRD), Mexico, 252
Penn-Kekana, L., 6
Pettifor, A., 312
Planned Parenthood clinics, 235
Population and Reproductive Health
Initiative (PRHI), 73. *See also* Centre for
Girls Education program
Population Council, 85, 94, 96; Adolescent
Data Guides from, 98
poverty, 93; abortion decriminalization in
Mexico City and, 184, 258–59; HIV,
IPV and, 211–12; microfinance for
women in, 212; in Safe Spaces Program,
102
power, 2, 239; contextualized understand-
ing of, 201; definition of, 219; gender,
health and, 5–7. *See also* gendered
power relations
PRD. *See* Partido de la Revolución
Democrática